Children and Young People's Mental Health

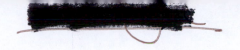

D0303455

Children and Young People's Mental Health equips nurses and healthcare professionals with the essential skills and competencies needed to deliver effective assessment, treatment and support to children and young people with mental health problems and disorders as well as to their families. Drawing on McDougall's *Child and Adolescent Mental Health Nursing* and taking the Cavendish Report and Willis Commission into account, this new textbook has been designed to ensure those working in child and adolescent mental health services (CAMHS) can continue to provide a high-quality, evidence-based service.

The book explores best practice in a variety of settings and addresses issues such as eating disorders, self-harm, ADHD, forensic mental health and misuse of drugs and alcohol in children and young people, as well as looking at child protection, clinical governance, safeguarding and legal requirements. Furthermore, with young people contributing directly to several of the chapters, the book reflects the importance of involving them in planning, delivering and evaluating CAMHS services.

It is essential reading for all health and social care professionals and students working with children and young people, particularly those working in specialist child and adolescent mental health settings.

Tim McDougall is Deputy Director of Nursing at Greater Manchester West NHS Foundation Trust, UK. He has over 100 journal and book publications in relation to child and adolescent mental health and nursing practice.

Children and Young People's Mental Health

Essentials for nurses and other professionals

Edited by Tim McDougall

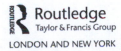

Routledge
Taylor & Francis Group

LONDON AND NEW YORK

First published 2017
by Routledge
2 Park Square, Milton Park, Abingdon, Oxon OX14 4RN

and by Routledge
711 Third Avenue, New York, NY 10017

Routledge is an imprint of the Taylor & Francis Group, an informa business

British Library Cataloguing-in-Publication Data
A catalogue record for this book is available from the British Library

Library of Congress Cataloging in Publication Data
Names: McDougall, Tim, editor.
Title: Children and young people's mental health : essentials for nurses and other professionals / edited by Tim McDougall.
Description: Abingdon, Oxon ; New York, NY : Routledge, 2017. | Includes bibliographical references and index.
Identifiers: LCCN 2016013852| ISBN 9781138915442 (hardback) | ISBN 9781138915459 (pbk.) | ISBN 9781315690223 (ebook)
Subjects: | MESH: Psychiatric Nursing--methods | Mental Disorders--nursing | Child | Adolescent
Classification: LCC RC440 | NLM WY 160 | DDC 616.89/0231--dc23
LC record available at http://lccn.loc.gov/2016013852

ISBN: 978-1-138-91544-2 (hbk)
ISBN: 978-1-138-91545-9 (pbk)
ISBN: 978-1-315-69022-3 (ebk)

Typeset in Goudy
by Saxon Graphics Ltd, Derby

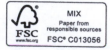

Printed and bound in Great Britain by
TJ International Ltd, Padstow, Cornwall

To the very many young people, parents and professionals who I have had the privilege of working with over 20 years in CAMHS. You have inspired and motivated me, and you taught me much of what I know and hold to be important as a nurse.

Contents

Contributing authors

Marie Armstrong (RMN, BA [Hons], PG Dip, MA, ENB 603, 998) is Nurse Consultant leading the Child and Adolescent Mental Health Service (CAMHS) Self-harm Team in Nottinghamshire Healthcare NHS Trust. With over 28 years of experience in CAMHS, Marie has worked in a variety of settings including adolescent inpatient care, children's day services, community mental health teams and primary care liaison. Marie was the first CAMHS nurse consultant in the UK and has been in post since 2000. Her current role involves 50 per cent clinical practice as well as research, leadership, consultancy, teaching and service development. Marie has developed and implemented good practice guidelines for young people who self-harm, and she contributed to the development of National Institute for Health and Care Excellence (NICE) guidelines on self-harm. Marie provides training and speaks at conferences about self-harm and young people. As well as being trained in child and adolescent mental health nursing, Marie is a qualified systemic family psychotherapist registered with the United Kingdom Council for Psychotherapy.

Laurence Baldwin is Senior Lecturer in Mental Health Nursing at Coventry University. He was previously Nurse Consultant (CAMHS) at Derbyshire Healthcare NHS Foundation Trust, where he was involved in service development and leading clinical practice, setting up the dedicated CAMHS Liaison team, and the introduction of CYP IAPT as a first-wave provider service. Laurence trained in Nottingham and worked there and at Mansfield CAMHS before moving to Derby. He has had secondments to the Department of Health and the National Institute for Mental Health in England/Care Services Improvement Partnership. In 2008, he completed his PhD at Nottingham University. He was previously the Chair of the Royal College of Nursing (RCN) Child and Young People's Mental Health Forum and presented two motions at Congress about child mental health. He was part of a Skills for Health working group that developed the CAMHS National Occupational Standards in 2014, and he represented the RCN on the Ministerial CAMHS Taskforce 2014–15. He is also an independent prescriber and a registered nurse teacher. Laurence has published articles in a variety of media and presented at national and international conferences. Currently, he chairs the Children and Young People's Integrated Research Group in the Centre for Social Futures at the Institute of Mental Health (University of Nottingham). He tweets as @drljbaldwin.

Fred Ehresmann has worked in the field of children and young people's mental health since qualifying as a mental health nurse in 1993. His practice experience has taken him across a wide range of settings and roles, including secure care, CAMHS Tier 2 and Tier 3 services, schools and local authority safeguarding children services. Fred is currently Senior Lecturer in Mental Health Nursing at the University of the West of England, and he also provides consultancy and training to local authorities, special schools and third sector providers of mental health provision for children and young people.

Lina Gatsou is Child and Adolescent Psychiatrist and Psychodynamic Psychotherapist for Children and Adolescents. Lina's special clinical interests are child and adolescent depression, personality disorders, attachment disorders and gender identity disorders, and the wellbeing and safeguarding of children and families. Lina holds the post of Honorary Professor with De Montfort University. She is Named Doctor for Safeguarding Children for Leicestershire Partnership NHS Foundation Trust and is responsible for the strategic and organisational development and implementation of safeguarding, particularly in families affected by parental mental illness. Lina and her colleagues were awarded a HIEC (Health, Innovation and Education Cluster) grant from the Department of Health in 2011/2012 and have developed and delivered the knowledge- and skills-based Think Family – Whole Family Multi-agency Training and Intervention programme for families affected by parental mental illness; this has had encouraging results, which have been presented at a number of national and international conferences with the first papers being published in peer-reviewed journals.

Rachel Hadland (RMN, MSc, PG Dip) is Senior Lecturer in Mental Health Nursing at the University of the West of England alongside working as a Specialist CAMHS Nurse in Bristol. She has prior experience of working in a national specialist inpatient CAMHS unit in London. Rachel led on the development of CAMHS-specific modules for both pre- and post-registration nursing programmes, introducing shared learning opportunities between children's and mental health nurses. Rachel also provides specialist consultation to new and developing CAMHS inpatient units. Rachel has key research interests in CAMHS service development, CAMHS workforce and CAMHS education and training.

Tim McDougall is Deputy Director of Nursing at Greater Manchester West NHS Foundation Trust. Tim spent 15 years as CAMHS Nurse Consultant and several as Clinical Director in CAMHS at the Cheshire and Wirral NHS Foundation Trust. Tim has worked in a range of CAMHS settings including community child mental health teams, adolescent inpatient services and secure adolescent forensic services. With a national profile in CAMHS and over 100 book and journal publications, Tim has spoken at national and European conferences about the mental health of children and adolescents. Tim was formerly Nurse Advisor for CAMHS at the Department of Health in England and has been a member of several National Advisory Councils. Tim chaired the Quality Network for Inpatient CAMHS (QNIC) Executive Committee for four years and has been involved in the development of several NICE guidelines affecting children and young people. Tim is currently part of the Mental Health Taskforce Safe Staffing Group.

Paul Mitchell is Senior Nurse in the Adult and Youth Specialised Services Directorate at Great Manchester West NHS Trust. He currently leads a project on police-mental health pathways and is also one of the Clinical Leads for the National Secure Forensic Mental Health Service for Young People. Until last year, he was the Clinical Lead for the mental health team at Hindley Young Offender Institute. Paul has worked in a range of CAMHS settings but primarily within adolescent forensic services and with young people in the youth justice system. He has undertaken research on pathways and interventions for young people in secure settings, and he worked on the NICE Guideline Development Groups for antisocial behaviour and conduct disorders and attachment disorder.

Terri-Anne Nolan is a Registered Mental Nurse (RMN) who has been working in Tier 4 CAMHS in Chester for the past 11 years. She has undertaken a wide range of training and research including on dialectical behavioural therapy (DBT) for adolescents. She completed a CAMHS degree at the University of Lancashire and a foundation course in Systemic Practice at the University of Leeds. Terri-Anne has a passion for working with young people who display aggressive or challenging behaviours, and part of her research for her CAMHS degree was looking at how nursing staff manage this.

Dawn Rees (MA, CQSW, FInstM) has 40 years of experience working in the public sector as a nurse and a social worker. She was a senior manager in health and local authorities. She led national improvement programmes in CAMHS sponsored by the Department of Health and the Department of Education, and she has been a member of a National Service Framework expert working group, the Northern Ireland Bamford Advisory Group, other national delivery boards and policy development groups and the National Advisory Council for CAMHS. She is an entrepenueur and independent consultant and undertakes high-level CAMHS reviews, develops and delivers leadership programmes and has a thriving executive coaching practice. Dawn was nominated as European Coach of the Year 2014 by the European Mentoring and Coaching Council.

Noreen Ryan is Consultant Nurse at Bolton Foundation NHS Trust. Noreen trained as a general nurse and worked as a staff nurse in neurosurgery for 12 months before training as a RMN, initially working on an elderly ward and then in CAMHS. She worked in a CAMHS inpatient service before holding the post of Community Psychiatric Nurse (CPN) in CAMHS in inner-city Manchester for eight years. Noreen then moved to Bolton CAMHS where she began her interest in working with children and families with attention deficit hyperactivity disorder (ADHD). She has further training in family therapy, in relationship work with mothers and children, and as an independent and supplementary nurse prescriber. Noreen has been a member of the Guideline Development Group for the NICE guideline on the treatment and assessment of ADHD that applies to children, adolescents and adults, and she also helped develop the NICE quality standards on ADHD.

Ben Samata is 14 years old and is in Year 10 at school. Ben is involved in a variety of projects related to mental health involving a charity and his local CAMHS. He has featured in a national television documentary about bereavement through suicide and is passionate about reducing stigma associated with mental health. He was pivotal in the development of the peer mentor project at Wirral CAMHS. Ben is diagnosed with ADHD and autism spectrum disorder. He is massively interested in gaming, his favourite food ever is ravioli and he enjoys the cinema.

Sally Sanderson is currently working with NHS Vale Royal and NHS South Cheshire Clinical Commissioning Groups on a series of service redesign projects and is General Manager for mental health and learning disability services across Central and Eastern Cheshire for Cheshire and Wirral Partnership NHS Foundation Trust. Sally has worked in adult mental health for over 30 years, primarily with people who have severe mental health problems but more recently with psychological services including Improving Access to Psychological Therapies (IAPT). Due to a belief that there must be more to treatment than the traditional medical models and high levels of medication, Sally became attracted to the growing body of evidence supporting the use of psychosocial approaches to treatment. Having completed her BSc (Hons), Sally developed a specific interest in the emergent early psychosis interventions, becoming involved in the planning and implementation process of early intervention in psychosis services.

Jasmine Scarisbrick is a musician who is working towards her degree in composition, French horn and piano performance. She is currently involved in writing the music and sound for a visual art project that presents the controversies and impacts of social, cultural and national identity, exploring how this affects personal development. Alongside her studies, Jasmine is completing a teaching diploma and facilitating music outreach workshops in disadvantaged areas. She believes passionately that working with children and young people is a privilege. When she is not in an orchestral rehearsal, Jasmine finds time for skydiving. Jasmine has been a service user in CAMHS and has three generations of family who have used mental health services. She is passionate about reducing mental health stigma and promoting participation and involvement with professionals and young people. Jasmine's key belief is that through participation, young people can take ownership and discover within themselves some form of self-resilience and self-belief that contributes to their health and wellbeing.

Angela Sergeant (MSc, RMN, RGN, ENB 603) is Consultant Nurse in Tier 4 CAMHS. Angela has worked in a wide range of CAMHS inpatient settings, and she has been a key player in the development and commissioning of inpatient units. She has a national profile in CAMHS, having conducted numerous reviews for the Health Advisory Service, Quality Network for Inpatient CAMHS (QNIC) and Royal College of Psychiatry external consultancy service in the UK and overseas. She was a QNIC executive member for nine years, part of the NHS Confederation CAMHS subgroup and a member of the Tier 4 policy implementation group. Angela has a passionate interest in the professional development of CAMHS nurses and led work on the nationally recognised *Working with Child and Adolescent Mental Health Inpatient Services* handbook. As part of her Consultant Nurse role, Angela is a Responsible Clinician for a number of young people within the inpatient service, and she became an approved clinician in 2013. Angela has developed a specialist interest in the treatment of young people with eating disorders, attachment difficulties and therapeutic engagement.

Fiona Smith (RGN/RSCN, Diploma in Professional Nursing Studies, BA [Hons] Health Studies, MBA [Health]) is the Royal College of Nursing Professional Lead for Children and Young People's Nursing. She provides professional support to 423,000 members, RCN staff and a range of forums and communities in the field of children and young people's nursing, including children's and neonatal intensive care, community nursing, emergency care, cardiac nursing, adolescent health, school nurses, health visiting, palliative care, mental health, looked after children and safeguarding children. Fiona is an Honorary Fellow of the Royal College of Paediatrics and Child Health and a member of the Royal College of Paediatrics and Child Health Council. Prior to taking up her position in the RCN, Fiona was Associate Director of Nursing/Named Nurse for Child

Protection and Paediatric Adviser across Leicestershire. During her time at the RCN, Fiona has participated in numerous research advisory groups including those related to commissioned research for Department for Children, Schools and Families/Department for Education about safeguarding/child protection. More recently, Fiona was one of the independent panel members for the Child Sexual Exploitation Inquiry in Northern Ireland and is currently the chairperson for the NHS England child health safety group. Fiona also works nationally and internationally, collaborating with other organisations in relation to health, social care and education to actively shape policy and service provision for children and young people. She is Coordinator of the Paediatric Nursing Associations of Europe Network and has been instrumental in the development of standards across Europe, working with the Council of Europe.

Amanda Tuffrey works with Great Involvement, Future Thinking (GIFT), and throughout her time there, she has commented on various documents for the National Institute for Health and Care Excellence, the Children's Mental Health Taskforce and the CAMHS Health Select Committee. She was Co-chair of the service development group that steers national service transformation through the Children's Improving Access to Psychological Therapies (IAPT) programme. Amanda is also an ambassador for the Time to Change charity, tackling stigma and discrimination in mental health.

Leanne Walker is studying geography and criminology at Keele University. She works for the GIFT (Greater Involvement, Future Thinking) consortium, improving standards of participation in CAMHS. Leanne has lived experience of CAMHS and is also a part of the Derbyshire CAMHS participation group, which works on improving the service locally, tackling stigma and raising awareness. Through this, Leanne is leading on the development of an outcomes monitoring application. Leanne is currently a member of several groups focused around improving integrated working and CAMHS nationally at the Department of Health in England. Leanne has presented on her personal experiences of using outcome measures on several occasions, and alongside other professionals, she has developed a young person's guide to using outcome measures.

Fiona Warner-Gale has over 28 years' experience working within the NHS and with other public sector organisations at a clinical, strategic and policy level. She has specific expertise in service review and redesign, service transformation, strategic leadership and professional development, and research and evaluation with a focus on children's mental health. Over the last 15 years, she has led service reviews and improvement and redesign projects using whole systems change methodology, and she has been key in toolkit and product development on a regional and national basis. She is also a senior academic and has published widely around primary mental health and mental health stigma – she is an Honorary Research Fellow in Mental Health at the University of Northampton.

Elaine Williams (RMN, BSc [Hons], PG Cert [DBT], PG Dip [social entrepreneurship and innovation], NMP, MSc, and Queen's Nurse) has worked in charitable, statutory and non-statutory services for adults, children and young people in the south-east and north-west of England. Elaine has specialised in substance misuse, youth offending and child and adolescent mental health. Elaine has extensive experience of service development and is passionate about addressing stigma and absolutely having service users at the forefront of service development.

Scott Yates is Reader in Psychosocial Studies and Lead for Youth Research at De Montfort University, Leicester. He obtained his PhD in psychology in 2002, and since 2004, he has been involved in interdisciplinary research and teaching across the fields of psychology, sociology, youth studies and health studies. He has undertaken work for a variety of funders, including local and national government, the NHS and national charities. He has published more than 20 book chapters and journal articles and spoken at numerous national and international conferences and events on young people, focusing on the subjects of employment and unemployment, disability and chronic illness, mental health and research methods. His most recent work examines the impacts of parental mental illness on families, its interactions with families' social and economic contexts, and the potential for developing effective family-focused programmes.

Foreword

I am delighted to write the foreword to this much-needed text. This book brings together a unique body of knowledge about the mental health of children and young people for nurses and other professionals across the UK, charting developments, reflecting on the past and providing inspiration for the future. Nursing in this field has developed considerably over the last 20 years with nurses leading and influencing both national and international policy and practice. Today, nurses participate as equal members of the team, providing care to children and young people and leading service provision, education programmes and research activities across the speciality.

This is undoubtedly a practical textbook, applying both policy and theory to day-to-day nursing practice and service provision using case exemplars. The book is divided into three parts. Part 1 focuses on policy and strategy, highlighting children and young people's participation and engagement, role development and service transformation. This part highlights the crucial role of education and training to underpin clinical developments, role expansion and new ways of thinking and doing. The lack of specific education in many instances has acted as a key inhibitor preventing nurses from pushing the boundaries of their practice. Part 2 considers some of the common mental health and psychosocial disorders, such as self-harm, eating disorders and attention deficit hyperactivity disorder (ADHD). In particular, the importance of prevention, recognition and early intervention is acknowledged along with the need to build children and young people's emotional resilience. Part 3 provides an insight into service provision, highlighting the positive impact of school-based mental health services, challenges of behaviour management, therapeutic engagement, restrictive practice and care provision within secure and forensic settings. The book concludes with a chapter about nurse entrepreneurship, which notes that enabling nurses and other health professionals to innovate and act in 'intrepreneurial' roles is a very cost-effective strategy.

Overall, the text clearly highlights the challenges for nursing leaders and practitioners within the field of child and adolescent mental health services over the coming months and years. Meeting the needs of young people will continue to be a challenge for practitioners and managers alike. The future is likely to encompass new models of service provision, and nurse leaders should be active in determining the shape of services to meet the specialist needs of their client group. The need to address mechanisms for practitioners to access underpinning education programmes in order to acquire specialist skills and knowledge in support of clinical developments is also a key challenge, particularly in view of today's time pressures and workforce constraints. Of vital importance is the need to clearly demonstrate the impact that skilled nursing care has upon outcomes for the child or young person, as well as their family. While this text is quite rightly practice based, the need for in-depth, clinically focused research cannot be overemphasised, particularly as future resources and services will undoubtedly be influenced by the available evidence to underpin decision-making.

It was a pleasure to be invited to write this foreword and to have the opportunity to acknowledge the immense contribution the authors have made over the years to child and adolescent mental health services. It is only due to their undoubted commitment and enthusiasm that initiatives, developments and improvements have occurred.

Fiona Smith
Professional Lead for Children and Young People's Nursing
Royal College of Nursing

Acknowledgements

The authors wish to thank the following people for their help and support in writing this book:

Dr Fiona Pender and Lesley Dougan from Cheshire and Wirral Partnership NHS Foundation Trust for inspiring Jasmine Scarisbrick; John Brooke, Librarian at Greater Manchester West NHS Foundation Trust for so helpfully sourcing articles and research papers; Dr Tony Morrison for his advice on attenuated psychotic symptoms; and Dr Gemma Trainor for being interviewed about her career in CAMHS.

Abbreviations

AC	approved clinician
ADD	attention deficit disorder
ADHD	attention deficit hyperactivity disorder
AHP	allied health professional
AMHS	adult mental health services
ARMS	at risk mental state
BME	black and minority ethnic
BMI	body mass index
BNF	British National Formulary
CAF	Common Assessment Framework
CAMHS	child and adolescent mental health services
CAPA	Choice and Partnership Approach
CASR	Conners Adolescent Self Report
CBT	cognitive behaviour therapy
CCG	clinical commissioning group
CHAT	Comprehensive Health Assessment Tool
CIC	community interest company
CoPMI	children of parents with mental illness
CORC	CAMHS Outcome Research Consortium
CPA	Care Programme Approach
CPD	continuing professional development
CQC	Care Quality Commission
CQSW	Certificate of Qualification in Social Work
CRHT	crisis resolution and home treatment
CYP IAPT	Children and Young People's Improving Access to Psychological Therapies
DBT	dialectical behaviour therapy
DSM	Diagnostic and Statistical Manual of Mental Disorders
EARL	Early Assessment Risk List
EBPU	Evidence Based Practice Unit
EIP	early intervention in psychosis
FaPMI	families with parental mental illness
FFA	free fatty acids
GIFT	Greater Involvement, Future Thinking
GP	general practitioner
HEE	Health Education England
HMRC	Her Majesty's Revenue and Customs

IAPT	Improving Access to Psychological Therapies
ICD	International Classification of Diseases
LASCH	local authority secure children's home
LiA	Listening into Action
LLP	limited liability partnership
MARSIPAN	Management of Really Sick Patients with Anorexia Nervosa
MVA	management of violence and aggression
NCCMH	National Collaborating Centre for Mental Health
NHS	National Health Service
NICE	National Institute for Health and Care Excellence
NIP	nurse independent prescriber
NMC	Nursing and Midwifery Council
NSF	National Service Framework
NWW	New Ways of Working
OCC	Office of the Children's Commissioner
ONS	Office for National Statistics
PMHW	primary mental health worker
PMI	parental mental illness
PMVA	preventing and managing violence and aggression
PSHE	Personal, Social, Health and Economic
QNIC	Quality Network for Inpatient CAMHS
RC	responsible clinician
RCN	Royal College of Nursing
RCP	Royal College of Psychiatrists
RCT	randomised controlled trial
ROM	routine outcome monitoring
SAVRY	Structured Assessment of Violence Risk in Youth
SDQ	Strengths and Difficulties Questionnaire
SEAL	Social and Emotional Aspects of Learning
S-NASA	Salford Needs Assessment for Adolescents
TaMHS	Targeted Mental Health in Schools
YJB	Youth Justice Board
YOI	young offender institution

List of figures, tables and boxes

Figures

Tables

Boxes

Note

All the case vignettes used in this book are real. However, the names of the young people concerned and some of their details have been changed. This is to protect their identity and respect their confidentiality.

Introduction

A lot has changed since a version of this book was published in 2006. So much so that it would not be appropriate to update this to a second edition and it has been necessary to start with a blank canvas. The political climate has changed dramatically, the nomenclature of emotional wellbeing and mental health has overtaken that of psychiatry and mental disorder, and there has been somewhat of a shift in the power base relating to involvement and participation.

However, it is unfortunate that some things have remained largely unchanged, such as attitudes to young people who self-harm and the system of organising child and adolescent mental health services (CAMHS), which has now become tired and out of date. It is positive that we see some change in the wind with a policy intention to move away from the tiered model and proposals to review the complicated commissioning arrangements for highly specialised CAMHS.

Worse still, some things have stood still. This includes the development of professional practice guidance and a career structure to recruit, retain and develop nurses who work in CAMHS. These are key areas of concern that we see illustrated in almost every chapter of this book.

What do we mean by CAMHS and the other terms we are using?

Part of the challenge in writing this book was deciding what to call it. There has been debate about the terminology we use to describe the interventions we offer in CAMHS and even whether we should be referring to CAMHS at all. Therefore, some qualifications are required before going any further. Confusingly, the terms 'mental health' and 'mental health problems' are often used interchangeably; this can be misleading and probably fuels the ongoing problem of stigma. All children and young people have mental health needs; many less develop mental health problems, and fewer still suffer from a mental disorder.

Mental health, or emotional health and wellbeing as it is becoming more commonly known as, is used to refer to psychological building blocks such as emotional resilience, good self-esteem and the skills to resolve conflict and to cope in the face of stress and adversity. Sedgewick et al. (2005) remind us that many people do not like to apply the term 'mental health' to children and young people as the first thing that can spring to mind is 'mental illness' and all the stigma that comes with that. This is explored and debated in detail in Chapter 6 and more generally throughout the book.

Emotional health, wellbeing and resilience

At a time when children and young people are facing many economic and social challenges, the concept of wellbeing has never been more important. Resilient children and young people live healthier, happier and more successful lives. They do better in school, college or vocational training and are more likely to form and sustain positive personal and social relationships. *The Good Childhood Report* (The Children's Society 2015) is based on the most extensive and coherent research programme on children's subjective wellbeing in the world. The latest survey ranks England bottom for a number of aspects of children's wellbeing, including those relating to school life, bullying and, especially for teenage girls, feelings about themselves. England ranks in second last place for happiness with life as a whole, with only children in South Korea faring worse. This is a worrying situation given that research shows that as children move into adolescence, their overall wellbeing is likely to decline.

The authors of the influential Foresight report on wellbeing (Foresight Mental Capital and Wellbeing Project 2008) describe resilience as emotional or mental capital. By this, they mean the buffer or cushion against which children and young people can be protected from the most serious effects of adversity. They suggest that interventions which optimise children's learning, promote their social development and enhance their wellbeing could have substantial economic and social implications over many decades. This includes protecting against cognitive decline in older age, which is one of the biggest challenges facing today's NHS.

In contrast to emotional health and wellbeing, the terms 'mental health problems' and 'mental disorders' describe difficulties that may be impairing and sometimes need addressing. Mental health problems are often not serious and most are temporary. Whilst they can interfere with the development and functioning of children or young people, they are different to mental disorders. These are more severe, complex or persistent and cause impairment in functioning. Young people experiencing serious mental disorders usually require professional intervention from CAMHS or early intervention in psychosis (EIP) teams.

The importance of prevention and early intervention

The latest of many compelling reports illustrating the costs and benefits of increased and early service provision in CAMHS was published as the finishing touches were being put to this book (see Centre for Mental Health 2016). Amongst other things, the authors of that report stated that many interventions for common childhood mental disorders are not only effective in improving outcomes but also good value for money. In some cases, they are outstandingly cost-effective, as measured by the surplus of measurable economic benefits over the costs of intervention. It is therefore of great concern that funding for mental health services continues to be cut.

In some areas of the UK, children and young people are waiting far too long to receive mental health support, and many continue to receive an inadequate or substandard service. This is despite numerous national reports highlighting the problems and suggesting solutions that will save the country a lot of money. The evidence that early intervention in the lives of troubled children improves outcomes and reduces costs down the line is compelling. However, this 'invest to save' approach has not gained traction with politicians or commissioners. Chief executives and directors of children's services know very well that lifespan strategies to improve health and wellbeing will be economical in the long term, but they are faced with the unenviable challenge of balancing the books in the short term.

Indeed, many local authorities and clinical commissioning groups (CCGs) have axed universal and targeted programmes for children and families recognised to be at risk of poor outcomes (YoungMinds 2014). A recent King's Fund (2016) analysis shows that around 40 per cent of mental health trusts experienced reductions in income in 2013/14 and 2014/15. This seriously undermines any long-term prevention and early intervention strategies to help ensure children grow up with good mental health and stay well. Unfortunately, this will bear out in the future, and the failure to properly invest in CAMHS will manifest for many years to come.

However, it is not all about money. There is much that nurses and other professionals can do to help make the vision set out in the *Five Year Forward View* (NHS England 2014) a reality. It is important that nurses remain optimistic and creative in times of austerity – this is as much about the positive mental health and resilience of the workforce as it is about determination that things will change for the better.

The structure of the book

This book is written in three parts. In Part 1, the focus is on policy and strategy, and authors navigate an important historical, political and professional practice landscape.

Part 2 comprises a discussion of the practical management of some common mental health problems and disorders affecting children and young people.

Finally, Part 3 explores the changing service provision context and how nurses can play important clinical, managerial and strategic roles to help transform CAMHS services.

Policy and strategy

Changing roles

It is fair to say that the history and evolution of CAMHS has taken an organic rather than a strategic course. Chapter 1 explores some of the origins of policy and discusses how this has influenced the practice of nurses in CAMHS.

Participation and involvement

Children and young people tell us that they want help before things reach crisis point. They want us to listen to them and involve them in decisions about care, treatment and the kind of help we offer. Meaningful participation in healthcare services is crucial in improving outcomes. It is also consistent with the Department of Health's spirit and intention of equity and excellence, which states that there should be 'no decision about me without me' (2010: 6).

Parents or carers also want to develop ongoing trusting relationships with us and to be given the necessary information and support to help their children recover. They remind us of the importance of citizenship, personalisation and social inclusion. Children, young people and families expect to be treated as individuals with a range of strengths and needs and as members of their wider communities. These important messages are not new, and it is essential that nurses and other professionals pay close attention to these basic principles of good practice. As Laing and Nolan (2015) point out, the nurse's proximity to service users enables them to have unique insights into the status and efficacy of services. Chapter 2 discusses the importance of meaningful participation and involvement of children and young people in planning, delivering and evaluating CAMHS. To illustrate this, the chapter has been written by two young people and a professional.

CAMHS transformation

In 2007, the UK government introduced dedicated funding for access to psychological therapies for those presenting with common mental health problems. A project called Improving Access to Psychological Therapies was launched for working-age adults but excluded CAMHS. This was reviewed for use with children and young people and funding for Children and Young People Improving Access to Psychological Therapies (CYP IAPT) was available from 2011 until 2015 when the programme was replaced with a broader CAMHS transformation strategy.

The learning from CYP IAPT was that involving children and young people in the redesign of CAMHS must be at the heart of the transformation agenda. It is crucial that the voice of children and young people is at the centre of service design and that success is evaluated against delivery of the outcomes that matter to them. Chapter 3 focuses on modernising therapeutic interventions and outcomes associated with the CAMHS transformation agenda.

Safeguarding children and families

Nurses and other professionals must not only help protect children from abuse and neglect, but they must also help safeguard them from mental and physical ill health, educational failure and antisocial behaviour. Chapter 4 explores how we can support and safeguard families where a parent is suffering from a mental health problem or disorder.

New roles in CAMHS

Chapter 5 discusses the main new and extended roles in CAMHS. The development of these roles 'has lagged behind many other specialities. The Royal College of Nursing (RCN) has published a range of guidance on the scope and application of new and extended roles including assistant practitioner, advanced practitioner, modern matron and nurse consultant' (see p. 57). Together, these may provide a framework for developing these roles and a career framework within CAMHS.

Challenging stigma

It is a poor reflection on society as a whole that many people including children and young people with mental health problems experience shame, ostracism and social exclusion. All too often they describe the consequences of mental health stigma as worse than those of the condition itself. Interventions to address stigma aim to educate people about mental illness and to overcome the stereotypes that are maintained by prejudice and fear. Along with pharmacological and psychological therapies, stigma interventions have emerged as valuable tools in modern mental health services (Horton 2016). The media and press have a universal role to play to reduce stigma and promote mental health through more sensitive and positive reporting of issues such as self-harm, suicide and behaviour problems. Chapter 6 reminds us of the important roles nurses and other professionals play, working in partnership with children and young people, to tackle mental health stigma.

Workforce development

Not only has demand for services increased as funding has been cut, but the workforce is shrinking as providing organisations have had to make efficiency savings. Between 2003 and 2013, there was a 2 per cent decline in the number of full-time equivalent mental health nurses, with some trusts cutting staff levels by more than 10 per cent (RCN 2014). There is also concern about the quality of the mental health workforce for children and young people. Education and training programmes for nurses and other professionals must ensure that practitioners emerge as competent, capable practitioners. They must be fit for practice and purpose in constantly evolving services. There is debate about whether they finish training with all the skills to do the job.

The education, training and workforce development needs of nurses working in CAMHS have been neglected during the last 20 years. Several high-profile reviews have recognised that the workforce requires better training, support and supervision. All those who work with children and families require basic training in child development and emotional health and wellbeing. They should also have access to specialist CAMHS for consultation and advice.

The evidence base for interventions and practice that improves mental health and psychological wellbeing is rapidly expanding. Nurses and other professionals can now make better use of the growing number of easily accessible evidence-based resources to help children and young people with significant mental health problems and disorders. This enables identification and sharing of best practice across agencies and professions and challenging of poor or substandard practice. This can only improve as the focus on mental health and wellbeing in children and young people moves up the political agenda. Chapter 7 discusses the history and future of CAMHS nurse education, training and workforce development.

Common mental health and psychosocial disorders

Self-harm

Nurses and other professionals come across children and young people who self-harm in a range of settings. These include Accident and Emergency departments, children's wards, community and prison settings and schools. But despite National Institute for Health and Care Excellence (NICE) guidelines and a growing body of research, nurses and other professionals struggle to provide compassionate care for young people who self-harm.

We avoid referring to deliberate self-harm in this book. This is not because young people have no control over their self-harm, which they often do; rather, it is because the intent of young people is frequently changeable or unclear and the term 'deliberate' is more often used to attribute blame rather than to be helpful or compassionate. Understanding and managing self-harm by nurses requires careful engagement and the ability to listen respectfully and non-judgementally to what the young person is trying to communicate. Chapter 8 discusses the importance of thorough assessment and a clear understanding of the context in which it is taking place as well as a number of strategies to help and support young people who self-harm.

Eating disorders

Chapter 9 discusses the challenging topic of nursing care for children and young people with eating disorders. These are serious, often persistent, mental health disorders associated with high levels of impairment to everyday functioning and development. They place a high degree of burden on families and carers and are associated with lifelong physical, psychological, educational and social impairment. In some cases, eating disorders can be fatal.

Nursing a young person with an eating disorder can be a challenging and demanding task that we suggest requires much compassion, patience and resilience on the part of the nurse. It is easy to become overwhelmed by the young person's battle with the eating disorder, and training, supervision and support are an essential part of providing effective care and treatment.

ADHD

Attention deficit hyperactivity disorder (ADHD) is one of the most commonly diagnosed behavioural disorders in children and young people. It is a complex and debated condition with conflicting schools of thought about what causes it and how it should be managed or treated. For some, ADHD is a neurodevelopmental disorder of the brain that can impair a child's day-to-day functioning. For others, it is a product of Western society where children and young people are too often labelled with psychiatric diagnoses or special educational needs.

Storebø et al. (2015) recently published a Cochrane systematic review on the efficacy and tolerability of stimulants for children and adolescents for the treatment of ADHD. Amongst other things, this challenges the quality of the evidence used by NICE to make first-line treatment recommendations. Chapter 10 navigates through the controversial evidence base for ADHD, incorporating and expanding on NICE guidelines to steer nursing practice. It is evident that nurses are in key roles to intervene early and help reduce the costs and burden of impairment of ADHD and improve quality of life. They can also help the treatment and management of ADHD become more holistic and focused on outcomes.

Psychosis and schizophrenia

Another important area in which nurses and other healthcare professionals can help limit the negative effect of mental health disorders on young people is in the early detection and treatment of psychosis. There is evidence that access to early treatment for young people who are at risk may reduce the transition to serious mental illness such as schizophrenia (McGorry et al. 2002). Chapter 11 discusses the role of the nurse in CAMHS, Early Intervention in Psychosis services and inpatient hospital care as well as the importance of care and crisis planning and family or carer involvement.

Service provision

School-based services

Nurses are the single biggest workforce specifically trained and skilled to deliver public health interventions for school-age children (Department of Health and Public Health England 2014). Unlike many other professionals, they work across education, health and social care boundaries, which puts them in a privileged place with children and in key positions of leadership and influence with colleagues in different agencies. Chapter 12 discusses the contribution of school nursing to the emotional health and wellbeing of pupils and students in school, college or higher education. In particular, the important role that primary mental health workers (PMHWs) perform in supporting schools and linking universal and primary services with specialist CAMHS teams is explored.

Challenging behaviours

There is growing interest in reducing the use of restrictive interventions with children and young people in residential care and hospital settings. This is because children are still in a process of physical and emotional development and because restraint can cause psychological and physical harm. Chapter 13 explores the management of aggressive or violent behaviours that challenge nurses and encourages them to consider a range of psychological interventions to prevent or minimise these behaviours. This chapter covers the importance of therapeutic engagement, the need for thorough assessment and collaborative care planning, the principle of 'least restrictive practice' and the government's Positive and Proactive Care strategy (Department of Health 2014), which is becoming more important and topical within CAMHS inpatient settings.

Young offenders

More children are imprisoned in the UK than in any other country in Western Europe. However, there has been a reduction in the last decade or so of more than 60 per cent in the number of young people placed in the secure estate. The reasons for this are not fully clear, but early intervention and diversion as well as better case management and interventions for those young people who do enter secure care or custody all likely play a major role. In the penultimate chapter, the role of the mental health nurse in the youth justice and juvenile prison system is explored. This is a growing area of service provision and clinical practice within the UK. Guidance exists for health and nursing care in the criminal justice system (RCN 2009), but this does not include a specific focus on children and young people in secure units or prisons.

CAMHS nurses as entrepreneurs

Finally, Chapter 15 considers the role of CAMHS nurses as entrepreneurs. The author of this chapter argues that '[c]ombined with a permissive environment and pursuing opportunities inside and outside the health system, nurses with entrepreneurial qualities have already established themselves as formidable change agents, leading healthcare reform and innovation' (see p. 226). She calls on nurses who are open to innovation and uncertainty and who have experience leading change to realise their potential in the health and business markets.

Using this book

It is necessary to qualify a few issues for those who wish to read any further, even if dipping into chapters without reading the whole book. Although it is nearly all about nursing and almost all chapters are written by nurses, we do not mean to be precious about this. Nurses in general are proud to practise as part of multidisciplinary and multi-agency teams and have much to learn from and share with their colleagues in different areas. Authors reinforce this philosophy throughout the chapters. The book is also very much practice based and arguably no less important than the growing number of resources one might call evidence-based. The authors discuss the art of the science of nursing as well as the research contribution of nurses to CAMHS.

Finally, the book has been written primarily for a UK audience. Some of the legal and professional practice issues do not apply any further afield than this, but some of the underpinning principles may be transferable to a worldwide readership. We aim to set a number of challenges to nurses and other professionals who read this book. These are to play their own important part in helping to improve the emotional health, wellbeing and resilience of children and young people, and to plan and deliver care and support that is easily accessible and based on the best available evidence.

References

Centre for Mental Health (2016) *Investing in Children's Mental Health: A Review of Evidence on the Costs and Benefits of Increased Service Provision.* London: Centre for Mental Health.

Children's Society, The (2015) *The Good Childhood Report.* London: The Children's Society.

Department of Health (2014) *Positive and Proactive Care: Reducing the Need for Physical Intervention.* London: Department of Health.

Department of Health (2010) *Achieving Equity and Excellence for Children: How Liberating the NHS Will Help Us Meet the Needs of Children and Young People.* London: Department of Health.

Department of Health and Public Health England (2014) *Health Visiting and School Nurse Programme: Supporting Implementation of the New Service Offer: Promoting Emotional Wellbeing and Positive Mental Health of Children and Young People.* London: Department of Health and Public Health England.

Foresight Mental Capital and Wellbeing Project (2008) *Mental Capital and Wellbeing: Making the Most of Ourselves in the 21st Century. Final Project Report: Executive Summary.* London: The Government Office for Science.

Horton, R. (2016) The health crisis of mental health stigma (editorial). *The Lancet,* 387(10023): 1027.

King's Fund, The (2016) *Mental Health Under Pressure.* London: The King's Fund.

Laing, K. and Nolan, P. (2015) Nurses' perceptions of mental health nursing. *British Journal of Mental Health Nursing,* 4(3): 116–21.

McGorry, P., Yung, A. and Phillips, L. (2002) Randomized controlled trial of interventions designed to reduce the risk of progression to first-episode psychosis in a clinical sample with sub-threshold symptoms. *Archives of General Psychiatry,* 59(10): 921–8.

NHS England (2014) *Five Year Forward View.* London: NHS England. Available at: www.england. nhs.uk/wp-content/uploads/2014/10/5yfv-web.pdf (accessed 23 June 2015).

Royal College of Nursing (2014) *Frontline First: Turning Back the Clock? Mental Health Services in the UK.* London: RCN.

Royal College of Nursing (2009) *Health and Nursing Care in the Criminal Justice Service: RCN Guidance for Nursing Staff.* London: RCN.

Sedgewick, J., Jones, N. and Turner, P. (2005) *Short Child and Adolescent Mental Health Programme (SCAMHP).* London: Care Services Improvement Partnership.

Storebø, O. J., Krogh, H., Ramstad, E., Moreira-Maia, C. R., Holmskov, M., Skoog, M., Nilausen, T. D., Magnusson, F. L., Zwi, M., Gillies, D., Rosendal, S., Groth, C., Rasmussen, K. B., Gauci, D., Kirubakaran, R., Forsbøl, B., Simonsen, E. and Gluud, C. (2015) Methylphenidate for attention-deficit/hyperactivity disorder in children and adolescents: Cochrane systematic review with meta-analyses and trial sequential analyses of randomised clinical trials. *British Medical Journal,* 351: h5203.

YoungMinds (2014) Devastating cuts leading to children's mental health crisis, 21 June [online]. Available at: www.youngminds.org.uk/news/blog/2480_devastating_cuts_leading_to_childrens_mental_health_crisis (accessed 20 July 2016).

Part 1

Policy and strategy

Chapter 1

Changing roles in changing times

Laurence Baldwin

Key points:

- Although children (and young people up to the age of 18) make up a quarter of the UK population, services to meet their mental health needs have historically been neglected, poorly coordinated and underfunded. Currently, child and adolescent mental health services receive 6–8 per cent of the mental health spend in the NHS budget despite increased awareness of need. Across the UK, this increased awareness of mental health issues has not been matched with greatly increased resources or the parity of esteem that policy suggests is needed.
- The increased awareness and understanding is crystallised in the *Future in Mind* report (Department of Health 2015). While this is a good resource, the change in government has reduced its potential impact. Nonetheless, some increased funding has been made available in England although much of it will be spent on preventative measures rather than directly on healthcare provision. The emphasis on resilience and prevention is also evident elsewhere in the world; for example, in the Australian Headspace projects.
- The growth in the evidence base for child mental health, the greater access to guidance from the National Institute for Health and Care Excellence relating to child and adolescent mental health, and the introduction of a children and young people's version of Improving Access to Psychological Therapies (via CYP IAPT) has brought an increased use of particular forms of therapies. It also brings a new emphasis on the use of routine outcome monitoring and other metrics that fit better with the way in which the NHS is commissioned and funded, but has some issues for professional practice and workforce planning.

Introduction

It is in the nature of publications like this that any attempt to look at policy necessarily becomes dated very quickly. Thus, this chapter looks at developments leading up to the current situation and draws some conclusions from the themes that have developed across the English-speaking world. Within the UK, the devolution of healthcare to the different administrations in England, Scotland, Wales and Northern Ireland has led, for example, to broadly similar services but with some differences in speed of implementation and emphasis. Across England, the commissioning arrangements through local clinical commissioning groups (CCGs) mean that there are variations in local provision whereas inpatient services are separately commissioned by NHS England and have been subject to a separate review.

This chapter also fails to do justice to the history and heritage of child and adolescent mental health services (CAMHS). The roots in the (social work-led) child guidance movement across the world and the rise of child psychological services and child psychiatry as a speciality in medicine and other professions has been covered elsewhere (see Black 1993; Cottrell and Kraam 2005; Williams and Kerfoot 2005). We do, however, try to draw out some of the implications of current changes for professional practice in nursing, social work, psychotherapies and the allied health professions in particular.

Background

In the past, very little policy attention was paid to the provision of services for child and adolescent mental health. An early UK report, *Bridges Over Troubled Waters* (Horrocks 1986), addressing deficits in provision of inpatient wards for young people was an exception to this, but it was not until a research report by Kurtz *et al.* (1994) led to the report by the NHS Health Advisory Service (1995), *Together We Stand*, that a four-tier model for CAMHS provision was proposed. The Health Advisory Service model was heavily based on Kurtz's research-based description of existing CAMHS delivery, although it codified that provision and made the important suggestion of a link worker role between health-provided CAMHS and primary care, or universal services. This link worker role was called a primary mental health worker (PMHW) with no explicit reference to the CAMHS element, so it has been easily confused with other primary care staff and other health roles. *Together We Stand*, whilst being seen as very influential now, actually took a while to have any widespread traction on policy or service development.

It was not until the *National Service Framework for Children, Young People and Maternity Services* (Department of Health 2004) was published that the four-tiered model was recognised nationally and used by commissioners to describe the provision of community services and to recognise the need for PMHWs as part of the service. More influential at the time was the Mental Health Foundation (1999) publication *Bright Futures*, which introduced the idea that rather than coming under neither mental health nor paediatric services, children and young people's mental health was 'everybody's business'. This concept helped change the prevailing culture so that more services started to consider emotional wellbeing as an important aspect of wider health and social care, and it was adopted as the title of a Welsh Assembly strategy for CAMHS (National Assembly for Wales 2001). Indeed, the title and the concept were taken up in other service areas, such as older adults (Department of Health 2005), but this led to loss of its distinctiveness and dilution of the idea's effect.

Another thread in the development of CAMHS policy in the UK and elsewhere involves debate as to the degree to which CAMHS is part of a wider mental health policy or part of policy for children's services. This can lead to confusion over which elements of policy (as with law) take priority. For example, when the *National Service Framework for Mental Health* was published (Department of Health 1999), it covered services for 'working age adults' – so this included young people aged 16 and 17 if they were working but not if they were in school or some other form of further education. The National Service Framework (NSF) for children (Department of Health 2004) specifically put CAMHS as the lead agency for young people's mental health up to their eighteenth birthday (Standard 9), thus setting up conflicting policies for some young people, at least for a while. Likewise, workforce policy has not always coincided with or has set out different aspirations for the children's workforce (Department for Children, Schools and Families 2008) whilst mental health workforce policy has followed a different pathway.

Current themes in policy and workforce

Rather than detailing exact policy moves across England, we look at different themes present in current policy and how they have influenced service delivery, or at least the policy that guides policy delivery, which may well be devolved across countries and regions, leading to different interpretations and implementations of policy locally.

Recognition of the existence of child mental health need and the importance of making provision

Within the competing world of healthcare funding, it has often been difficult for children and young people's mental health to make its voice heard and to stake a claim on the limited resources that are available under any system for provision of care. Falling between mental health and paediatric services has led to CAMHS being seen as a 'Cinderella service' (YoungMinds 2014), and there remains a struggle for recognition that is only now being addressed. The YoungMinds submission to the House of Commons Health Select Committee noted that whilst one in ten young people have some form of mental health issue, only a quarter of those young people access services; it also drew attention to the fact that the CAMHS budget is around 7 per cent of mental health funding, which itself does not have parity of esteem with physical healthcare provision.

As with the Mental Health Foundation's *Bright Futures* report (Mental Health Foundation 1999), it has often been for the third sector (voluntary and charity providers) to make the argument for increased provision and recognition of mental health and emotional wellbeing needs. Pressure from YoungMinds and others led to a review of inpatient CAMHS provision in 2014 (CAMHS Tier 4 Steering Group 2014) from which followed the Health Select Committee review of all CAMHS services in England (House of Commons Select Committee 2014). From this was developed the Children and Young People's Mental Health and Wellbeing Taskforce, set up by the then Care Minister Norman Lamb, to make recommendations for future services. This expert reference group brought together a wide range of professional and service user representatives who reported in early 2015 with the *Future in Mind* document and accompanying resources (Department of Health 2015).

The *Future in Mind* report was clear in pointing out an economic argument for investment in CAMHS. In addition, because of an awareness that in the past, good words and high intentions have not always been followed by action, the report looked at how implementation might take place. It also highlighted that access to information which might drive change has been difficult within CAMHS. Part of this problem is to do with reliable prevalence data. The last general survey of mental health across the country was conducted by the Office for National Statistics (ONS) more than a decade ago (Green *et al.* 2005), and whilst there have been partial attempts at large-scale census since then, these have not been comprehensive. The Durham CAMHS mapping exercise (see National Child and Maternal Health Intelligence Network 2015), for example, was based on clinician-reported samples, whilst the Centre for Mental Health cohort study has only been able to focus on a younger age group (a millennial cohort who are still growing up) (Gutman *et al.* 2015). Recommendations for better data collection may be irksome for those who have to collect and input the data (usually the clinicians), but it strengthens the case for increased provision of resources. Similarly, increased collection of data on outcomes gives quantitative evidence for efficacy of services as well as demonstrating the level of need.

The importance of early intervention and the role of resilience

Whilst the importance of early intervention has been known about and advocated by various schools of thought for a long time, it has rarely been included in health policy, which has concentrated largely on secondary care. Community psychology, for example, has long stressed the need for dealing in a more systemic way with the conditions that lead to poor mental health (Casale *et al.* 2015). Bowlby's theories of attachment (1988) – although criticised for putting excessive blame on the role of the mother (and not including fathers) – have been influential in helping understand infant mental health development, as have the psychodynamic models of Anna Freud and Melanie Klein. Developmental theories have always informed our understanding of young people's psychological functioning but, again, have not strongly influenced how much importance we give to enabling children to develop healthy minds. The recent focus, however, on the function of resilience has helped to make people think more carefully about why some children and young people seem to survive and flourish when others in similar circumstances develop serious mental health conditions (e.g. Gilligan 2004).

In particular, this renewed interest has led to a greater focus on the role of schools in promoting and sustaining mental health from a public health and primary prevention viewpoint. There is not complete agreement on how best this should be done, however, and there are different solutions proposed for different settings. In Australia, a major study of school-based interventions (URBIS 2011) concluded that there was no 'one size fits all' solution, and schools should be careful in selecting the right approach for their setting based on their own demographics and needs. In the UK, the skills deficit (or often the lack of confidence to deal with mental health issues) has been addressed in part with the establishment of an online resource called MindEd, which is an electronic learning resource that is free to access and provides a range of teaching for professionals (see www.minded.org.uk).

The development of increased evidence-based practice within child mental health

As CAMHS have developed over the last few years, the practice has been increasingly informed by the rise of evidence-based practice. Mostly, this change is because the evidence base was previously very poor and finding research funding to develop evidence within this speciality has often been difficult. The importance of being able to justify the rationale for what we deliver to young people is well understood, but in the past, this had not been effectively developed.

Whilst, historically, departments of child psychiatry and child psychology have followed their disciplinary lines in developing research, the CAMHS Evidence Based Practice Unit (EBPU) was established in 2006 at the Anna Freud Centre, University College London. Their initial projects included the CAMHS Outcome Research Consortium (CORC), which recruited a group of four CAMHS services to routinely collect outcome measures in order to start developing metrics; this aimed to inform commissioning and embed the concept of regularly use of metrics to inform practice. Since 2004, its membership has spread across the UK, and there are now over 70 member organisations. CORC also created a baseline of evidence with the publication of a review of findings relating to CAMHS (Wolpert *et al.* 2006) and built on the work by Professor Fonagy on developing evidence-based approaches (see Fonagy *et al.* 2014).

Alongside this, the number of National Institute for Health and Care Excellence (NICE) guidelines that include elements of child mental health have increased. With NICE guidelines come the evidence base and practice-based recommendations that are relevant to CAMHS, and within healthcare, the rightful expectation is that this will be followed where possible. NHS governance has an expectation that guidelines reflect good practice, but what is often overlooked is that NICE always now provides a tool for calculating the costs of implementing this best practice (e.g. NICE 2015). Tools like these have been used to calculate staffing implications for a full implementation of guidelines (Royal College of Psychiatrists [RCP] 2013). This work has also informed the CYP IAPT programme, based on the adult Improving Access to Psychological Therapies (IAPT; examined in more detail in Chapter 3) that is now the dominant model within England for a transformation of CAMHS.

Increased importance of participation of young people

The importance of including children, young people and families in developing services is the subject of Chapter 6 and is discussed in detail there. CAMHS was late to adopt participatory methods, mostly because of perceived difficulties in doing so. Whilst adult mental health services have included service users in planning for a long while, simple logistical issues of working with children and young people made this more complex. Healthcare provider meetings usually take place in office hours, for example, when children and young people are legally required to be in school. Adult service user organisations often rely on a core group of people who have had experience of services whereas, by definition, children and young people move on from CAMHS; for example, they are often away at university soon after finishing their CAMHS experience. Tribute should be paid then to the efforts which have been made to ensure that their voices are now more prominent in CYP IAPT and elsewhere. This move has been mirrored in research circles where ethical approval for studies, including CAMHS studies, requires some user involvement in developing appropriate and useful research projects. This area is examined in more detail in Chapter 2.

Service delivery models and age ranges

As we have previously noted, the history of CAMHS has evolved from the child guidance movement, and initially the staffing and operational management of services was almost haphazard with no central direction as to how services should be provided. In some ways, this suited professionals who were left to provide services as they saw fit. As child psychiatry overtook social work as the dominant force within service provision (alongside child psychology in some areas), the name changed to reflect this. The concept of child and adolescent mental health reflected the child and adolescent psychiatry speciality, for example, and is rooted in the developmental stage approach to this age group. It is fair to say that most young people prefer not to think of themselves as 'adolescents' and, given a choice, would think of a different name for the service (as is increasingly happening with greater participation and involvement).

Alongside this move, the model of implementation also reflected contemporary practice in mental health services during the early eighties when the emphasis was on community care and multidisciplinary teamwork. As multidisciplinary teams were set up, they were based on an unfounded assumption that the correct skill set came with the right combination of disciplines. Most teams included child and adolescent psychiatrists, nurses, social workers (either as local authority employees or as healthcare workers using their original social work training as their main method of working, more in the tradition of 'hospital social worker') and clinical psychologists and then a range of other therapeutic modalities dependent on local need or preference. These might have included art psychotherapists, child psychotherapists, drama therapists, play therapists and occupational therapists.

Efforts to more precisely map team composition started with *Together We Stand* (NHS Health Advisory Service 1995), which mentions in passing which professional groups should be in a CAMHS team. As we have seen though, this report was based on descriptive research that reflected contemporary practice and so included the groups mentioned above but without specifying what each group contributed, thus continuing the 'taken for granted' multidisciplinary team concept. It was only really with the New Ways of Working (NWW) project (Department of Health 2007a) that attention shifted to team composition and a clearer concept of skills necessary for achieving the outcomes that were required within the service. In this respect, NWW was reflecting the overall move towards outcomes-based and evidence-based practice. It was also, however, a project with some political motivation, in its broadest sense.

Originating from the RCP, there was a motivation within NWW to look at the work all psychiatrists were doing and to manage that work in a way which best used the skills of the profession. The movement led to psychiatrists being able to shift the burden of case managing large outpatient numbers to other professions (largely nurses) in adult mental health settings and making the psychiatrist role much more focused on diagnostics, medication management and other high-level skills. NWW soon expanded to become a multidisciplinary project as psychologists and other professional groups joined the working groups to explore the effects that changing one professional role had on the rest of the multidisciplinary team. It also looked more broadly across the age ranges to include CAMHS and other specialities.

In line with the start of more service user-focused participatory methods, NWW also included a tool called the Creating Capable Teams Approach (Department of Health 2007b) that looked at what skills were needed to achieve the aims and commissioned purpose of each team. This movement towards skills-based team building in mental health, rather than assuming that a multidisciplinary team would automatically provide the correct range of skills, had been foreshadowed by The Sainsbury Centre for Mental Health's (2001) work on the 'capable practitioner'.

The capable practitioner model had started to challenge the concept that professional training would automatically provide what people needed from a mental health worker and focused instead on what service users found useful in the people who try to help them. Sadly, service users' experience was often that professionals failed to provide what they really needed or wanted, and this experience continued to be reflected in some of the CYP IAPT participation feedback exercises that followed a few years later (Lavis and Hewson 2011). Whilst this is hard to swallow for many professionals who do not generally come to work each day thinking that they will do a bad job, it does come across consistently that people are unsatisfied with what they get from CAMHS and other mental health services.

A search of YouTube or Twitter with the keyword 'CAMHS' will quickly find some often graphic examples of this. Of course, there are also large numbers of people who have been helped and who are very grateful, and they may be less likely to express their views on social media or when given opportunities within participation exercises. However, service failures cannot be denied or fully blamed on financial cuts, when a lot of what service users are unhappy with are failures in basic skills of engagement or how care or treatment was delivered.

A common theme of discontent is difficulty in accessing services. Waiting times in particular can be difficult, despite national targets, as well as understanding what services CAMHS have commissioned and able to provide. The commissioning arrangements for CAMHS services haven't always helped with this, initially being extremely vague and latterly becoming overly precise. In many cases, commissioning arrangements were vague because there were not the resources to match demand. Within the children's NSF, for example, there was an evidence-based staffing level for CAMHS (Kelvin 2005), but this was never achieved in any area according to the Durham mapping exercises (National Child and Maternal Health Intelligence Network 2015).

According to the more recent report of the RCP (2013), this level of staffing should be almost doubled if services are to actually implement all the NICE guidelines relevant to CAMHS practice. In some ways, these reports further highlight the need to increase collection of accurate figures that reflect both need and the work done within CAMHS as a tool for allowing more effective commissioning and a more equitable distribution of funding. The development of CYP IAPT data collection from routine outcome monitoring (ROM) and a full implementation of a national minimum dataset expected in 2016, whilst difficult, should provide the evidence on which to base better decisions.

One other development within CAMHS service delivery has been the adoption in some services, in the UK and elsewhere, of a model of service that aims to look at demand management and more effective use of existing resources to overcome bottlenecks and reduce waiting times. The Choice and Partnership Approach (CAPA; York and Kingsbury 2013) is used widely in the UK, Ireland, Belgium, Holland, New Zealand, Australia and Canada. This is in CAMHS, adult mental health, and child and adult learning disability services. CAPA uses industry models to map demand and capacity in order to allow a more effective system of early access to assessment (the 'Choice' appointment) and then initial treatment on a short-term basis (a short series of 'Partnership' appointments) with the option of further specialist treatment pathways if needed. The focus of CAPA is on quick and effective treatment, throughput and not keeping people in service any longer than is needed. This has been further developed in the THRIVE model (Wolpert et al. 2014) that also focuses on what can be provided, is evidence-based and can be demonstrated to be producing good outcomes, thus fitting well with the CYP IAPT approach. It does leave a couple of issues where there are questions unanswered, or the answers are presumed.

One issue is that the skill set for delivering the outcomes under CYP IAPT is based on the preferred therapeutic modalities that the project is delivering (and we look below at what this means for professional practice). The second issue arises because a large part of CAMHS work up until recently has included addressing the mental health needs of young people with neurodevelopmental issues such as attention deficit hyperactivity disorder (ADHD) and autism spectrum condition/disorder. NICE guidelines for each of these conditions (NICE 2008, 2011, 2013) specify the need for ongoing monitoring of medication either by psychiatrists, paediatricians or specialist practitioners. These longer-term interventions do not fit well with the THRIVE model, and there has been some movement towards developing separate neurodevelopmental teams, often across community paediatric services and CAMHS, which can offer a more targeted service to this group. By removing this user group from CAMHS, there will necessarily be a change in the culture of CAMHS, but in many ways, this is precisely what the CYP IAPT programme is aiming for in its transformational approach.

Implications for nursing and professional practice

What does this overall direction of travel mean for professional practice? So far, we have examined the way in which evidence-based practice is increasingly influencing policy and slowly being implemented in services. The previous lack of evidence and the evolutionary development of services, rather than there being much central planning, meant that there had been a reliance on professional judgement to provide a service which was fit for local need. Mostly this worked, but individual differences in the development of services led to what the media and politicians call a 'postcode lottery'. So depending on where you lived, there would be certain therapies available or approaches to different conditions might vary. For example, if one had a child psychiatrist who didn't 'believe' in ADHD a few years ago then it would be difficult to get a diagnosis and treatment with medication. In theory, this move to evidence-based practice is a good thing, but there is also an argument to be made that these developments have been made at the expense of important elements of mental health care which children and young people, as well as their parents, always highlight in their feedback to services. Ironically, given the importance attached to engaging young people and their families in developing services, the evidence of participatory projects in respect of these elements is usually not given the credence that theoretically it ought to receive.

In large part, the evidence on which we are building new CAMHS services is driven by two main professional groups – psychiatrists and psychologists. Relatively little of the research within child and adolescent mental health comes from the other professional groups who make up the face-to-face staffing of child mental health services, such as nurses, social workers and allied health professionals (AHPs). Cognitive behaviour therapy (CBT), for example, has developed a better evidence base, though a lot of that evidence has been gathered by clinical psychologists whose core professional orientation fits with this method. Moreover, building an evidence base for some therapies relies much more on qualitative research methods, which are often less influential and technically cannot claim generalisability in the same way as quantitative studies usually do. So while there is an evidence base for psychoanalytically based therapies and systemic family therapies, this largely relies on methods specific to those therapies – like case studies and phenomenological approaches – rather than 'gold standard' randomised controlled trials (RCTs).

For nurses, social workers and AHPs, there is not as strong an emphasis within their core training on developing the evidence base or on research training and involvement as there is in medicine (and therefore psychiatry) and in clinical psychology. Each of these disciplines, within their core training as well as their continuing professional development (CPD) requirements, highlight the need for ongoing involvement in research activities and ensure that job planning includes time for such activities. The initial training is at higher levels and involves research training as a core element. Medical doctors in the UK train to at least master's level, and membership of the Royal Colleges (which allows access to consultant-level posts) is arguably at doctorate level.[1]

A few years ago, clinical psychology moved qualification-level training through a Doctorate in Clinical Psychology (DClinPsych). Whilst AHP training has been at bachelor's degree level for a while, both social work and nursing have been slow to move into this academic range. Social workers formerly completed a Certificate of Qualification in Social Work (CQSW), and until very recently, nursing registration was also usually at diploma level. Though both of these professions now train and qualify at bachelor's degree level – which includes some research awareness training and understanding of the importance and development of evidence-based practice – this shift has not been without considerable challenge. In part, this is because of the practical nature of the disciplines, each of which pride themselves on their relatedness to their patients (or clients in social work), and because they have used an apprenticeship approach to skills development. In nursing, the debates have often reflected concern about excluding those with good practical skills but lacking academic abilities, and this has led at times to an inverse snobbery about degree-level nurses who are seen as 'too posh to wash'.

The Royal College of Nursing (RCN), where many of these debates have been hotly contested, has come down in favour of the all-graduate workforce, in part because of the lost ground in developing evidence-based approaches that highlight nursing skills (RCN 2015). The Agenda for Change formulas used in the NHS for determining pay have also been an influence as they lay great store by the level of qualification required for a post, thus directly affecting remuneration levels for different disciplines. Pay is not everything, but it is a concrete way of demonstrating value as Salvage (1985) points out. Lesser-paid professional groups are often valued less by society and by the professional groups themselves.

Bachelor's-level degrees ought to give nurses the skills to understand what good clinical evidence is so that they can critically appraise the value of new developments and to grasp the reasoning behind NICE guidelines, but they do not necessarily give access to the means to develop new evidence. Although there are an increasing number of nurses, social workers and AHPs with master's-level degrees and above, this level of qualification – which would include skills to lead and develop research projects and, crucially, to attract the funding to complete the projects – remain rare amongst these groups. In nursing, for example, it is only at nurse consultant level that a master's degree is considered essential.

The result is a lack of good practice-based research on the essential attributes of these disciplines. Much of the research that is completed is done by those whose careers have moved into education within universities, and this influences what is being researched. Whilst there is a lot of good nursing research on nursing education, for example, there is less on nursing practice.

Within mental health nursing, the essential paradigm of the therapeutic relationship (as developed by Peplau, Altschul, Skillern and latterly by Barker) has remained in the realms of nursing theory; its value within CAMHS is not showing through in current policy, however. The lack of an evidence base for what CAMHS nurses do that is actually distinctive to nursing has been noted in the past (Baldwin 2002). As long ago as 2000, Limerick and Baldwin examined the roles of CAMHS nurses and warned that unless nurses were able to clearly articulate and identify the specific contribution they made, there was a danger of the role being filled by generic workers. Still, there has been little focus on the therapeutic roles and responsibilities of CAMHS nurses or how they use their nursing skills, theory and experience to implement current CAMHS policy. If pushed, it is possible for practitioners to think about this, but the nature of fast-paced practice and lack of research time and funding means that this area remains underdeveloped, and there remains a risk that nurses, social workers and AHPs face a loss of professional identity within a generic skills base in CAMHS.

What nurses in CAMHS do sometimes highlight is that the emphasis they place on the need to develop relationships with children, young people and their families is strongly influenced by their original training within mental health nursing (Baldwin 2008). This is exactly what children and young people highlight as being what they want from the people they see (Lavis and Hewson 2011). What is important to them is feeling listened to, being valued as people and not having their views dismissed. Not one of them talks about wanting particular modalities of therapy or the latest meds. They may understand the need for these things but they don't want to be 'fobbed off with more tablets' at the expense of being listened to.

Some of these skills which are highlighted in modern policy developments were available to nurses in the past, but as a profession, we seem to have clung to the central ethos of getting on with the practical tasks, privileging our time with patients over developing the rationale for how and why we do this. Smoyak (1975), for example, wrote about family therapy for nurses before family therapy developed into systemic psychotherapy with a distinct training, advanced levels of training and a membership structure.

Systemic thinking fits well with the holistic approach that nursing uses, so a distinctively systemic approach is also the basis of family systems nursing (Wright and Leahey 2000). In the UK, this is not a well-known theory and has not been widely adopted by CAMHS nurses in their practice despite the obvious overlay of nursing theory and structural and strategic family therapy theory inherent in their writing. This risk to professional identity is not exclusive to nurses. AHPs such as occupational therapists also have a long history of working in CAMHS, although again using more generic mental health skills rather than their core training. This reflects the general move within CAMHS during the eighties and nineties for all professionals to use a fairly common set of core skills that merged and blurred their identities towards a single CAMHS practitioner approach, risking the loss of some of the essence of their professional skill sets. Occupational therapists have moved towards reclaiming their strengths in sensory assessment for young people with autistic spectrum disorders (and in meaningful occupation for the older age group), for example.

Summary

These are exciting times for the development of CAMHS services with unprecedented awareness of the issues and a concrete direction of travel, in England at least, through the evidence-based CYP IAPT programme and the developing THRIVE model. The increased involvement of children, young people and their families in developing new services should mean a much closer alignment between provision and what is wanted and needed. Joined-up commissioning across health, social care and the third sector also aims to prevent silo thinking and encourage everyone to think of children and young people's mental health and emotional wellbeing as truly being 'everybody's business'. Yet there are dangers which may be overlooked. In particular, there is the potential for professional skills to be lost in the current drive despite what we know about what children and young people value – human skills in therapeutic relationships, which are part of the core training of nurses, social workers, AHPs and psychotherapists.

Note

1   Most medical doctors in the UK have an honorary doctorate, rather than the MD (which is common in the US), or a university PhD (Doctor of Philosophy) or a professional doctorate such as the DClinPsych or DNursing. This can be confusing when clinical psychologists refer to themselves as 'Dr Smith', and so on because they have a professional doctorate or when some nurses or AHPs with PhDs or professional doctorates are also 'Dr Baldwin', etc. because of their academic qualification. Vernacular use of the title outside of university circles almost always assumes a medical doctor.

References

Baldwin, L. (2008) *The Discourse of Professional Identity in Child and Adolescent Mental Health Services*. PhD thesis, University of Nottingham. Available at: http://eprints.nottingham.ac.uk/10504/ (accessed 30 August 2015).

Baldwin, L. (2002) The nursing role in out-patient child and adolescent mental health services. *Journal of Clinical Nursing*, 11(4): 520–5.

Black, D. (1993) A brief history of child and adolescent psychiatry. In D. Black and D. Cottrell (eds) *Seminars in Child and Adolescent Psychiatry*. London: Gaskell, pp. 1–5.

Bowlby, J. (1988) *A Secure Base*. London: Routledge.

CAMHS Tier 4 Steering Group (2014) *Review of CAMHS Tier Four Services*. London: NHS England. Available at: www.england.nhs.uk/wp-content/uploads/2014/07/camhs-tier-4-rep.pdf (accessed 14 November 2015).

Casale, L., Zlotowitz, S. and Moloney, O. (2015) Working with whole communities: delivering community psychology approaches with children, young people and families. *The Child and Family Psychological Review*, 3(Summer): 84–94.

Cottrell, D. and Kraam, A. (2005) Growing up? A history of CAMHS (1987–2005). *Child and Adolescent Mental Health*, 10(3): 111–17.

Department for Children, Schools and Families (2008) *2020: Children and Young People's Workforce Strategy*. London: Department for Children, Schools and Families.

Department of Health (2015) *Future in Mind: Promoting, Protecting and Improving Our Children and Young People's Mental Health and Wellbeing*. London: Department of Health.

Department of Health (2007a) *Mental Health: New Ways of Working for Everyone. Creating and Sustaining a Capable and Flexible Workforce. Progress Report*. London: Department of Health.

Department of Health (2007b) *Creating Capable Teams Approach: Best Practice Guidance to Support the Implementation of New Ways of Working (NWW) and New Roles*. London: Department of Health.

Department of Health (2005) *Everybody's Business: Integrated Mental Health Services for Older Adults: A Service Development Guide*. London: Department of Health.

Department of Health (2004) *National Service Framework for Children, Young People and Maternity Services*. London: Department of Health.

Department of Health (1999) *National Service Framework for Mental Health*. London: Department of Health.

Fonagy, P., Cottrell, D., Phillips, J., Bevington, D., Glaser, D. and Allison, A. (2014) *What Works for Whom? A Critical Review of Treatments for Children and Adolescents* (second edition). London: Guilford Press.

Gilligan, R. (2004) Promoting resilience in child and family social work: issues for social work practice, education and policy. *Social Work Education*, 23(1): 93–104.

Green, H., McGinnity, A., Meltzer, H., Ford, T. and Goodman, R. (2005) *Mental Health of Children in Great Britain 2004*. London: Office of National Statistics.

Gutman, L. M., Joshi, H., Parsonage, M. and Schoon, I. (2015) *Children of the New Century: Mental Health Findings from the Millennial Cohort Study*. London: Centre for Mental Health. Available at: www.centreformentalhealth.org.uk/children-of-the-new-century (accessed 14 November 2015).

Horrocks, P. (1986) *Bridges Over Troubled Waters: A Report from the NHS Advisory Service on Services for Disturbed Adolescents*. London: NHS Health Advisory Service.

House of Commons Health Select Committee (2014) *Children's and Adolescents' Mental Health and CAMHS: Third Report of Session 2014–5*. London: House of Commons Health Select Committee.

Kelvin, R. (2005) Capacity of Tier 2/3 CAMHS and service specification: a model to enable evidence based service development. *Child and Adolescent Mental Health*, 10(2): 63–73.

Kurtz, Z., Thornes, R. and Wolkind, S. (1994) *Services for the Mental Health of Children and Young People in England: A National Review*. London: Maudsley Hospital and South West Thames Regional Health Authority.

Lavis, P. and Hewson, L. (2011) How Many Times Do We Have To Tell You? A Briefing from the National Advisory Council about What Young People Think about Mental Health and Mental Health Services [online]. Available at: www.chimat.org.uk/resource/item.aspx?RID=110049 (accessed 14 November 2015).

Limerick, M. and Baldwin, L. (2000) Nursing in outpatient child and adolescent mental health. *Nursing Standard*, 15(13–15): 43–5.

Mental Health Foundation (1999) *Bright Futures: Promoting Children and Young People's Mental Health*. London: Mental Health Foundation.

National Assembly for Wales (2001) *Child and Adolescent Mental Health Services: Everybody's Business*. Cardiff: National Assembly for Wales.

National Child and Maternal Health Intelligence Network (2015) Data Atlas [online]. Available at: http://atlas.chimat.org.uk/IAS/ (accessed 14 November 2015).

National Institute for Health and Care Excellence (NICE) (2015) Depression in Children and Young People: Identification and Management – Tools and Resources [online]. Available at: www.nice.org.uk/guidance/cg28/resources/ (accessed 30 August 2015).

National Institute for Health and Care Excellence (NICE) (2013) *Autism in Under 19s: Support and Management (CG170)*. London: NICE.

National Institute for Health and Care Excellence (NICE) (2011) *Autism in Under 19s: Recognition, Referral and Diagnosis (CG128)*. London: NICE.

National Institute for Health and Care Excellence (NICE) (2008) *Attention Deficit Hyperactivity Disorder: Diagnosis and Treatment (CG72)*. London: NICE.

NHS Health Advisory Service (1995) *Together We Stand: The Commissioning, Role and Management of Child and Adolescent Mental Health Services*. London: HMSO.

Royal College of Nursing (RCN) (2015) *Registered Nurses and Health Care Support Workers: A Summary of RCN Policy Positions*. London: RCN.

Royal College of Psychiatrists (RCP) (2013) *Building and Sustaining Specialist CAMHS to Improve Outcomes for Children and Young People (CR182)*. London: RCP.

Sainsbury Centre for Mental Health, The (2001) *The Capable Practitioner*. London: The Sainsbury Centre for Mental Health.

Salvage, J. (1985) *The Politics of Nursing*. Oxford: Butterworth-Heinnemann Ltd.

Smoyak, S. (1975) *The Psychiatric Nurse as a Family Therapist*. New York: John Wiley & Sons.

URBIS (2011) *Literature Review on Meeting the Psychological and Emotional Well-Being Needs of Children and Young People: Models of Effective Practice in Educational Settings. Final Report*. Australia: URBIS Pty Ltd. Available at: www.det.nsw.edu.au/media/downloads/about-us/statistics-and-research/public-reviews-and-enquiries/school-counselling-services-review/models-of-effective-practice.pdf (accessed 14 November 2015).

Williams, R. and Kerfoot, M. (2005) *Child and Adolescent Mental Health Services: Strategy, Planning, Delivery and Evaluation*. Oxford: Oxford University Press.

Wolpert, M., Harris, R., Jones, M., Hodges, S., Fuggle, P., James, S., Weiner, A., McKenna, C., Law, D. and Fonagy, P. (2014) *THRIVE: The AFC-Tavistock Model for CAMHS*. London: Anna Freud Centre. Available at: www.annafreud.org/media/2552/thrive-booklet_march-15.pdf (accessed 14 November 2015).

Wolpert, M., Fuggle, P., Cottrell, D., Fonagy, P., Phillips, J., Pilling, S., Stein, S. and Target, M. (2006) *Drawing on the Evidence: Advice for Mental Health Professionals Working with Children and Adolescents*. London: CAMHS Evidence Based Practice Unit.

Wright, L. and Leahey, M. (2000) *Nurses and Families: A Guide to Family Assessment and Intervention*. Philadelphia, PA: F. A. Davis & Co.

York, A. and Kingsbury, S. (2013) *The Choice and Partnership Approach: A Service Transformation Model* (fourth edition). London: CAMHS Network.

YoungMinds (2014) *Submission to the Health Select Committee of the House of Commons on Child and Adolescent Mental Health Services*. London: YoungMinds.

Chapter 2

Increasing participation and involvement

Elaine Williams, Jasmine Scarisbrick and Ben Samata

Key points:

- There is a long-documented history of a commitment to involving people in their treatment and care.
- There is compelling evidence that highlights the impact and value of meaningful involvement.
- Involve the people who use your service in order to ensure everyone's vision is aligned.
- It is important to be clear about what will happen with the information you receive during participation and involvement events.

Introduction

This chapter sets out to explore participation theory in practice and provide health professionals with the opportunity to critically reflect on what participation and involvement means to them. Innovative examples of participation and involvement are described by the authors as case examples throughout the chapter.

The participation and involvement agenda is contextualised below into an easy-to-follow timeline. This chapter does not present an academic overview but, rather, hopes to provide a platform to develop critical analysis of one's own position and that of the healthcare service the reader is interested in.

Background

The aspiration to involve people and give them more control over their health and care has a long history within nursing and health services, and patient involvement can be traced back to the roots of the NHS. Morse (1991) describes the value of involvement in the nurse–patient relationship, and making sure a young person is fully involved in their care is one of the good practice principles for working with young people identified by the Royal College of Nursing (2008).

Over time, this has evolved from being able to choose your own general practitioner (GP), as outlined in the White Paper *Working for Patients* (Department of Health 1989), to the introduction of the personalisation agenda in 1997. *The NHS Plan* published at the turn of the century called for services to be redesigned to be patient-centred within ten years (Department of Health 2000).

More recently, there has been increasing emphasis on individuals being involved in all aspects of healthcare from commissioning to every level of provision, incorporating prevention and health promotion through to self-management of long-term conditions (Foot *et al.* 2014).

The NHS aspires to put patients at the heart of everything it does. It should support individuals to promote and manage their own health. NHS services must reflect, and should be coordinated around and tailored to, the needs and preferences of patients, and their families and carers, where appropriate, will be involved in and consulted on all decisions about their care and treatment. The NHS should actively encourage feedback from the public, patients and staff, welcome it and use it to improve its services. The NHS Constitution, which aspires to uphold the principles that guide the NHS, was updated in 2013, and this strengthened the commitment to patient involvement (see excerpts in Box 2.1). This update was published partly in response to the report into the failings at Mid Staffordshire NHS Foundation Trust by Francis (2013).

Box 2.1 NHS Constitution (2013)

Working together for patients.

Patients come first in everything we do. We fully involve patients, staff, families, carers, communities, and professionals inside and outside the NHS. We put the needs of patients and communities before organisational boundaries. We speak up when things go wrong.

Commitment to quality of care.

We earn the trust placed in us by insisting on quality and striving to get the basics of quality care – safety, effectiveness and patient experience – right every time. We encourage and welcome feedback from patients, families, carers, staff and the public. We use this to improve the care we provide and build on our successes.

Source: National Health Service, England (2013)

Charitable organisations have long been pioneers of the participation agenda. Examples of this exist within adult substance misuse services, adult mental health services, and as discussed within Street and Herts (2005), this is established within children's services.

Key policy framework in relation to children and young people's services

The last two decades have seen a number of programmes come and go that were intended to improve outcomes for children. These included Quality Protects (Department of Health 1998) and the Healthy Schools agenda that was part of the wider public health strategy in *Saving Lives: Our Healthier Nation* (Department of Health 1999). Overarching policies such as *Every Child Matters* (Department for Education and Skills 2003) and the *National Service Framework for Children, Young People and Maternity Services* (Department of Health 2004) had emotional health and wellbeing at their core.

Comprehensive approaches to improving emotional health and wellbeing have become increasingly common over the years. These include the Targeted Mental Health in Schools (TaMHS) project (Department for Children, Schools and Families 2008), Targeted Youth Support (Department for Children, Schools and Families 2007) and the Social and Emotional Aspects of Learning (SEAL) programme (Department for Education 2005).

Table 2.1, though not a comprehensive guide, identifies some of the key milestones for child and adolescent mental health services (CAMHS) policy and strategy, some of which have been discussed in Chapter 1. Some of these, but not all, contain declarations related to participation and involvement.

Table 2.1 Key milestones in relation to CAMHS policy and strategy

Year	Milestone
1991	UN Convention on the Rights of the Child
1995	*Together We Stand: The Commissioning, Role and Management of Child and Adolescent Mental Health Services* (NHS Health Advisory Service thematic review)
1998	*Quality Protects* (Department of Health)
1999	*Children in Mind: Child and Adolescent Mental Health Services* (Audit Commission)
	NHS Modernisation Fund and Mental Health Grant for Child and Adolescent Mental Health Services (Department of Health)
	Bright Futures: Promoting Children and Young People's Mental Health (Mental Health Foundation)
2001	*Special Educational Needs Code of Practice* (Department for Education and Skills)
	Health and Social Care Act 2001
	Promoting Children's Mental Health Within Early Years and School Settings (Department for Education and Skills)
2002	Education Act 2002
2003	*Every Child Matters* set out a core framework for reform of children's services, including five outcomes – being healthy, staying safe, enjoying and achieving, making a positive contribution and achieving economic wellbeing (Department for Education and Skills)
	Framework for developing a comprehensive CAMHS, one of the underlying principles being that the commissioning and delivery of services should be informed by stakeholder views with those of children and young people being key
	The Victoria Climbie Inquiry by Lord Laming
2004	Children Act 2004 and the development of children's trusts, requiring local authorities and other agencies concerned with children and young people to work collaboratively and be informed by the views of local children, young people and families
	Choosing Health: Making Healthier Choices Easier (Department of Health)
	The Chief Nursing Officer's Review of the Nursing, Midwifery and Health Visiting Contribution to Vulnerable Children and Young People (Department of Health)
2005	The first Children's Commissioner for England was appointed with the expectation that they oversee plans to involve children in the inspection of local services alongside a specific remit to act as an independent voice for children and young people
	Transition: Getting it Right for Children and Young People – Improving the Transition of Children with Long-Term Conditions to Adult Services (Department of Health)
	Chief Nursing Officer's Review of Mental Health Nursing (Department of Health)
2007	*Pushed Into The Shadows: Young People's Experience of Adult Mental Health Facilities* (Office of the Children's Commissioner)
	Transition Guide for All Services: Key Information for Professionals about the Transition Process for Disabled Young People (Department for Children, Schools and Families)

Table 2.1 Continued

Year	Milestone
2008	First Children's Plan published and Think Family initiative launched (Cabinet Office)
	Launch of Targeted Mental Health in Schools project (Department for Children, Schools and Families)
	Final report of the National Advisory Council for Children's Mental Health and Psychological Wellbeing (Department for Children, Schools and Families/Department of Health)
	Transition: Moving On Well: A Good Practice Guide for Professionals and Their Partners on Transition Planning for Young People with Complex Health Needs or a Disability (Department of Health)
	The National CAMHS Support Service: Learning Perspectives from the National Child and Adolescent Mental Health Service Improvement Programme (Department of Health)
	Turning what Young People Say into What Services Do: Quality Standards for Children and Young People's Participation in CAMHS (Health and Social Care Advisory Service)
2009	The mental health strategy New Horizons was published, setting out a vision for improving the mental health of the whole population regardless of age range
	You're Welcome Quality Criteria: Self-assessment Toolkit (Department of Health)
2010	Age-appropriate environment duty under Section 131a of the Mental Health Act (1983) took effect
	Involving Young People in the Development of Health Services (Department of Health/ Association for Young People's Health)
	Liberating the NHS: No Decision About Me Without Me (Department of Health)
	Getting it Right for Children and Young People: Overcoming Cultural Barriers in the NHS so as to Meet Their Needs (Department of Health)
2011	*No Health without Mental Health: A Cross-governmental Outcomes Strategy for People of All Ages* (HM Government/Department of Health)
	Government provided a commitment to expand Improving Access to Psychological Therapies (IAPT) to children in *Talking Therapies: A Four-year Plan of Action* (Department of Health)
	£20 million investment in Time to Change to continue their work on tackling stigma; the second phase of work aimed at children and young people
2012	The Health and Social Care Act 2012 provided a legislative framework for a number of changes to the way health services were arranged in England; established the NHS Commissioning Board; and required every local authority to have a Health and Wellbeing Board and also a local Healthwatch to act as a champion for health and social care
	The NHS Constitution: The NHS Belongs to Us All sets out the principles and values of the NHS in England as well as the rights and responsibilities of patients, the public and staff
	Positive for Youth: A New Approach to Cross-government Policy for Young People Aged 13 to 19 (HM Government) – the Government urged every local area to establish and maintain arrangements for ensuring that the voice of young people is heard in local decision-making and that young people have a role in inspecting and reporting on the quality of service delivery (Cabinet Office and Department for Education)

Year	Milestone
2013	Government responded to the Children and Young People's Health Outcomes Forum and committed to doing everything they could to improve the health of children and young people, setting up a new Children and Young People's Health Outcomes Forum to provide ongoing expertise and constructive challenge to the next phase of work (Department of Health)
2014	The *Mental Health Crisis Care Concordat* was signed by 22 national bodies, resulting in a national agreement between services and agencies involved in the care and support of people in crisis (Department of Health and Concordat signatories)
	The Health Select Committee held an inquiry into CAMHS services following a report highlighting major problems with children waiting for beds, cuts to early intervention services and waiting times for CAMHS
	A taskforce was announced to look at how CAMHS can be improved; as a result, *Future in Mind: Promoting, Protecting and Improving Our Children and Young People's Mental Health and Wellbeing* (Department of Health and NHS England) was published, providing the vision for children and young people's mental health and clearly setting the agenda for reform within CAMHS (Department of Health and NHS England)

Source: adapted from Street and Herts (2005) and expanded.

Pause to reflect

So far, you have read about some political drivers for involving people primarily in their own, or their family's, care and treatment.
What are your values in relation to participation and involvement?
Do you know what the values are for the organisation you are involved with?

Participation and involvement: what is the difference?

In 1969, Sherry Arnstein published 'A ladder of citizen participation' (see Figure 2.1). Arnstein's model has been widely used, criticised and adapted to fit a variety of modern healthcare agendas. It was redeveloped by the National Youth Agency and renamed the ladder of participation.

Roger Hart (1979) created the ladder of young people's participation (see Table 2.2) as a means of expressing the different levels of youth involvement and as a tool to help organisations map their youth participation activity. Although there is debate about which of Hart's ladder rungs are the most meaningful, it demonstrates that involvement can take place on a variety of levels.

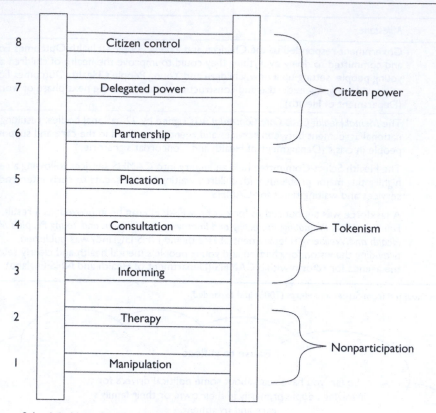

Figure 2.1   A ladder of citizen participation
Source: Arnstein (1969).

Table 2.2 Roger Hart's ladder of young people's participation

Rung 8	Young people and adults share decision-making
Rung 7	Young people lead and initiate action
Rung 6	Adult-initiated, shared decisions with young people
Rung 5	Young people are consulted and informed
Rung 4	Young people are assigned and informed
Rung 3	Young people are tokenised
Rung 2	Young people are decoration
Rung 1	Young people are manipulated

Source: adapted from Hart (1979).
Note: Hart explains that rungs 1–3 represent non-participation.

The Office of the Children's Commissioner in conjunction with the National Children's Bureau Research Centre carried out research to identify how health systems and services proactively engage with children and young people in decisions about health service design and delivery. They utilised the Wheel of Participation (Figure 2.2) and suggested that participation by young people took place in one of three ways: informing, consulting or involving.

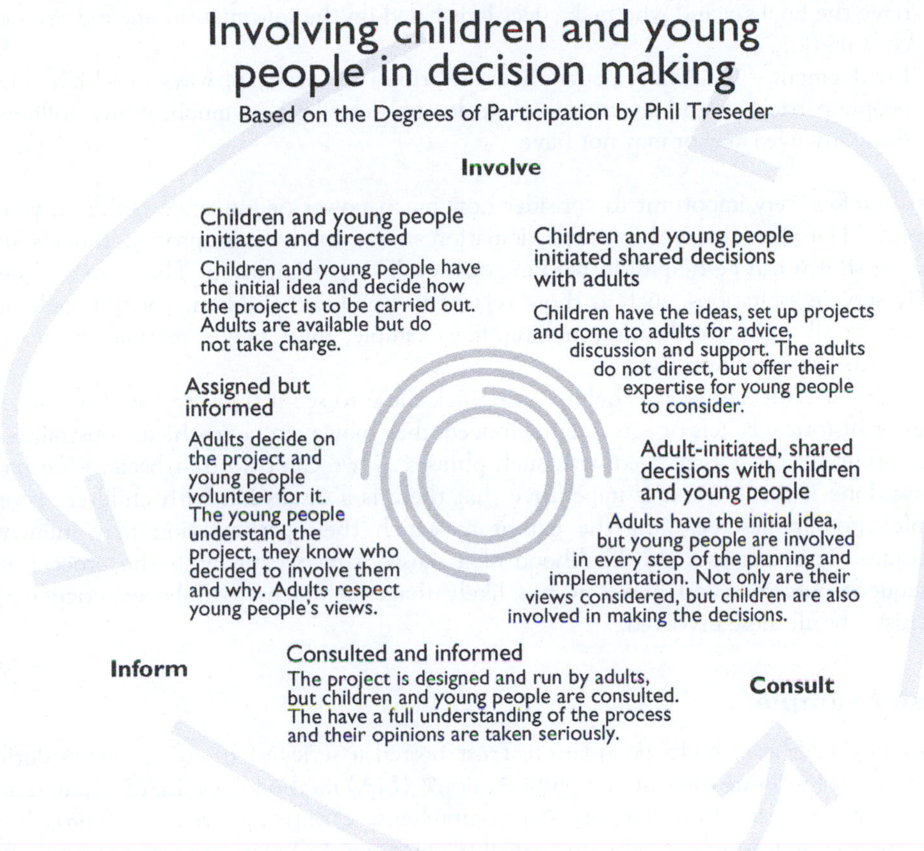

Involving children and young people in decision making

Based on the Degrees of Participation by Phil Treseder

Involve

Children and young people initiated and directed

Children and young people have the initial idea and decide how the project is to be carried out. Adults are available but do not take charge.

Children and young people initiated shared decisions with adults

Children have the ideas, set up projects and come to adults for advice, discussion and support. The adults do not direct, but offer their expertise for young people to consider.

Assigned but informed

Adults decide on the project and young people volunteer for it. The young people understand the project, they know who decided to involve them and why. Adults respect young people's views.

Adult-initiated, shared decisions with children and young people

Adults have the initial idea, but young people are involved in every step of the planning and implementation. Not only are their views considered, but children are also involved in making the decisions.

Inform

Consulted and informed

The project is designed and run by adults, but children and young people are consulted. The have a full understanding of the process and their opinions are taken seriously.

Consult

Figure 2.2   Wheel of participation
Source: Office of the Children's Commissioner (2012: 13).

Models by Roger Hart and the Children's Commissioner each provide helpful guidance on the levels to which children, young people and families can engage in meaningful participation. The models also challenge the organisers of participation events to consider and establish what weight is being given to the outcomes from the participation events.

'Involvement' tends to be used as an umbrella term that encapsulates anything from consultation with children, young people and families through to active participation in the decision-making process. When planning any project, it is useful to consider the following key terms as discussed by Street and Herts (2005):

- Participation – refers to young people taking an active role in a project or a process. By participating, young people have the power to help shape a process. It doesn't define whether or not the children or young people participating have any influence on the outcomes.
- Consultation – broadly means listening to young people's voices and views and giving them appropriate feedback. Consultation can be on a large or small scale and is often equated with participation. However, following consultation, it is often adults who

have the final say and who make decisions based on the information elicited from the consultation.

- Involvement – used more generally to describe the variety of ways in which young people participate and are consulted. It doesn't describe how much, if any, influence those involved may or may not have.

It is therefore very important to consider how much power or influence children, young people and families have within the participation and/or involvement process. Models such as those shown can be helpful in working out levels of participation. They can also help clarify service aspirations, such as those related to involving children, young people and families in all aspects of decision-making. For example, there may sometimes be service constraints that may limit this.

If there are constraints, it is helpful to unpick these to see if they are based on current issues or historical beliefs or agreements. Indeed, they may even be mythical constraints or blocks that are often associated with such phrases as 'we can't do that because we have always done it this way!' It is imperative that there is a discussion with children, young people and families regarding the extent to which their participation may influence outcomes. This increases the likelihood of a sense of ownership with the process and subsequent outcomes and makes it less likely that the process will be experienced as tokenistic by all those involved.

Case example

Berkshire Healthcare NHS Foundation Trust hosted a series of listening events during October 2014 utilising the Listening into Action® (LiA) methodology. LiA® is a national change management initiative; it is a comprehensive outcome-oriented approach to engaging the right people in relation to quality outcomes. LiA® is designed to engage and empower clinicians and staff in conjunction with any challenge. Within the trust, this model has been utilised since 2012, affecting a groundswell of change that resulted in a number of initiatives to improve patient experience and clinical outcomes. Staff who attended the trust's internal 'Big Conversations' earlier in 2014 were asked two questions:

1 What are the main things that get in the way of staff proactively listening, hearing and acting on what patients and their carers are saying?
2 What practical steps should we take to improve the patient and carer experience?

Responses from this exercise led to Berkshire Healthcare NHS Foundation Trust's aspiration to explore what helps and hinders engagement of patients, carers and members of the public with the organisation. It reaffirmed their commitment to put patients, carers and employees at the centre of developing quality services.

The trust hosted six listening events that were open to people who use its services and the general public. Three events were open for people aged 18 years and over; one event was for families; one was for people who use the learning disability service; and one was for young people who had been involved with CAMHS. The trust used an adaptation of the LiA® method. This simple framework poses a question to the audience about a problem, and then the audience is asked to generate solutions. The question asked was: 'How do we better involve service users, families, carers and the general public in the development of our services?' Young people suggested one solution would be to use Twitter. This could be used to ask a question or to send a link to a questionnaire that young people could answer straight away with very limited interruption to their day-to-day activities. The young people who attended said they would be much more willing to answer questions in this way than to respond to a paper questionnaire that would require time and organisation to complete.

As a result of the event, the children and young people's service in Berkshire Healthcare NHS Foundation Trust have consulted more widely with people who use the services and are changing how the service communicates with them.

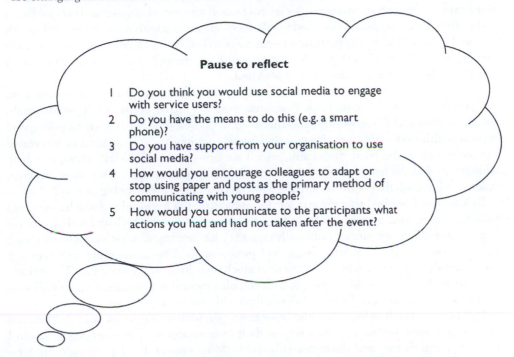

Pause to reflect

1   Do you think you would use social media to engage with service users?
2   Do you have the means to do this (e.g. a smart phone)?
3   Do you have support from your organisation to use social media?
4   How would you encourage colleagues to adapt or stop using paper and post as the primary method of communicating with young people?
5   How would you communicate to the participants what actions you had and had not taken after the event?

When thinking about service user participation and/or involvement, it is important to consider what it is you are actually aiming to achieve. For example, are you thinking about how best to involve a young person in their treatment plan? Or are you hoping to increase completion rates for a questionnaire, aimed perhaps at informing treatment? Are you aiming to consult with young people about how to develop a service? The complexity of the intention can be placed on a continuum, from posing a simple question (e.g. we would like to paint the waiting room – which colour do you prefer on the paint chart provided?) to aiming for real and meaningful participation (Bell 2004) at the opposite end of the spectrum (e.g. we would like to invite all our key stakeholders to redesign our mental health services starting with a blank piece of paper).

Experiences and reflections from the authors

Jasmine

I am a young person who has previously been involved in contributing to the MyMind website, which has been developed directly by CAMHS and young people (www.mymind. org.uk). If you're not familiar with the website, you should go online and check out their resources. It is aimed at anyone interested in the mental health and wellbeing of children and young people across Wirral and Cheshire. There are interactive resources to help improve mental health, a Twitter feed, a blog by young people written for young people and lots of important information that is vital for reducing mental health stigma in the community.

MyMind has helped me a lot. A few years back, when I was studying for my A levels, I started therapy with CWP. I was full of angst and anxiety, which is something I think all teens experience to a certain degree. Social interaction was overwhelming, and my childhood had been a little complicated as I had family members coping with complex mental health illness. Luckily, I had the opportunity to get involved with the MyMind website and help develop its resources while I was in therapy, and I got through my issues with help from CWP and through using resources from MyMind.

My therapist was absolutely inspirational and a pivotal figure in creating the website from the ground up. My therapist helped organise workshops that consisted of professionals, young people and children working together as equals, developing materials to help integrate mental health work with a new dynamic and innovative approach. Through this, we created resources such as the Next Step cards, which are now used in CAMHS therapy to help adolescents and children have a more patient-centred treatment. It is giving them an active voice in what goals they want to achieve while in treatment, however big or small.

By the time I finished therapy and left for university, the MyMind website had evolved into something quite extraordinary. Indeed, the great thing about MyMind is that it never stops evolving. The website is continually growing with new resources; it's constantly giving help to young people, parents, carers and professionals. The community can access it anonymously and engage with the website as much or as little as they need to. The website and Twitter feed is accessible to people with complex mental health difficulties as well as to people who might just need a bit of help dealing with day-to-day stresses.

MyMind is about building a healthy communication with young people and children and encouraging them to take an active role in their own treatment. The most crucial lesson I learnt through therapy and through seeing the MyMind project develop is that there is no magical cure for mental health difficulties. I have learnt that life is a continually changing journey, and it is about learning a set of coping skills to help one get through any adversities that may be presented.

What I really want to tell you is how the whole ethos that has grown from this website and spread throughout the CAMHS services has benefited so many young people. The therapists and professionals I have collaborated with are recognising that young people have important opinions and that young people and children are valuable and rather stable citizens in this chaotic society. As well as that, in times when there is not much funding for youth services, all of the resources on the website are teaching young people and children to take ownership and to learn self-resilience and new coping strategies. MyMind is a true example of how participation in health services can have such a positive impact on patient-centred care.

If you are reading this as a mental health professional, I want you to know just how important it is to treat a young person as an equal and to value their opinions, as my therapists did. The one thing a psychology degree will not teach you is people skills and how to have a real conversation with someone. That is something all of us seem to learn gradually throughout our intricate lives, and it is a skill greatly admired by those experiencing mental turmoil. Have empathy, have patience and have compassion. It goes a long way in helping young people and children through treatment.

As a young person and previous service user, I feel very passionate about the development of mental health services so that they are catered towards adolescents and children, not just adults. I believe the only way mental health services can be of any use to young people is if professionals are prepared and willing to engage and to let adolescents and children take ownership. If professionals are able to engage like this then young people will be far more likely to take an active role in their treatment, and their personal growth will be far greater.

I find it scandalous that so little of our budget is spent on young people's mental health. If we tackle poor mental health early on, the outcome is often far more positive. In times of austerity, we can no longer keep relying on the notion that the NHS will always be able to fund continuous treatment. That is why we need to invest more in projects like MyMind and in resources that help integrate the community, break down mental health stigma and engage young people and children.

Attending the Health Service Journal Awards in November 2014 for the MyMind website was a real highlight for me, mainly because I realised how much I had progressed since beginning therapy. Five years ago, I had dreaded using public transport due to anxiety; yet last month, I managed to get a train to London, use the tubes in rush hour, dress appropriately for a black tie awards evening and actually enjoy the whole night. The MyMind website got 'highly commended' for innovation in mental health at the awards evening – a well-deserved achievement.

Early in 2015, I had the pleasure of attending the CYP IAPT participation conference, which brought together young people, children and professionals. The conference really was a true example of professionals listening to young people's voices and working together in participation and promoting involvement with our mental health services. It was a real privilege to attend the conference because I was able to see just how much work young people had contributed to our health service. One great example was that of two young people from CWP who have become young advisors. They are now advising the trust on aspects of the services that could be improved. It was also great to see their hard work in creating projects used to reduce stigma and integrate the service into the community.

Another example of participation given at the conference was the work done by young people on communication in schools. The young presenters showed how they had developed a strong link with schools in terms of working through wellbeing issues that adolescents and children may have to cope with. The young people explained how they had created lesson plans regarding mental health and also designed a wellbeing pledge for schools to sign. This really signified how much of a difference schools can make in reducing mental health stigma and why it is so important that school staff need to have a strong awareness of young people's wellbeing.

As a young person, I am really proud of CWP, proud of all the work from inspirational professionals such as Elaine Williams, Dr Fiona Pender and Lesley Dougan, whom I've had the privilege to work with over the past few years. I am grateful to CWP CAMHS for all their help and hard work. Through involvement with MyMind, my life has been transformed from being gripped by anxiety and depression to being able to pursue my goals as a classical musician and study music at university. Finally, I want to say how amazing it is to see so many young people, children and families benefiting from MyMind, and I am pleased to see the CWP mental health services continually go from strength to strength. Here's to the future!

Ben

Book-a-Leaf transformed a simple story about how involving young people, families, referrers and team members can shape the development of a service, whilst still meeting its commissioning targets.

From 2012 to 2013, the CWP Columbia Team developed a number of resources following the Columbia Connected event which took place in 2012. Young people, parents and referrers took part in a planning day which led to a number of helpful resources and events being developed. The Columbia Connected report is available on www.mymind.org.uk.

When I was 11 years old, I joined the Columbia Team away day with my stepdad. I'm now 15 years old and have remained involved with the CAMHS service, both as a service user and as someone who has helped shape the development of services over the last few years. I wrote a blog post for www.mymind.org.uk to showcase what we started.

Since then, I have remained involved with CAMHS. However, I am finding it much more difficult to attend during school hours or in the evenings because of GCSE work. The Columbia away day was held during school holidays and was just for a day.

Elaine

Ben, aged 11, suggested that we develop Book-a-Leaf. This was information that was halfway between a leaflet and a booklet. Ben wanted young people who were coming to the service to have more information about who the young person might see and what type of questions might be asked. The challenge for us was to ensure there was information for adults and information for children or young people in order for them to prepare for coming to CAMHS and also to ensure consent was obtained.

Over the last 12 months, a number of resources have been developed that in some way incorporate Ben's Book-a-Leaf idea. Ben wanted to show children, young people and parents/carers how to find information within www.mymind.org.uk. For information about what may happen when you come to CAMHS, have a look at the 5–12 section, where you will meet Max who will tell you all about this. Or have a look at the *Life is a Journey* animation in the 13–19 section. All of this information has been developed by children and young people who have been in CAMHS.

Ben said it can be quite difficult to set goals, but staff in CAMHS can help with this using the Next Step cards. These have also been developed by children and young people and help to keep the focus on you without you being in the spotlight. Ben thinks the Next Step cards could help you get to your goal. He says they are especially useful for young people with ADHD as they keep their attention because they are bright and colourful.

Summary

The participation and involvement of the people who use health services has been a core element of government reforms of the health service in recent years. These reforms have been set nationally with the intention that local services develop their participation and involvement agendas to best suit the needs of their local population. There are many ways to undertake participation and involvement, however the reader must first carefully explore the question of who am I doing this for? Do the children and young people have any authority, influence or power to positively affect change?

References

Arnstein, S. (1969) A ladder of citizen participation. *Journal of the American Planning Association,* 35(4): 216–24.

Bell, B. (2004) *Practice Standards in Children's Participation.* London: Save the Children.

Department for Children, Schools and Families (2008) *Targeted Mental Health in Schools Project. Using the Evidence to Inform Your Approach: A Practical Guide for Headteachers and Commissioners.* Nottingham: Department for Children, Schools and Families.

Department for Children, Schools and Families (2007) *Targeted Youth Support: A Guide.* Nottingham: Department for Children, Schools and Families.

Department for Education and Skills (2005) *Excellence and Enjoyment: Social and Emotional Aspects of Learning: Guidance.* London: Department for Education and Skills.

Department for Education and Skills (2003) *Every Child Matters.* Cm 5860. London: The Stationery Office.

Department of Health (2004) *National Service Framework for Children, Young People and Maternity Services.* London: Department of Health.

Department of Health (2000) *The NHS Plan: A Plan for Investment, A Plan for Reform.* Cm 4818-I. London: The Stationery Office.

Department of Health (1999) *Saving Lives: Our Healthier Nation.* Cm 4386. London: The Stationery Office.

Department of Health (1998) *Quality Protects.* London: The Stationery Office.

Department of Health (1989) *Working for Patients.* London: HMSO.

Kings Fund (2014) *People in Control of their Own Health and Care: The State of Involvement.* London: The King's Fund.

Francis, R. (2013) *Report of the Mid Staffordshire NHS Foundation Trust Public Inquiry.* London: The Stationary Office.

Hart, R. (1979) *Children's Participation: From Tokenism to Citizenship.* New York: UNICEF.

Morse, J. M. (1991) Negotiating commitment and involvement in the nurse–patient relationship. *Journal of Advanced Nursing,* 16(4): 455–68.

National Health Service, England (2013) The National Health Service (Revision of NHS Constitution–Principles) Regulations 2013 [online]. Available at: www.legislation.gov.uk/uksi/2013/317/contents/made

Office of the Children's Commissioner (2012) *Participation Strategy, Ensuring Children and Young People's Voices Are Embedded in the Work of the Office of the Children's Commissioner.* London: Office of the Children's Commissioner.

Royal College of Nursing (2008) *Adolescent Transition Care: Guidance for Nursing Staff.* London: Royal College of Nursing.

Street, C. and Herts, B. (2005) *Putting Participation into Practice: A guide for practitioners working in services to promote the mental health and well-being of children and young people.* London: YoungMinds. Available at: www.youngminds.org.uk/training_services/publications/21_putting_participation_into_practice (accessed 20 July 2016).

Chapter 3

CAMHS transformation

Modernising therapeutic interventions and outcomes

Tim McDougall

Key points:

- The Children and Young People's Improving Access to Psychological Therapies programme (CYP IAPT) is organised around nine key principles that focus on how children and young people can be supported to feel good, how professionals can do the right job and how services can be run well.
- *Future in Mind* (Department of Health 2015) and the local child and adolescent mental health service (CAMHS) transformation planning process to deliver this strategy will involve a national roll-out of CYP IAPT by 2018. CAMHS services across England will be expected to deliver a choice of evidence-based treatments and interventions, adopt routine outcome monitoring and work collaboratively with children and young people and their families.
- Commissioners and providers across the whole CAMHS system need to work together to develop bespoke integrated care pathways that facilitate timely access to effective evidence-based treatments and interventions. CYP IAPT done properly requires that children and young people should be involved in the commissioning, procurement, design and evaluation of services.
- There is now widespread agreement that the values and qualities embodied in the CYP IAPT programme should be part of a wider drive for change in improving children and young people's access to timely, high-quality mental health provision. Indeed, the principle of collaboration is the backbone of the CAMHS transformation programme.
- There seems to be no question at all that CYP IAPT has been successful in changing the culture of CAMHS to be more collaborative, less medical in focus and more systematic in monitoring and evaluating outcomes to improve care and services for children, young people and families.

Introduction

Psychological therapies refer to a wide range of talking therapies, the most common of which are cognitive behaviour therapy (CBT), dialectical behaviour therapy (DBT), interpersonal therapy and family therapy. These have been shown to be effective for some children with mental health problems and disorders, but the evidence base is far from comprehensive.

This chapter summarises the history of the Children and Young People's Improving Access to Psychological Therapies (CYP IAPT) programme, which ran from 2011 until 2015 when it was expanded and became part of a bigger CAMHS transformation strategy to deliver *Future in Mind* (Department of Health 2015), commencing in 2016.

It is important to note that not all children and young people want or benefit from talking therapies. This may be because of their age, development stage or disposition. For example, very young children will not be able to work with the abstract concepts involved in CBT and may engage better with non-verbal therapies such as those based on play, music or dance. However, the evidence base for these so-called creative therapies is similarly lacking. Deciding which psychological therapy to use depends on the developmental status of the child, the evidence base for use and the choices of the child and their parents or carers. It is also important to take account of developmental considerations in the design, implementation and evaluation of interventions (McDougall 2011).

What do we mean by transformation?

Future in Mind describes an integrated whole system approach to delivering further improvements in children and young people's mental health outcomes. This requires joint commitment by the NHS, public health, voluntary and community services and local authorities to adopt some key principles for joint working (see Box 3.1).

Box 3.1 Key principles underpinning CAMHS service transformation

- Place emphasis on building resilience, promoting good mental health and wellbeing, prevention and early intervention.

- Deliver a step change in how care is provided, moving away from a system defined in terms of the services that organisations provide towards one built around the needs of children, young people and their families.

- Improve access so that children and young people have easy access to the right support from the right service at the right time and as close to home as possible. This includes implementing clear evidence-based pathways for community-based care to avoid unnecessary admissions to inpatient care.

- Deliver a clear joined-up approach, linking services so care pathways are easier to navigate for all children and young people, including those who are most vulnerable.

- Sustain a culture of continuous evidence-based service improvement delivered by a workforce with the right mix of skills, competencies and experience.

- Improve transparency and accountability across the whole system, being clear about how resources are used in each area and providing evidence to support collaborative decision-making.

Source: adapted from Department of Health (2015).

The concept of transformation is not new in the NHS. The King's Fund (2016) points out that mental health services in England have a history of transformation. This is through replacing long-stay institutions with care in the community, diversifying services to focus support on people with specific needs and extending access to evidence-based mental health treatment to those in primary care.

In recent years, modern health transformation programmes have emerged that aim to move away from a 'medicalised' system of delivering care and treatment to one that focuses on the principles of recovery, with services and the workforce redesigned to reflect that focus. In recent years, mental health providers have embarked on transformation programmes to implement large-scale changes to services, workforce and corporate infrastructure (The King's Fund 2016).

Local CAMHS Transformation Plans

In 2015, the Department of Health issued guidance for commissioners and their strategic partners on the development of Local Transformation Plans to support improvements in children and young people's mental health and wellbeing. This set out a five-year vision for delivering improvements, as defined in *Future in Mind* (Department of Health 2015), which is effectively the most up-to-date national CAMHS strategy. This states that commissioners and providers across the whole system need to work together to develop integrated, bespoke care pathways that incorporate effective, evidence-based interventions for vulnerable children and young people, ensuring those with protected characteristics such as learning disabilities receive an appropriate service.

To achieve these ambitious aims where previous strategies have failed to produce meaningful change requires radical service transformation. Furthermore, to do so effectively requires transformation to be embedded within shared partnership governance arrangements. This approach is consistent with the spirit and intention of the Transforming Care programme, which is jointly delivered by the Association of Directors of Adult Social Services, the Care Quality Commission, the Department of Health, Health Education England, the Local Government Association and NHS England.

Children and Young People's Improving Access to Psychological Therapies (CYP IAPT)

CYP IAPT began in 2011 with a target to work with CAMHS serving 60 per cent of the 0–19 population by 2016. By August 2015, nearly three-quarters of English CAMHS partnerships in the NHS, local authorities and the voluntary sector were involved with the CYP IAPT programme (NHS England 2015). *Future in Mind* (Department of Health 2015) and the local CAMHS transformation planning process for delivering this will involve a national roll-out of CYP IAPT and access for 100 per cent of the 0–19 population by 2018. CAMHS across the country will be expected to deliver a choice of evidence-based treatments and interventions; to adopt routine outcome monitoring (ROM) and feedback to guide treatment and service design; and to work collaboratively with children and young people and their families.

What does CYP IAPT provide?

The CYP IAPT programme and curriculum was developed by learning collaboratives comprising higher education institutions, local CAMHS partnerships and commissioners. Trainees are required to cover a number of key areas as part of the core curriculum. These are:

1   expectations for students
2   core values of CYP IAPT
3   collaborative care model
4   young people's and parents' participation
5   active outcomes framework

6   evidence-based practice/practice-based evidence
7   the process of organisational change.

Additionally, the CYP IAPT core training programme includes a summary of the clinical knowledge base required to work in CAMHS. This involves:

1   ensuring the delivery of services that support equality of access, respect diversity and minimise disadvantage or discrimination
2   fundamentals of therapy adapted to CYP IAPT principles
3   shared aspects of evidence-based practice with children.

The core training also introduces trainees to the key therapeutic modalities used in CAMHS, which are based on National Institute for Health and Care Excellence guidance. This includes CBT for children and young people, covering basic CBT skills for parenting work, anxiety disorders and depression. Also included is parent training for conduct problems, interpersonal psychotherapy for adolescents and systemic work with families.

   To help embed CYP IAPT principles into clinical practice, there is a curriculum for supervisor training. This addresses:

1   understanding CYP IAPT
2   principles of supervision
3   promoting psychological knowledge in supervision
4   the use of outcomes data in supervision
5   facilitating therapeutic processes in supervision
6   delivering modality-specific supervision.

Nine key areas

CYP IAPT is organised around nine key areas that focus on how children and young people can be supported to feel good, how professionals can do the right job and how services can be run well (see Box 3.2). Each are discussed in this chapter, and some have been translated into quality standards to assist organisations to make specific and measurable improvements.

Box 3.2 Nine key areas of the CYP IAPT programme

1   Initial assessments
2   Session-by-session monitoring
3   Complaints and advocacy
4   Staff training
5   Recruitment and selection
6   Supervision and appraisal
7   Commissioning
8   Leadership
9   Shared values

Initial assessments

One of CYP IAPT quality standards is that children, young people and their parents or carers are offered an initial assessment without significant delay. They set the standard that an initial assessment or choice appointment is offered within six weeks for 90 per cent of all non-urgent referrals. YoungMinds have been working closely with the national CYP IAPT team, and they make a number of important recommendations to help ensure initial assessments are effective and acceptable to young people. They stress the importance of co-production and of letting the child or young person know what to expect from the assessment.

It is important that children and young people are enabled to express what the issues are in their own words rather than being bombarded with questions. Young people tell us that continuity is important and that they do not like being passed from one person to the next. There should be constant feedback so that points can be checked continually for accuracy and agreement that the right information is being shared if this is necessary (YoungMinds 2011).

There is evidence that time between referral and assessment decreased by 73 per cent and number of days between assessment and discharge decreased by 21 per cent during the lifespan of the CYP IAPT programme. In some areas, there has also been improved access through self-referral routes, a single point of access, outreach services, and evening and weekend appointments (Pugh et al. 2016). However, in other areas of England, services are still restricted to between 9 a.m. and 5 p.m. from Monday to Friday, referrals are made through traditional channels and there is no option of outreach to young people in crisis.

Session-by-session monitoring

One of the key successes of CYP IAPT has been the introduction of session-by-session monitoring. This is where children and young people, and their parents or carers as appropriate, are asked to give feedback about the therapies they are receiving. This helps keep the intervention on the right track and promotes adherence to the treatment modality or evidence base. The feedback from children and young people about their involvement in session-by-session monitoring has been generally positive (Hall et al. 2014). The approach was reviewed in 2012 and a number of new measures were introduced to further improve flexibility and effectiveness.

Complaints and advocacy

CYP IAPT recommends that each CAMHS service has available a complaints procedure and independent advocacy service that is accessible, well signposted and sufficiently resourced.

Staff training

CYP IAPT programme designers recognise that professionals need access to up-to-date skills and knowledge. They recommend that training for CYP IAPT trainees and existing CAMHS staff systematically includes young people in its design, delivery and evaluation. This is a valuable way to explore how treatments are offered as well as what they involve.

Recruitment and selection

Priority 5 of the CYP IAPT programme is to involve young people in the recruitment and selection of staff. To support this process, GIFT (Greater Involvement, Future Thinking) have produced a guide to involving children and young people in interviews. This emphasises the importance of early planning and use of the participation model. It is important that children and young people are prepared with necessary information and are aware of issues such as confidentiality, equality and diversity and equal opportunities.

Supervision and appraisal

CYP IAPT suggests that the supervision and appraisal of staff includes children and young people through a range of accessible and appropriate methods. It also recognises that in order to deliver evidence-based treatments, there needs to be rigour and monitoring of the therapy process and fidelity to the treatment model. Law and Wolpert (2014) state that the practice of reflecting on service user feedback and session-by-session outcomes in supervision allows young people's voices to be represented within supervision case discussions – it serves as a reminder to keep the service user at the centre of supervision.

Through CYP IAPT, there is a commitment to careful monitoring of clinical progress and data-based supervision of practice. Reflection and treatment planning can be kept focused, and therapeutic drift is reduced. This approach can be recognised as practice-based evidence, and it is an important part of the treatment model and process. For example, the use of Goal Based Outcome measures allow therapists and young people to monitor how well they are doing in tackling the goals that were identified at commencement of treatment. These are highly appropriate for use in CAMHS as they can help measure outcomes across a broad spectrum of interventions, across a variety of settings, and with a variety of service users (Law 2009). Other monitoring tools include the Outcome Rating Scale and the Session Rating Scale.

Commissioning

Good information is the foundation for good commissioning. In order to run services well, systems and structures need to be clear. CYP IAPT done properly requires that children and young people should be involved in the commissioning, procurement, design and evaluation of services.

For commissioners wishing to adopt CYP IAPT-based principles and values, the CYP IAPT national programme team has developed model service specifications for targeted and specialist CAMHS (Tier 2/3). We are also seeing the start of CYP IAPT principles being embedded in accreditation processes for professional bodies, education and training courses, and contracts to help ensure quality assurance.

Leadership

The CYP IAPT programme includes a Transformational Leadership curriculum, which is designed for service managers and clinical leaders. This supports them to embed sustainable cultural change in order to deliver evidence-based, high-quality, outcomes-focused services. According to Pugh and colleagues (2016), teams in the five-year CYP IAPT programme had more proficient organisational cultures and more functional organisational climates than a comparison sample of mental health services for children and young people in the US.

Shared values

We have heard that CYP IAPT aims to improve collaborative practice between professionals and children, young people and their families. In other words, the approach encourages young people and those working with them to agree key problems and identify goals together. The CYP IAPT values can be organised into those that services demonstrate in their interactions with young people and their parents or carers and those that are required to deliver services well. There is now widespread agreement that the values and qualities embodied in the CYP IAPT programme should be part of a wider drive for change in improving children and young people's access to timely, high-quality mental health provision. Indeed, the principle of collaboration is the backbone of the CAMHS transformation programme.

Routine outcome monitoring (ROM)

It is important to measure outcomes across several domains. Improving functioning in one domain may have a positive effect in another. As illustration, treating a young person's ADHD may improve their educational attainment at school or addressing a young person's depression may improve their social functioning (McDougall 2014). Through the work of the Evidence Based Practice Unit (EBPU), Law and Wolpert (2014) identify a number of outcome measures that can assist practitioners to help identify problems as part of a wider assessment (see Table 3.1).

Table 3.1 Tools to help identify problems

Tool	Age range	Reported by
Goal Based Outcomes	All	Child, parent, family, teacher, professional
Health of the Nation Outcome Scale	3–18	Professional, child, parent
Revised Children's Anxiety and Depression Scale	8–18	Child, parent
Children's Global Assessment Scale	4–18	Professional
Strengths and Difficulties Questionnaire (SDQ)	3–16	Child, parent, teacher
Current View	All	Professional
Children's Outcome Rating Scale	All	Child, parent
Short Warwick-Edinburgh Mental Well-being Scale	13+	Child

Source: adapted from Law and Wolpert (2014).

Involvement and participation

Children and young people's participation is at the heart of the CYP IAPT, and through GIFT, young people have been involved from the outset. There is a golden thread of young people's focus on the key principles of feeling good, doing the job right and running the service well. These have been carried forward through to the CAMHS transformation programme.

Summary

The CYP IAPT programme has been successful in transforming CAMHS over the last five years. It has had a key influence on *Future in Mind* (Department of Health 2015) and, in turn, on the *Five Year Forward View for Mental Health* (Mental Health Taskforce 2016). This has been during a period of significant cuts to CAMHS that has impacted on the ability of some services to take full advantage of the programme.

The next phase of CAMHS transformation will build on the foundations of CYP IAPT and will expand psychological therapies to children and young people with eating disorders, learning disabilities and autism spectrum conditions. There will also be a curriculum on counselling interventions, working with under-5s and combination treatments comprising medication and psychological therapies.

There seems to be no question at all that CYP IAPT has positively influenced the culture of CAMHS. This has been to be more collaborative, less medical in focus and more systematic in monitoring and evaluating outcomes to improve care and services for children, young people and families. The future is exciting if the gains made in the modernisation of CAMHS during the last five years extend into the *Five Year Forward View*.

References

Department of Health (2015) *Future in Mind: Promoting, Protecting and Improving Our Children and Young People's Mental Health and Wellbeing*. London: Department of Health.

Hall, C., Taylor, J., Moldavsky, M., Marriot, M., Pass, S., Newell, K., Goodman, R., Sayal, K. and Hollis, C. (2014) A qualitative process evaluation of electronic session-by-session outcome measurement in child and adolescent mental health services. *BMC Psychiatry*, 14(1): 113.

King's Fund, The (2016) *Mental Health Under Pressure*. London: The King's Fund.

Law, D. (2009) Mind the gap: evidence based interventions for children and families with more complex mental health needs. *Psychological Therapies in the NHS*, New Savoy Partnership Conference, 27 November 2009. Available at www.newsavoypartnership.org/2009presentations/28_Duncan_Law_day_two_workshop_two.pdf (accessed 20 July 2016).

Law, D. and Wolpert, M. (eds) (2014) *Guide to Using Outcomes and Feedback Tools with Children, Young People and Families* (second edition). London: CAMHS Press.

McDougall, T. (2014) What do we mean by specialist hospital, intensive community and home based services? In T. McDougall and A. Cotgrove (eds) *Specialist Mental Health Care for Children and Adolescents: Hospital, Intensive Community and Home Based Services*. Abingdon: Routledge, pp. 6–22.

McDougall, T. (2011) Mental health problems in childhood and adolescence. *Nursing Standard*, 26(14): 48–56.

Mental Health Taskforce (2016) *Five Year Forward View for Mental Health*. London: Mental Health Taskforce.

NHS England (2015) *Local Transformation Plans for Children and Young People's Mental Health and Wellbeing: Guidance and Support for Local Areas*. London: NHS England.

Pugh, K., O'Herlihy, A. and Fonagy, P. (2016) *What Next for CYP IAPT?* London: NHS England.

YoungMinds (2011) *My Access to Psychological Therapies*. London: YoungMinds.

Chapter 4

Supporting and safeguarding families with parental mental illness
Issues, challenges and possibilities

Lina Gatsou and Scott Yates

Key points:

- It is important that nurses and other professionals understand how parental mental illness can affect children and young people and how they can help to safeguard their mental health and wellbeing.
- The most serious concerns for the welfare of children of parents with mental illness are the potential for them to experience violence and neglect. However, the vast majority of parents with mental illness do not harm or neglect their children.
- Anxiety and fear are common in the lives of children whose parents have mental illness. This can be about their own future mental health and concern about the degree to which they might be responsible for the illness of their parent. Children may also be worried they may be separated from their parent through hospitalisation, through the intervention of social services, or by suicide.
- Whilst there is evidence that children and families in which there is mental illness can benefit from psycho-educational interventions, non-stigmatising family-focused support and family therapy, there are some major gaps in services and generally patchy provision, both in the UK and overseas.
- There are challenges for nurses and other professionals to balance the need to identify children and young people at significant risk with those associated with compounding mental health and other forms of stigma and discouraging help-seeking and engagement with services.

Introduction

Parental mental illness (PMI) is a growing area of concern for mental health and social care researchers and services. One of the most important factors establishing it as a serious public health priority is its high prevalence. In the UK, between 10 per cent and 23 per cent of children live in a household in which a parent has a mental illness (Falkov 2011; Maybery *et al.* 2009). Fifteen per cent of dual-parent families and 20 per cent of single-parent families have a parent with a mental illness (Cleaver *et al.* 1999), and a study in the US indicates that around 68 per cent of women and 55 per cent of men with psychiatric disorders are parents at any given time (Nicholson *et al.* 2004). The stress of parenting itself is in fact liable to increase risk of serious psychiatric symptoms, especially in those caring for multiple young children (Oyserman *et al.* 2000). In a recent audit of mental health services in one county in the UK, it was found that around 60 per cent of children and young people accessing child and adolescent mental health services were children of parents with mental illness (CoPMI) and that almost 40 per cent of patients in adult mental health services

(AMHS) had dependent children (Gatsou *et al.* 2016). It is therefore important that nurses and other professionals understand how PMI can affect children and young people and how they can help to safeguard the mental health and wellbeing of this group.

Although it is important to resist the implication that PMI is axiomatically associated with abuse, neglect or other child protection concerns, there are associations between the presence of PMI and a range of negative experiences and outcomes, including behavioural, interpersonal and academic difficulties, poverty, discrimination, stigma, bullying, social exclusion and children developing their own mental health problems over time (see, for example, Rutter and Quinton 1984; Mowbray *et al.* 2000; Farahati *et al.* 2003; Cunningham *et al.* 2004). In terms of safeguarding, PMI features in one-third of serious case reviews and is associated with between 10 per cent and 42 per cent of child protection cases across Europe, the UK, Australia, Canada and the US (Reupert *et al.* 2012). It is a significant factor in the likelihood of children being take into care (Social Care Institute for Excellence 2011).

Oyserman *et al.*'s (2000) review of the literature on PMI suggests that there is a high heritability risk for a range of psychiatric disorders, being as high as 80 per cent in the case of borderline personality disorder, 75 per cent for schizophrenia and 34–48 per cent for depression; although there remains debate as to which disorders carry risk of passing on a genetic predisposition, what 'resilience' factors might protect children in different cases and how other contextual factors exacerbate or mitigate the risk of intergenerational transmission (Seifer *et al.* 1996; Reupert and Maybery 2007; Boursnell 2011). Our recent audit of mental health services found that 40 per cent of CoPMI themselves presented with mood disorders (Gatsou *et al.* 2016).

It is a challenge for safeguarding and undertaking protective and supportive work with families that a mental illness diagnosis for a parent does not alone represent a protective concern (Reupert *et al.* 2012). Moreover, some evidence actually suggests that parenting can be a key positive and motivating force in the lives of women with serious psychiatric disorders, increasing their engagement with treatment, providing an otherwise lacking valued social role and providing strong motivation to achieve or maintain normal lives for their children (Oyserman *et al.* 2000; Reupert and Maybery 2007).

Thus, there is a need for services and policymakers to understand the risks and challenges associated with PMI and the context in which they operate. This chapter presents evidence from existing literature and from a recent research project undertaken with families with parental mental illness (FaPMI) and multi-agency professionals who work with them in order to: summarise what is known about the potential mechanisms through which PMI impacts the lives of children and families; consider ways that services can undertake family-focused work to promote recovery and reduce the burden on children and young people; and consider some challenges to recovery and safeguarding presented by socio-economic factors and current social policy.

Research study

The study discussed and used to supplement evidence from existing literature was carried out with families and professionals in 2011 and 2012. One hundred professionals including nurses in one region of the UK were given two days of knowledge- and skills-based training in family-focused work on PMI (for full details of the training programme and evaluation, see Gatsou *et al.* 2015). Over the course of the study, these nurses and other professionals worked with 31 families where at least one parent had a diagnosed mental illness.

Evaluation and research data were collected through questionnaires and interviews with family members and professionals and in focus groups with professionals. Overall, 94 pre- and post-training questionnaires were completed by professionals; 61 pre- and post-intervention questionnaires were completed by family members (34 by parents and 27 by children and young people); 17 interviews were carried out with family members across 6 families; and 20 interviews and 5 focus groups were carried out with professionals.

The impact of PMI on children and families

The most serious concerns for the welfare of CoPMI are around the potential for them to experience violence and neglect. Pritchard *et al.* (2012), in their decade-long study of child homicide assailants, found that whilst still extremely rare, mentally ill parents were the most frequent category of child assailants, with mothers with children on the Child Protection Register and men with previous convictions for violence also presenting significant risks. There are also risks of neglect as parents with mental illness may have reduced capacity to meet the needs of their children. In some cases, this neglect can constitute a serious child protection concern. Risk for harm and neglect increases in cases where multiple adverse situations and experiences are present alongside PMI, notably poverty, lack of affordable housing, social isolation, domestic violence, substance and alcohol misuse and the presence of men with previous violent convictions (e.g. Chaffin *et al.* 1996; Cleaver *et al.* 2011; Pritchard *et al.* 2012). It should be emphasised, however, that whilst cases where these issues occur can be very serious, prevalence remains very low and the vast majority of parents with mental illness do not harm or neglect their children.

Much concern about the impact of PMI additionally focuses on its effect on parents' capacity to nurture and support their children and on the quality of family relationships. Whilst acknowledging that most parents with mental illness are motivated to be good parents, researchers have identified that mentally ill parents experience a strain between the demands of coping with their illness and the needs of their children and families (e.g. Nicholson *et al.* 1998; Oyserman *et al.* 2000, 2005; Reupert and Maybery 2011). There are a number of ways that parents' abilities to meet the needs of their children might be thwarted by the difficulties of living with a mental illness. These include the interplay between a child's needs and limited parental capacity or interaction effects between clinical and other contextual factors in families' lives. Notable mechanisms by which children's emotional and mental wellbeing might be threatened are shown in Box 4.1.

The lack of confidence that mentally ill parents have of their own ability to be effective parents is especially well noted (e.g. Nicholson *et al.* 1998; Oyserman *et al.* 2005; Reupert and Maybery 2011); and this emerged as an important issue in the research described earlier (Gatsou *et al.* 2015). This can interact with aspects of mental illness symptomatology to the detriment of parent–child relations as in, for example, misinterpreting normal childhood behaviours and experiencing emotional reactions to them (Gatsou *et al.* 2015) and increasing difficulty setting boundaries for children and using discipline (Nicholson *et al.* 1998; Oyserman *et al.* 2005).

Further challenges can emerge where parents' symptomology includes delusional thinking. Cooklin (2013) points out that whilst it is relatively rare for full and fixed delusions to be transmitted to children, children are liable to be closely caught up in a parent's delusions and invaded by their delusional thinking at moments of stress and uncertainty. The content

---

Box 4.1 *Threats to children's emotional health and wellbeing*

- Low self-esteem and blunted emotion leading the parent to experience mood swings and exhibit irritability, hostility or unresponsiveness.

- Parents having difficulty organising their lives and failing to sustain key routines that children need (Cleaver *et al.* 2011).

- Mothers with mental illness being less emotionally available, less involved and less positive in their interactions with their children.

- Mentally ill parents being less able to differentiate their own needs from those of their children and less able to maintain good interpersonal relationships with their children.

- Threats to attachment arising from parents' reduced responsiveness and their low confidence in their own parenting skills.

- Parents being uncertain about infants' needs and more tense and less communicative in interactions with them, creating less optimal conditions for infants to learn social communication skills (Oyserman *et al.* 2000).

- Poor parent–child relationships can manifest in hostility and blaming from parents that can be psychologically damaging for the children involved (e.g. Dunn 1993; Barlow and Schrader 2010).

---

of delusions is often frightening and foreboding and can cause considerable distress and anxiety for children. There is also an increased risk of violence where children become the targets of parents' delusions (Cleaver *et al.* 2011).

Children living with a parent with mental illness are also more likely to experience heightened levels of fear and anxiety on other dimensions – particularly fear for their own future mental health, anxiety over the degree to which they might be responsible for a parent's illness, fears that their relationship with their ill parent will deteriorate, concern that they may be separated from their parent through hospitalisation or through the intervention of social services, and even fear that their parent might take their own life (see, for example, Reupert and Maybery 2007; Cooklin 2013; Gatsou *et al.* 2015).

Young carers

The lives of CoPMI can be further impacted by the need to take on caring responsibilities. The 2001 census of young carers estimated that nearly one-third were caring for a parent with a mental illness. Cooklin (2010) extrapolates from other research to suggest that as many as 55,000 to 60,000 children in England and Wales are affected by the need to care for a parent with a mental illness. It is known that whilst some level of caring during childhood can be routine and even highly valued, children undertaking exaggerated levels of caring for an ill parent can risk a range of negative outcomes including limited involvement with peers, curtailed recreation and play, and impacts on education and personal growth (see Atkin 1992; Aldridge and Becker 1999, 2003). Young people caring for mentally ill parents can face particularly onerous experiences given the especially debilitating effects of serious mental illness and the demands for emotional as well as domestic caring responsibilities, the episodic nature of mental illness itself and the associated caring needs, and the lack of sufficient respite care (Aldridge and Becker 2003; Reupert and Maybery 2007; Gatsou *et al.* 2015).

Stigma

The impacts of PMI on and within families are complicated by mental health stigma. The powerful effects of mental illness stigma and their negative impacts on self-esteem and recovery are well known (e.g. Link *et al.* 2001; Whitley and Campbell 2014). For mentally ill parents, concerns over the stigma of mental illness overlap with fears of being judged negatively as a parent and potentially even losing custody of their children (e.g. Nicholson *et al.* 1998; Falkov 2011). There is also liability for children to suffer what Goffman called 'courtesy stigma', or stigma by association, by virtue of their family connection to stigmatised mentally ill parents (e.g. see Hinshaw 2005; Larson and Corrigan 2008).

Aside from the direct effects of public stigma and self-stigma on the self-esteem, wellbeing and mental health of parents and children, these issues also contribute to a tendency for mentally ill parents to minimise the impacts of their illness and fail to acknowledge the need for support, even actively resisting interacting with professional services and coping alone, thus hindering their recovery. We observed that this desire to hide and minimise the illness also extended to intra-familial relationships such that parents tried to hide the existence of the illness from their children, either failing to acknowledge their symptomology or creating alternative explanations (such as back pain or physical illness) when symptoms became observable (see Gatsou *et al.* 2015). This contributed further to the commonly noted misunderstandings and misconceptions that children often held about their parents' illness, leaving them more vulnerable to anxiety about their parents' wellbeing and more liable to blame themselves for their parents' low mood, lack of engagement or hostility (on this, see also Reupert and Maybery 2007).

The lives of FaPMI in context

Without wishing to downplay the importance of the mechanisms discussed above in generating challenges for children and parents in FaPMI or to understate the potential impact of them on later developmental stages of children's lives, it is important not to overlook a number of other important issues. These include the ways that systematic neglect and deprivation and discriminatory economic and social barriers can prevent people with mental illness from securing an acceptable quality of life (Reupert and Maybery 2007; see also Boursnell 2011). As Oyserman *et al.* (2000) note in their influential review, most studies into the impacts of PMI fail to include socio-economic factors or experiences of discrimination in their analyses. This is despite Rutter's (1981) early discovery that direct effects of PMI are less significant than the social and economic deprivation and adversity that are usually associated with mental illness. There is thus a pressing need to consider not only the family context for those families affected by PMI, but also their wider social and economic contexts.

Poverty and disadvantage

It is well established that mental illness is disproportionately represented amongst the poorest off, and that economic hardship and precarity themselves have negative impacts on the mental and physical health of adults and children (e.g. Patel *et al.* 2010; Knapp 2012). It has additionally been noted that poverty and poor housing are themselves additional factors interacting with PMI in generating risks to children's wellbeing (e.g. Chaffin *et al.* 1996) and that families' resources and socio-economic status mediate the impact of PMI (e.g. Hammen *et al.* 1987). Our research study demonstrated, as Rutter (1981) argued, a complex interplay between the symptoms and impacts of PMI and factors relating to families' social and economic situations, such as job loss or precarious employment, financial deprivation, poor housing and social isolation.

A common theme in the cases of families we worked with was the connection between job loss and job insecurity with the precipitation of mental health crises in families. This manifested both in situations where job loss and the resultant financial stress and loss of status played key roles in the decline of a parent's mental health and in those where a mental health crisis itself led to job loss, which compounded negative impacts for the parent and other family members.

Case example 1

A single mother of two teenage children had experienced a mental health crisis after a series of events that culminated in the breakup of her relationship, her resigning from her job and the family being forced to move home. The father of the family had been abusive and was eventually imprisoned. The siblings, one male and one female, had developed an antagonistic relationship, and the son, who had also been diagnosed with attention deficit hyperactivity disorder (ADHD), was threatened with expulsion from school due to poor behaviour and attendance. The mother had been in a well-paid and relatively high-status job, but her family situation and the stress of dealing with it had been taking a toll on her emotional state and she was occasionally called to her son's school during work hours. Her manager changed her work role a number of times and became bullying; this led to the mother raising a formal grievance but then taking sick leave due to stress and eventually needing to resign, which also led to the family having to move house. She later identified this bullying, stress and the fear of job loss (on top of existing family-related stress) as a key contributor to her going through a depressive episode:

> As a single parent trying to provide for your kids, trying to stay in a job when there are redundancies going … I am always first in line to be on the top of redundancy lists just because of how family life impacts on my work … I had gone through a couple of job changes that were really awful. I was signed off work with work-related stress. So I was suffering from depression and anxiety – it was just everything going wrong all at once; it was like the perfect storm.

Additional factors connected to families' marginal positions socially and economically are also liable to interact to produce very challenging environments for all members of the family. Notable examples from our study included families facing forced relocation after job loss, temporary homelessness, extreme economic hardship, shame associated with poverty and receiving benefits, stress and anxiety over benefit sanctions and dealing with local authorities, and poor-quality housing and overcrowding – with some instances of families with two or three generations having mental illness being forced to share inadequate accommodation.

Case example 2

Anne is a 16-year-old mother with depression and anxiety. Both her parents had mental health issues, and due to an antagonistic relationship with her mother, Anne and her baby lived with the family of the baby's father. However, the baby's paternal grandmother, Beth, had personality disorder, and the house was overcrowded with two of the father's siblings also living there. All of Beth's children had taken on caring roles. She self-harmed and was suicidal. Her children were aware of this and had deep fears for her safety. The youngest child was scared to leave her mother even to go to school in case her mother would kill herself and she would be to blame. She also began self-harming and she was getting into trouble at school. Beth saw herself only as a loving mother and did not have insight into the impacts of her illness on her children. She felt extreme shame about her mental health issues, which contributed to her isolating herself from the outside world, hiding her illness as much as possible and failing to seek help. Being in this environment was causing severe stress for Anne. It was overcrowded (six people in a three-bedroom house), relationships were characterised by anxiety, and Beth's mental health problems were having a powerful emotional impact on everyone in the house. Anne had been homeless in the past and anxiety about her housing situation exacerbated her own mental illness. The professional working with the family did manage to build a relationship with Beth and the rest of the family. Beth began to have greater insight into the impacts of her illness on her children and she sought help through her GP (although, unfortunately, the GP was initially dismissive and failed to recognise the severity of her illness, the ongoing safeguarding issues or the developing mental health problems of the children). An important factor in Anne's recovery was eventually being supported to move out of Beth's home into her own accommodation. As the professional said, 'the only way that [her mental health] could improve was by Anne being away from Beth's home'. After obtaining her own accommodation, Anne's mental health and her attitude towards it and her relationship with her baby 'changed radically'.

The compounding of PMI with other factors in situations like these was associated with a range of negative effects for the families in our study (see Box 4.2).

Box 4.2 Negative factors associated with parental mental illness

- Increased stress within the family, strained relationships and elevated levels of hostility and intra-familial conflict, especially in cases of poor or overcrowded housing and multigenerational mental illness.

- Parents being less able to provide economically for children's needs and wants; reduced peer group engagement for children; bullying by peers.

- Social isolation and families being removed from or unable to access important support networks (services, friends, family), presenting further threats to family members' mental health and challenges to recovery.

- School resistance or difficulties attending school; conflict with school and behaviour issues.

- Decreased self-esteem and self-confidence for all family members including the mentally ill parent, particularly impacting their confidence in their role as parents.

- Threats to children's mental and emotional wellbeing.

- Stigma and shame connected to poverty, unemployment, status loss and receiving benefits in addition to (and interacting with) mental illness stigma; reduced help-seeking and resistance to professional interventions.

There is thus a range of complex issues for services and professionals concerned with supporting families and safeguarding children in families affected by PMI (see also Peckover

2009). Whilst PMI alone is not a sufficient condition to constitute a safeguarding issue, our study supports what others have argued (e.g. Reader *et al.* 2003; Barlow and Schrader 2010; Forrester and Harwin 2011) – that complex interactions of PMI with familial and social and economic context can create environments in which a range of risk factors compound, family relations become strained and children's own mental health becomes at risk.

It is undoubtedly important to consider ways that services might more effectively support families and ensure that children's wellbeing is safeguarded (as we shall explore in the following section), but anyone concerned with these issues cannot but share our concern with problems connected to social policy and existing systems of practice that might exacerbate mental health difficulties present in families. In the UK context, for example, some recent policy initiatives might be seen as cause for concern in terms of their impact on the mental health of families (Peckover 2009). Proposals to limit the provision of housing benefit to young people, for example, risk removing the ability of young people in families like the ones discussed here to move out of environments that are threatening to their mental health, especially where multiple generations in the same house have enduring mental illnesses. In our research, we saw a number of cases in which the ability of young people to move away from the family home and live independently was recognised by families and professionals as instrumental in promoting their recovery and improving their mental and emotional wellbeing (see Gatsou *et al.* 2015).

Researchers and practitioners might also focus attention on the impacts of other policy issues, such as precarious, irregular and insecure work, the recent sharp increases in poorly paid self-employment, increased welfare conditionality and the growing prevalence of benefit sanctions for families that breach a range of government-imposed occupational and behavioural conditions. Each of these present challenges to families with a vulnerability to mental illness as they are liable to increase stress and put strain on intra-familial relationships and, as noted, to complicate the impacts of PMI on children and families and increase the burdens of disease on children and young people.

Supporting families and safeguarding

Whilst there is evidence that children and families in FaPMI can benefit from psycho-educational interventions, non-stigmatising family-focused support and family therapy (e.g. Owen 2008; Reupert and Maybery 2011; Cooklin 2013; Gatsou *et al.* 2015), there are some severe gaps in services and generally patchy provision, both in the UK and overseas. In the UK context, Ofsted, the national educational inspectorate, in collaboration with the Care Quality Commission (CQC) recently noted that responses to PMI from mental health services were often inadequate and that there was a general failure by services to adapt assessment or practice to identified need for FaPMI (Ofsted 2013). In our recent audit of services in one UK region, we also found that CAMHS were failing to record necessary information that would enable them to identify cases where their clients were members of FaPMI (Gastou *et al.* 2016).

Of course, as noted above, a PMI diagnosis alone is not enough to establish need for any specific intervention and, taken alone, does not represent a safeguarding issue. However, since interactions of PMI with other contextual, familial and socio-economic factors can create problematic situations for families – situations in which children's health and wellbeing can become at risk, including serious (but thankfully rare) cases of neglect or abuse – it is essential that nurses and other professionals can identify safeguarding issues where they do arise (see also Reader *et al.* 2003; Peckover 2009; Barlow and Schrader 2010).

Given current evidence, there is a need for mental health services to critically review their practice in identifying situations where existing and incoming service users might be members of FaPMI and in assessing where the impacts of PMI on children and young people might be especially troublesome and where they are co-present with other compounding risk factors. Pritchard *et al.* (2012) also make a convincing case for the need for children's services to show better awareness and focus on PMI in conjunction with other factors that raise the risk of abuse and neglect, particularly the presence of violence and violent individuals in the household and existing or previous child protection concerns – the so-called 'child protection-psychiatric-violence interface' (Pritchard *et al.* 2012: 1403).

Our study also affirmed that, as advocated by the UK's Social Care Institute for Excellence (2011), a 'no wrong door' approach to identifying need around PMI can provide an important element of successful support and safeguarding. Our research included nurses and other professionals from a broad spectrum of the multi-agency workforce (including but not limited to family support services, parenting services, primary mental health services, specialist child and adult mental health services, child behaviour services, health visitors and school nurses). Across this range of services, a common theme was professionals being aware of families who were affected by PMI, but failing to routinely assess its impact or to attempt to work on it with families (Gatsou *et al.* 2015). There was a range of factors behind this failure, many of which affirm points noted in other work (e.g. Social Care Institute for Care Excellence 2011; Reupert and Maybery 2014):

- Professionals lacked confidence to discuss mental illness with parents, make assessments and carry out work focusing on PMI. Concerns over the stigma of mental illness and how families would react to it being discussed contributed to this.
- Many services have relatively narrow single-issue remits such as to improve children's behaviour or school attendance, to teach parenting skills, to address drug use, and so on. Without an awareness of how PMI can interact with other issues, they are not likely to see it as part of their role to work with it or to offer support.
- Pressures on time and resources and an emphasis on client throughput prevented services from undertaking longer-term engaged work, including the necessary process of building trust and rapport with families. Lack of management understanding and support was a key factor in this.

Our experience shows that FaPMI often welcome family-focused work that addresses the impact of PMI on family members. Professionals and family members agreed that it was the flexible, voluntary and family-led nature of the intervention we employed that fostered such broad positive engagement (see Gatsou *et al.* 2015). The words of one mother from our study explaining the breakdown of her relationship with social services are illustrative. This mother argued that having raised three children who have achieved well, it should be recognised that she had 'done okay' as a parent; she felt that after only six months of experiencing an episode of mental illness that coincided with behavioural problems for her youngest daughter, her capabilities as a mother were unjustly maligned. She commented that she was made to feel judged as being 'crap' in terms of bringing up her children and that this 'got my hackles up, it got my defences up' to the extent that she resented and resisted further engagement.

This echoes points made by other researchers who note that there is a disproportionate focus on parental deficit and negative parent–child interactions for parents with mental illness that needs to be counterbalanced with a more supportive focus with recognition of the positive parenting by the majority of parents with mental illness in often very difficult circumstances (see, for example, Nicholson *et al.* 2009; Boursnell 2011). Given the known negative impacts of stigma on the self-esteem of people from stigmatised groups and taking into account the amount of high-profile work highlighting and challenging mental health stigma, policies and services concerned with supporting families and safeguarding children need to balance the real but rare risks associated with PMI with the danger of further stigmatising families, the majority of whom will not present formal child protection concerns.

Unfortunately, there is a trend in UK social policy to focus efforts on addressing the assumed deficits of 'problem' or 'troubled' families as they have become known – the criteria for which overlap with the multiple problems faced by FaPMI. There is an emphasis in these policies on enforcement and on preventing social problems that so-called 'troubled' families are assumed to cause. The persistent, assertive and challenging approach mandated in policy aimed at these families (Crossley 2015) overlaps with increased welfare conditionality and benefit sanctions aimed at eliciting desired (usually employment-focused) behaviour. This approach runs the real risk of compounding the negative impacts already discussed on mental health, self-esteem, help-seeking and access to support associated with a heavy deficit focus and stigma. We would argue that individuals and organisations concerned with the welfare of families should not shy away from taking a critical and engaged approach to the formation and implementation of policy and practice that has the potential to impact on the mental health and wellbeing of vulnerable families.

For the majority of families, for whom safeguarding is not a current concern but who face multiple challenges alongside a predisposition to mental illness, our study supports others in suggesting that non-stigmatising, supportive and flexible work with FaPMI can have positive impacts on the mental health of all family members (Nicholson *et al.* 2009; Boursnell 2011; Gatsou *et al.* 2015). In our experience, this includes not only direct work with families, but also professionals addressing a diverse range of actions including:

- supporting parents and intervening with employers in cases of public stigma in the workplace;
- tackling bullying or discrimination;
- supporting families experiencing confusion around welfare eligibility;
- liaising with schools where responses to children's absence and lateness are unhelpful;
- addressing young people's intermittent caring responsibilities.

In order for such approaches to gain traction, there is a need to: raise awareness across the workforce engaging with families of the potential challenges facing families as well as the potential causes of mental health crises, the impact of PMI and its interactions with family and social context; and to ensure workers acquire the necessary skills and confidence to undertake supportive and non-stigmatising work with families.

Conclusion

Parental mental illness is a public health issue with alarmingly high prevalence, and in extreme cases, it can present risks of harm to children through violence, abuse or neglect. There is a need for nurses and other professionals to ensure that they identify situations and assess impact where users of adult services are parents of dependent children and where users of child and adolescent services have parents with a mental illness. Children's services and social services also need to attend to the intersection of PMI with other key factors in families that increase the risk of abuse and neglect.

However, there are challenges for nurses and other professionals to balance the need to identify cases of significant risk against recognition both that cases of serious harm to children remain rare and that an overemphasis on the assumed deficits of FaPMI risks compounding mental health and other forms of stigma and discouraging help-seeking and engagement with services. Alongside focused risk assessment, there is the potential to improve support for FaPMI through ensuring a 'no wrong door' approach to family-focused support by upskilling the multi-agency workforce so that they can identify PMI, understand and assess its impacts and interactions with the family and social context, and offer supportive and non-stigmatising family-focused work. We argue also that it behoves academics, clinicians and professionals with a concern for the wellbeing of FaPMI to pay critical attention to the ways that social policy and service structures and protocols might inadvertently foster conditions that have negative impacts on mental health in families.

References

Aldridge, J. and Becker, S. (2003) *Children Caring for Parents with Mental Illness: Perspectives of Young Carers, Parents and Professionals*. Bristol: Policy Press.

Aldridge, J. and Becker, S. (1999) Children as carers: the impact of parental illness and disability on children's caring roles. *Journal of Family Therapy*, 21(3): 303–20.

Atkin, K. (1992) Similarities and differences between informal carers. In J. Twigg (ed.) *Carers: Research and Practice*. London: HMSO, pp. 30–58.

Barlow, J. and Schrader, A. (2010) *Safeguarding Children from Emotional Maltreatment: What Works*. London: Jessica Kingsley.

Boursnell, M. (2011) Parents with mental illness: the cycle of intergenerational mental illness. *Children Australia*, 36(1): 23–32.

Chaffin, M., Kelleher, K. and Hollenberg, J. (1996) Onset of physical abuse and neglect: psychiatric, substance abuse, and social risk factors from prospective community data. *Child Abuse and Neglect*, 20(3): 191–203.

Cleaver, H., Unell, I. and Aldgate, J. (2011) *Children's Needs – Parenting Capacity: Child Abuse: Parental Mental Illness, Learning Disability, Substance Misuse and Domestic Violence* (second edition). London: The Stationery Office.

Cleaver, H., Unell, I. and Aldgate, J. (1999) *Children's Needs – Parenting Capacity: The Impact of Parental Mental Illness, Problem Alcohol and Drug Use, and Domestic Violence on Children's Development*. London: The Stationery Office.

Cooklin, A. (2013) Promoting children's resilience to parental mental illness: engaging the child's thinking. *Advances in Psychiatric Treatment*, 19(3): 13–22.

Cooklin, A. (2010) 'Living upside down': being a young carer of a parent with mental illness. *Advances in Psychiatric Treatment*, 16(2): 141–6.

Crossley, S. (2015) *Realising the (Troubled) Family, Crafting the Neoliberal State: Families, Relationships and Societies*. London: Policy Press.

Cunningham, J., Harris, G., Vostanis, P., Oyebode, F. and Blissett, J. (2004) Children of mothers with mental illness: attachment, emotional and behavioural problems. *Early Child Development and Care*, 174(7–8): 639–50.

Dunn, B. (1993) Growing with a schizophrenic mother: a retrospective study. *American Journal of Orthopsychiatry*, 63(2): 177–89.

Falkov, A. (2011) *Parents as Patients*. London: Royal College of Psychiatrists.

Farahati, F., Marcotte, D. E. and Wilcox-Gök, V. (2003) The effects of parents' psychiatric disorders on children's high school dropout. *Economics of Education Review*, 22(2): 167–78.

Forrester, D. and Harwin, J. (2011) *Parents who Misuse Drugs and Alcohol. Effective Interventions in Social Work and Child Protection.* London: NSPCC/Wiley.

Gatsou, L., Yates, S., Hussain, S., Barrett, M., Gangavati, S. and Ghafoor, R. (2016) Parental mental illness: incidence, assessment and practice. *Mental Health Practice*, 19(5): 25–8.

Gatsou, L., Yates, S., Goodrich, N. and Pearson, D. (2015) The challenges presented by parental mental illness and the potential of a whole-family intervention to improve outcomes for families. *Child and Family Social Work*, online early view article. DOI: 10.1111/cfs.12254.

Hammen, C., Adrian, C., Gordon, D., Burge, D., Jaenicke, C. and Hiroto, D. (1987) Children of depressed mothers: maternal strain and symptom predictors of dysfunction. *Journal of Abnormal Psychology*, 96(3): 190–8.

Hinshaw, S. (2005) The stigmatization of mental illness in children and parents: developmental issues, family concerns, and research needs. *Journal of Child Psychology and Psychiatry*, 46(7): 714–34.

Knapp, M. (2012) Mental health in an age of austerity. *Evidence-Based Mental Health*, 15(3): 54–5.

Larson, J. and Corrigan, P. (2008) The stigma of families with mental illness. *Academic Psychiatry*, 32(2): 87–91.

Link, B., Struening, E., Neese-Todd, S., Asmussen, S. and Phelan, J. (2001) The consequences of stigma for the self-esteem of people with mental illness. *Psychiatric Services*, 52(12): 1621–6.

Maybery, D., Reupert, A., Patrick, P., Goodyear, M. and Crase, L. (2009) Prevalence of parental mental illness in Australian families. *Psychiatric Bulletin*, 33(1): 22–6.

Mowbray, C., Schwartz, S., Bybee, D., Spang, J., Rueda-Riedle, A. and Oyserman, D. (2000) Mothers with a mental illness: stressors and resources for parenting and living. *Families in Society*, 81(2): 118–29.

Nicholson, J., Albert, K., Gershenson, B., Williams, V. and Biebel, K. (2009) Family options for parents with mental illnesses: a developmental, mixed methods pilot study. *Psychiatric Rehabilitation Journal*, 33(2): 106–14.

Nicholson, J., Biebel, K., Katz-Levy, J. and Williams, V. (2004) The prevalence of parenthood in adults with mental illness. In R. W. Manderscheid and M. J. Henderson (eds) *Mental Health, United States*. Washington DC: US Department of Health, pp. 120–37.

Nicholson, J., Sweeney, E. and Geller, J. (1998) Mothers with mental illness: I. The competing demands of parenting and living with mental illness. *Psychiatric Services*, 49(5): 635–42.

Ofsted (2013) *What About the Children? Joint-Working between Adult and Children's Services When Parents or Carers Have Mental Ill Health and/or Drug and Alcohol Problems.* Manchester: Ofsted. Available at: www.ofsted.gov.uk/resources/130066 (accessed 20 July 2016).

Owen, S. (2008) *Children of Parents with a Mental Illness: Systems Change in Australia.* Adelaide: Owen Educational Consultancy.

Oyserman, D., Bybee, D., Mowbray, C. and Hart-Johnson, T. (2005) When mothers have serious mental health problems: parenting as a proximal mediator. *Journal of Adolescence*, 28(4): 443–63.

Oyserman, D., Mowbray, C., Meares, P. and Firminger, K. (2000) Parenting amongst mothers with a serious mental illness. *American Journal of Orthopsychiatry*, 70(3): 296–315.

Patel, V., Lund, C., Hatherill, S., Piagerson, S., Corrigall, J., Funk, M. and Flisher, A. (2010) Mental disorders: equity and social determinants. In E. Blas and A. S. Kurup (eds) *Equity, Social Determinants and Public Health Programmes*. Geneva: World Health Organization, pp. 115–34.

Peckover, S. (2009) 'Health' and safeguarding children: an 'expansionary project' or 'good practice'? In K. Broadhurst, C. Grover and J. Jamieson (eds) *Critical Perspectives on Safeguarding Children*. London: Wiley-Blackwell, pp. 149–70.

Pritchard, C., Davey, J. and Williams, R. (2012) Who kills children? Re-examining the evidence. *British Journal of Social Work*, 43(7): 1403–38.

Reader, P., Duncan, S. and Lucey, C. (2003) *Studies in the Assessment of Parenting.* Hove: Brunner-Routledge.

Reupert, A. and Maybery, D. (2014) Practitioners' experiences of working with families with complex needs. *Journal of Psychiatric and Mental Health Nursing*, 21(7): 642–51.

Reupert, A. and Maybery, D. (2011) Programmes for parents with a mental illness. *Journal of Psychiatric and Mental Health Nursing*, 18(3): 257–64.

Reupert, A. and Maybery, D. (2007) Families affected by parental mental illness: a multiperspective account of issues and interventions. *American Journal of Orthopsychiatry*, 77(3): 362–9.

Reupert, A., Maybery, D. and Kowolenko, N. (2012) Children whose parents have a mental illness: prevalence, need and treatment. *MJA Open*, 1(Supplement 1): 7–9.

Rutter, M. (1981) *Maternal Deprivation Reassessed* (second edition). London: Penguin.

Rutter, M. and Quinton, D. (1984) Parental psychiatric disorder: effects on children. *Psychological Medicine*, 14(4): 853–80.

Seifer, R., Sameroff, A., Dickstein, S., Gitner, G., Miller, I., Rasmussem, S. and Hayden, L. (1996) Parental psychopathology, multiple contextual risks and one-year outcomes in children. *Journal of Clinical Child Psychology*, 25(4): 423–35.

Social Care Institute for Care Excellence (2011) *Think Child, Think Parent, Think Family*. London: Social Care Institute for Care Excellence.

Whitley, R. and Campbell, R. (2014) Stigma, agency and recovery amongst people with severe mental illness. *Social Science and Medicine*, 107(April): 1–8.

Chapter 5

New and extended roles for CAMHS nurses

Angela Sergeant

Key points:

- In recent years, several high-profile reviews of the contribution of nursing to health, education and welfare services have brought new, extended roles for nurses in the UK. This has led to many service innovations including nurse-led clinics, transformational leadership through nurse consultant roles, and independent nurse prescribing.
- The Royal College of Nursing has published a range of guidance on the scope and application of new and extended roles including assistant practitioner, advanced practitioner, modern matron and nurse consultant, which together offer a framework for developing such roles within child and adolescent mental health services settings.
- The future workforce will likely be embedded in multi-agency teams with a core of generic skills, common across all the professional groups, with some more specialised skills matched to the demands of the population.
- Advanced nursing practice has provided new opportunities for nurses in terms of career pathways and professional development. These roles enhance patient user satisfaction and enable better self-management as well as providing a more holistic approach to assessment that leads to earlier diagnosis and interventions.
- It is the task of those currently in leadership positions to inspire and nurture the next generation of nurse leaders through a wide range of development opportunities.

Introduction

This chapter focuses on the new and extended roles for nurses that have been developed in recent years. The development of new and extended roles within inpatient settings has lagged behind many other specialities. The Royal College of Nursing (RCN) has published a range of guidance on the scope and application of new and extended roles including assistant practitioner, advanced practitioner, modern matron and nurse consultant, which together offer a framework for developing such roles within child and adolescent mental health services (CAMHS) settings. This is alongside practice standards for more traditional roles such as ward sister and charge nurse and for the clinical nurse specialist role, all of which are more common yet poorly defined within CAMHS (McDougall 2000, 2016).

Background

The mental health workforce has undergone significant transformation in recent years, teamwork being key to the delivery of a modern, flexible mental health service combined with service users and carers taking a more central role in their care and treatment. CAMHS are no exception to this because healthcare delivery to children and young people is evolving all the time. This dynamic is driven by service user demand and policy directives on integrated service provision alongside establishment of more home treatment teams and emphasis on improving access and shorter length of inpatient stay.

With this is mind, the traditional barriers between hospital and home treatment and health and social care are likely to reduce or vanish altogether in the decade ahead. Through the Integrated Personal Commissioning programme, individual care packages will be delivered by teams that carry out a wider range of functions. Alongside this, there will more integration between the CAMHS community and inpatient staff as intensive community services become located within or in close proximity to inpatient care. This will hopefully allow for the development of flexible or rotational posts that work across the care pathway and not in silos of either community or inpatient services.

There has been a flurry of activity in recent years concerning the review of CAMHS services, which has not always translated into change at grass-roots level. The publication *No Health Without Mental Health* (Department of Health 2011) outlined the plan to expand the front-line workforce and review the contribution that professionals make to developing the mental health of children and young people. The impact of the Health and Social Care Act 2012 will significantly change the health and social care landscape, and the government's mental health strategy will further develop CAMHS services.

Future in Mind (Department of Health 2015) sets out a clear vision for how we can all take responsibility for promoting children's psychological wellbeing and mental health, and how we can best achieve a step change in the quality and consistency of services at all levels. A key element of this relates to accountability, which in CAMHS is currently diffuse with a lack of clarity around lines of responsibility and a lack of leadership and effective joint working.

Further guidance is given by the Children and Young People's Outcomes Forum, which reinforces the importance of having staff with the right knowledge, skill and competence across the child's and young person's care pathway. The future workforce will likely be embedded in multi-agency teams with a core of generic skills, common across all the professional groups, with some more specialised skills matched to the demands of the population. In recognition of all these different components, it will be crucial that CAMHS services are well led with strong, experienced leadership as they respond to new commissioners with changing priorities. There will be a need for clear direction in CAMHS to guide children's emotional health, wellbeing and mental health practitioners through this process.

So without doubt, there is acknowledgement and consensus that child and adolescent services are becoming increasingly complex and will require a range of skills to deliver safe and effective care. The workforce is already changing in response to policy initiatives and professional requirements. Several roles have been extended and the deliberate blurring of boundaries between different professional roles is undoubtedly increasing and may continue to extend further.

Along with numerous policy directives and various CAMHS reviews, a number of wider workforce factors have influenced new and extended roles. These include the reduction in junior doctors' working hours as a result of the European Working Time Directive and changes in specialist medical training. At the same time has been a drive to create opportunities for expanding nurses' roles to advance professional autonomy, framed within the political agenda in the UK. As nursing roles, responsibilities and areas of practice have diversified and expanded, some of the boundaries of professional practice and competence have extended into the domain of what have previously been medically held roles.

Professional bodies can often be protective of their current boundaries and practice, and staff may fear that their professional roles will change; but strict adherence to traditional professional groupings may have to adjust due to future recruitment and retention challenges. The most difficult aspect is how to expand and extend roles whilst retaining the positive qualities and unique aspects of the various types of training without diluting all professional roles and responsibilities.

The RCN highlights that even when service developments have envisaged new ways of working that include nurses working at an advanced practice level, they 'have not invested in the training and development required to undertake such roles' (2014: 9). 'There has been an apparent dissonance between management and professional expectations and a lack of investment in the development, training and education, and continuing competency assessment required as nurses move on into roles such as children's advanced and specialist practitioners' (2014: 9).

So it is clear that the demand for services to grow and develop will provide us with opportunities for role development and service innovation. With the predicted shortfall in professionally qualified staff, traditional practices and roles must be reviewed to make the best use of highly trained professionals. We need to tackle this by providing good career opportunities to recruit and retain good-quality nursing staff in order to deliver the best care for service users and their families.

Responsibility and accountability

The emphasis on effective teamworking and distribution of responsibility has necessitated a re-evaluation of notions of accountability relating to particular roles and professions. Taken together with the changing patterns of healthcare, these factors are forcing commissioners and workforce planners to explore new service models – alongside expanding levels of autonomy, skill and decision-making – with staff that can adapt to the emerging technology. Positively, the broadening of the scope of practice for nursing has evolved in part to fill the gaps in the healthcare system. In particular, *Mental Health: New Ways of Working for Everyone* (Department of Health 2007) devolved authority and responsibility from psychiatrists to the wider multidisciplinary team, extended the boundaries of what nurses and other professionals are able to do and aimed to provide better and more efficient care and treatment for all service users including children, young people and their families.

New and extended roles

Matrons

The government's strategy for modernising all aspects of the National Health Service was set out in *The NHS Plan* (Department of Health 2000). The consultation exercise that preceded the plan found that patients and their relatives were often confused by lack of clear authority and nurse leadership at ward and unit level. In order to offer more clarity, guidance was given that every hospital should appoint 'modern matrons'. These were equivalent to senior sisters and charge nurses who could easily be identifiable and accountable for a group of wards. The three main strands of the modern matron role (Department of Health 2001) were to:

- provide leadership to professional and direct care staff, securing and assuring the highest standards of clinical care;
- ensure the availability of appropriate administrative and support services;
- provide a visible, accessible and authoritative presence in ward settings.

In *Modern Matrons: Improving the Patient Experience* (Department of Health 2003), the then Chief Nursing Officer spelt out the ten key responsibilities of modern matrons (Box 5.1).

Box 5.1 Modern matrons: ten key responsibilities

10   Leading by example

11   Making sure patients get quality care

12   Ensuring staffing is appropriate to patient needs

13   Empowering nurses to take on a wider range of clinical tasks

14   Improving hospital cleanliness

15   Ensuring patients' nutritional needs are met

16   Improving wards for patients

17   Making sure patients are treated with respect

18   Preventing hospital-acquired infection

19 Resolving problems for patients and their relatives by building closer relationships.

Source: Department of Health (2003: 5).

Inpatient CAMHS

The inpatient CAMHS nursing team has traditionally been led by either a matron or a ward sister, and both of these roles exist in some services. The terms ward sister and charge nurse are often used interchangeably, and these roles have been regarded as the backbone of the NHS and the hub of the wider clinical team (Department of Health 1999). With their 24-hour responsibility for care, the ward sisters are at the interface between management and clinical staff – at the point of care delivery where policy aspirations meet operational realities.

It is often the case that the modern matron role can overlap with the ward sister's responsibilities, and having a taller nursing hierarchy runs the risk of weakening the ward sister's position (RCN 2009). This could be due to systems of governance that involve the measurement and achievement of targets alongside financial penalties for failure to do so since both roles may be required to report against the measurement of performance. One way to meet the challenges posed by this situation is to create role delineation and clear division of labour among ward sisters, specialist nurses, modern matrons, bed managers and other managers (Doherty *et al.* 2010).

This is often easier said than done within CAMHS settings where the career structure has been described as 'difficult' (Morris *et al.* 2009). Having said that, the RCN (2009) report *Breaking Down Barriers, Driving Up Standards* found that roles can be difficult to delineate due to the demands of bureaucratic processes, the varying expectations of managers and other health professionals, and the expectations of patients and carers. The report concluded that the job of ward sister has become almost impossible to deliver as there remains so much conflict between its clinical and managerial functions.

New and extended roles in CAMHS

Turning now to extended roles that have already developed in CAMHS, the nurse practitioner, independent nurse prescriber, nurse specialist and nurse consultant have, to a greater or lesser extent, all been implemented to undertake tasks once viewed as being within the remit of doctors. The 'extension' of a nursing role usually refers to the inclusion of a particular skill or area of practice responsibility not previously associated with the role. In contrast, role 'development' tends to imply higher levels of clinical autonomy brought about by new demands and perceived shortcomings in the quality of patient care and healthcare resources.

Advanced nursing practice

'Advanced nursing practice' is an umbrella term used to describe a number of specialist roles including clinical nurse specialist and nurse practitioner. Advanced nursing practice roles have evolved significantly over the last 20 years with the emergence of increased autonomy, enhanced clinical decision-making, professional responsibility, nursing research and the expansion of traditional nursing roles.

As nursing roles, responsibilities and areas of specialist practice have diversified and expanded, some of the boundaries of professional practice and competence have become blurred. In order to provide clarity around the concept of advanced nursing practice, the Department of Health issued a position statement in 2010. This was to be used as a 'benchmark to enhance patient safety and the delivery of high-quality care by supporting local governance, assisting in good employment practices and encouraging consistency in the development of roles and posts' (2010: 4). This position statement made it possible for nurses to adopt additional clinical tasks or expand service provision provided they acquired the appropriate education or training and levels of competence and recognised their accountabilities in relation to their new practices.

Advanced nursing practice roles are not new. They were first introduced in the 1990s by the now defunct United Kingdom Central Council for Nursing, Midwifery and Health Visiting (1994). The Nursing and Midwifery Council ([NMC] 2007) has since updated the definition of advanced nurse practitioners, stating that the roles should be undertaken by highly skilled nurses with a range of competencies (see Box 5.2).

Advanced nursing practice has provided new opportunities for nurses in terms of career pathways and professional development. While the RCN acknowledges that advanced nursing practice is regulated by *The Code* (NMC 2008), they suggest further governance is needed. The introduction of local governance frameworks should be viewed as positive measures that seek to assure fitness for practice and consequent public protection, especially in light of numerous inquiries highlighting poor professional practice. This should help to overcome the *ad hoc* development of advanced nursing roles and the highly variable use of titles by nurses that infer levels of clinical expertise that cannot be verified.

The NMC intends to open a subpart of the nurses' part of the register – subject to Privy Council approval – with a definition of advanced nurse practitioner, which means that the

> **Box 5.2 What should advanced practitioners be able to do?**
>
> - Take a comprehensive patient history
>
> - Carry out physical examinations
>
> - Use their expert knowledge and clinical judgement to identify the potential diagnosis
>
> - Refer patients for investigations where appropriate
>
> - Make a final diagnosis
>
> - Decide on and carry out treatment, including the prescribing of medicines, or refer patients to an appropriate specialist
>
> - Use their extensive practice experience to plan and provide skilled and competent care to meet patient's health and social care needs, involving other members of the healthcare team as appropriate
>
> - Ensure the provision of continuity of care including follow-up visits
>
> - Assess and evaluate, with patients, the effectiveness of the treatment and care provided and make changes as needed
>
> - Work independently, although often as part of a healthcare team
>
> - Provide leadership
>
> - Make sure that each patient's treatment and care is based on best practice.
>
> Source: NMC (2007).

title will now be protected. However, this still does not prevent employers developing many varied posts and titles depending on local service configuration and need. So the career path towards being an advanced nurse is not clear. The abundance of advanced practitioner titles being used in the UK adds to the confusion. These include nurse specialist, nurse practitioner and nurse therapist. It is little wonder, therefore, that nurses are confused, let alone other professionals and the general public.

On a more positive note, Begley *et al.* (2013) evaluated the advanced practitioner role and found that it improves patient satisfaction and enables better self-care and management as well as providing a more holistic approach to assessment that leads to earlier diagnosis and interventions. Evaluating the impact of advanced nursing practice roles – whichever titles are used – remains difficult, and conceptual debate exists. However, there is a growing body of anecdotal evidence that these roles have a positive impact in the delivery of high-quality care.

Even more needs to be done to ensure that these types of roles are developed and are not lost as part of cost improvement plans in times of economic constraints. However, Rolfe (2014a) cautions against advanced nurse practitioner roles being developed just to 'plug the gap' in junior doctors' working hours. Rolfe also suggests that advanced nursing practice depends less on what nurses do than on how they do it. For example, some tasks on the list of competencies defined by the NMC (2007) can be performed well or poorly by either a nurse or a doctor. Rolfe (2014b) states that the advancement of nursing practice should concentrate on developing nurses' abilities in building relationships with patients and working with them to improve their care.

Independent nurse prescribing

The practice of non-medical prescribing in mental health comes primarily from the US, where nurse prescribing has been in place since the 1970s and this extended role for nurses has become embedded in practice. In the UK, the developing role of prescribing by nurses in general has been broadly supported. However, the uptake of non-medical prescribing by child and adolescent mental health nurses has been much slower than in the US, and it is mostly mental health nurses who work with adults of working age who are training to prescribe. As well as a raft of opportunities and benefits, non-medical prescribing in CAMHS creates many questions, challenges and dilemmas. Some have claimed that nurse prescribing is considerably quicker, much cheaper and more efficient than medical prescribing. They argue that it produces equivalent or better outcomes, more choice and flexibility, improved concordance with treatment and better quality of overall care.

According to the RCN (2012), over the last decade, nurse prescribing in the UK has grown significantly as professional bodies, legislative reforms and policy directives have encouraged nurses' prescribing roles in acute care and in community settings. The RCN (2012) reports UK figures of more than 54,000 nurse and midwife prescribers and over 19,000 nurse independent and supplementary prescribers.

Training requirements

Independent prescribing is a very challenging course to complete. In order to be an independent prescriber, nurses must complete a NMC-accredited prescribing course through an approved education institution. This requires a minimum of 26 days of teaching (and for distance-learning programmes, there must be a minimum of eight face-to-face taught days), which includes 12 days of supervised learning in practice. This training is provided at a minimum of first degree level (academic level 3) and is completed within one academic year (NMC 2006).

To be eligible to undertake an accredited nurse prescribing course, applicants must be a registered first level nurse, midwife and/or specialist community public health nurse with at least three years' practice experience. Additionally, they should be deemed competent by their employer in history taking, clinical assessment and diagnosing, and the employer must confirm support for the nurse to undertake the course. The nurse must also provide evidence via the Accreditation of Prior and Experiential Learning process that they are able to study at degree level. Agreement is required from a medical practitioner who meets eligibility to provide medical supervision of nurse prescribers and who will provide supervised practice. In the year immediately preceding the programme, the nurse must have been working in the clinical field that they will be prescribing in (NMC 2006).

Types of nurse prescriber

The RCN (2012) describes two types of nurse prescribers. First, nurse independent prescribers (NIPs) are specially trained nurses who are authorised to prescribe 'any licensed and unlicensed drugs within their clinical competence' (RCN 2012: 1). Since 2006 they have had full access to the *British National Formulary* (BNF) and this has 'put nurses on a par with doctors in relation to prescribing capabilities' (RCN 2012: 1). The legislative changes that came into effect in the UK with the Health and Social Care Act 2012 gave NIPs the power to prescribe Schedule 2–5 controlled drugs. NIPs were thereafter able to prescribe controlled drugs within their competence.

The RCN (2012) notes that community practitioner nurse prescribers are a distinct category of independent prescribers who are 'allowed to independently prescribe from a limited formulary called the Nursing Formulary for Community Practitioners, which includes over-the-counter drugs, wound dressings and applications' (RCN 2012: 1).

The second type is nurse supplementary prescribing. This is 'based on a voluntary prescribing partnership between a doctor (independent prescriber) and a nurse (supplementary prescriber)' (RCN 2012: 1). The patient is diagnosed by a doctor, and then the supplementary nurse prescriber can prescribe any drug included in the patient's clinical management plan. The supplementary prescriber is not limited legally to certain clinical conditions and 'this is most beneficial for nurses caring for patients with long-term conditions like diabetes or asthma' (RCN 2012: 1).

The evidence demonstrates that patients report a high level of satisfaction and confidence in nurse prescribing, and the benefits have been consistently reported in the literature. This is mainly through qualitative and anecdotal surveys, and further high-quality research is required. According to Latter *et al.* (2011), many believe that nurse prescribing in the UK improves access to medications for patients by increasing the availability of healthcare providers who can prescribe, thus facilitating a more efficient use of skills and experience within the nursing workforce.

Within CAMHS, one of the most common neurodevelopmental disorders in children is attention deficit hyperactivity disorder (ADHD). As a direct result of the 2012 legislative changes, nurses can now independently provide a complete and holistic package of care for individuals with ADHD, including prescribing medication. This has been happening in practice for some time now with well-established nurse-led ADHD clinics in the UK; however, data regarding the safety or clinical appropriateness is not yet available due to lack of trials (Mangle *et al.* 2014).

However, there have been criticisms of nurse prescribing in the UK, relating to professional identity, the training and skills needed and potential litigation. 'The passionately protected therapeutic relationship, central to the nursing role, and the changing emphasis from "caring" to "curing" has prompted some nurses to consider whether non-medical prescribing is a backward step for the profession' (McDougall and Ryan 2016).

Nurse consultant

The role of clinical nurse consultant has been in existence in Australia for almost 30 years, and in the UK, the role is more senior to nurse specialists and advanced nurse practitioners. Nurse consultants were first introduced into the NHS in England in 2000 as part of the government's strategy for nursing. This aimed to drive up quality by strengthening the nursing, midwifery and health visiting contribution to health and healthcare. The Department of Health specified that the role should compromise four core functions (see Box 5.3).

The nurse consultant role is unique in its capacity to provide clinical leadership across a range of contexts. However, the role has been plagued with confusion due to lack of clarity in some circumstances over the many applied titles, inconsistent role application, and function and appropriateness for purpose within health organisations across different contexts. Many nurse consultant roles have developed in an *ad hoc* manner – due to changes within the multidisciplinary team or as service gap fillers – without clear links to any nursing strategy.

Nonetheless, as well as the role being intended to achieve better outcomes for patients by improving quality and services, it offered the opportunity for nurses to remain in clinical

---

Box 5.3 Nurse consultant core functions

1 Leadership and consultancy

2 Education and training

3 Service development, research and evaluation

4 Expert clinical practice.

Source: adapted from NHS Executive (1999).

---

practice rather than moving into management. It had been clear that there was a need for a clinical career structure with financial rewards that would retain senior staff in clinical practice, thus encouraging recruitment and retention.

Case example of how the nurse consultant role helps improves outcomes

Gemma is one of three national nurse consultants who specialises in young people who self-harm. She has over 30 years' clinical experience and has spent the last 20 actively researching treatments. Gemma is the lead for a Tier 4 specialist day and outpatient service for young people aged 13 to 18 presenting with complex mental health difficulties. Gemma spends 50 per cent of her time in direct clinical practice and has gained national recognition in the field of self-harm with young people. She has been a panel member of two expert topic groups for National Institute for Health and Care Excellence (NICE) guidance on longer-term treatments of self-harm and depression in young people. Gemma has co-designed a group treatment known as 'developmental group psychotherapy', which has been the subject of three randomised controlled trials (RCTs) both in the UK and in Australia. The treatment is offered over a variety of Tier 3 services in the north-west of England. As well as being a busy clinician, Gemma has published in a variety of journals and books. She is particularly proud of her involvement in developing the service user and carer agenda. Some of the ex-service users are currently employed by the service where she works, and others have gone on to complete a variety of careers post volunteering at outpatient services. The following are examples of what the young people said about Gemma's involvement.

> I feel that the involvement of a nurse consultant in my care has been extremely beneficial. The training and qualifications that go beyond that of a staff nurse give more knowledge and a better ability to make decisions and advise the young people. Despite the amount of knowledge they possess, they still maintain personal relationships and see the young people more than medical staff for example. This gave me a lot more security in my care.
>
> Well, I attend a day service which is run by a nurse consultant. They are usually around and are very approachable. They seem to take time to understand my issues and never second-guess them, and especially they never ask me how I am feeling on a scale of 1 to 10, 10 being good and 1 being bad.

Attributes and motivations

One of the early studies on the characteristics and achievements of nurse consultants identifies some key characteristics. Woodward *et al.* (2005) suggest that clinicians who are highly experienced in practice, education, leadership and research on appointment were much more likely to be able to cope with the demands of the post. By contrast, Woodward *et al.* report that those who were finding the demands of the post difficult were often lacking in education, leadership and research experience. The study identified a number of attributes and motivational factors in postholders, many of whom were specialist nurses in their field, holding a master's degree and with research experience.

Attributes included:

- Expert practice – all nurse consultants had a history of expert practice in their specialist field, and many were innovative and proactive practitioners.
- Leadership – this was a quality that emerged with some practitioners working at a national level.
- Empowerment – empowering others was an important attribute that emerged in the study, and many saw this as one of the main missions of their role.
- Challengers of the status quo – most nurse consultants had demonstrated the ability to challenge the status quo of existing practice, service organisation or culture at a variety of levels.
- Determination – many identified that this was needed to achieve goals and assert views in situations that might be intimidating, such as at a trust level or at national level and often with managers or policymakers.
- Self-confidence – along with determination went high levels of self-confidence that enabled nurse consultants to challenge, achieve change and 'fight their corner' for what they perceived as being important.
- Collaboration – the final attribute was collaboration with others, needing to work and liaise with many others in a wide variety of situations locally, regionally and nationally within their field and at the margins.

Motivations reflected the following:

- Personal agendas and desire for change – most interviewees were highly motivated individuals who had areas of interest and a strong desire for change in their field of practice. They may also have been motivated by career progression and the 'kudos' of the post.
- Role achievement – all of those interviewed were aware of the importance of evidence-based practice and critical appraisal skills for all nurses working in the NHS. Some felt that they had achieved integration of the four domains of the role at strategic and national levels. Others described the phenomena of 'graphic equalisers', noting that across the period of the day, week or month, some areas would be more prominent than others.

'[T]he Nurse Consultant role differs from the Nurse Practitioner (NP) in that their expert knowledge base is more likely to be applied to the education and development of practice in others and they are more likely to be involved in leading practice change and research' (Giles *et al.* 2014). As McDougall (2003) points out, nurse consultants are in key positions to help raise the profile of research and define knowledge in nursing. As well as identifying, evaluating and implementing evidence in practice, nurse consultants undertake research projects and publish their work in order to develop innovative and creative ways of working with children and families. In line with the national strategy for nursing research and development, nurse leaders must help enable other nurses to maximise their contribution to nursing knowledge and research. This involves creating opportunities to access and critique research as well as helping nurses to maximise their potential and celebrate their success in the public arena.

Nurses must be encouraged to articulate their worth by writing for publication and speaking at conferences. Nurses who celebrate their successes, publish and speak about their work help raise levels of professional confidence. Kennedy *et al.* (2011), in evaluating the impact of the role, report that in the few existing studies, the nurse consultant roles were found to be often 'diverse and complex' (2011: 3); the findings also suggest a 'largely positive influence by nurse consultants on a range of clinical and professional outcomes' (2011: 721). As the role often lends itself to indirect rather than direct patient contact, it is often difficult to measure the impact on health outcomes. It is clear that further research is required that involves patients who receive care directly from nurse consultants to explore their experiences and the outcomes they value most.

Nurses as approved clinicians

The 2010 report by the Commission on the Future of Nursing and Midwifery in England, *Front Line Care*, emphasises that '[a]s the largest group of registered professionals in the NHS, [nurses have] great power and potential to influence health and healthcare' (2010: 14). Since the 1990s, 'nurses have acquired greater responsibility as autonomous and interdependent practitioners' (2010: 14); they have been leading programmes of care, independently prescribing.

Following changes to the Mental Health Act in 2007, non-medical clinicians were empowered to become approved clinicians (ACs). This was previously the exclusive domain of consultant psychiatrists. The responsible clinician (RC) role was also introduced. Once you gain AC status, you become eligible to be a RC.

How the approved clinician role helps improves outcomes

Box 5.4 Case example: Angela

Angela is one of the two national CAMHS nurse consultants who has acquired the status of approved clinician. She has 25 years' CAMHS experience, and her specialist areas are inpatient CAMHS and treatment of young people with eating disorders. She is the lead for the specialist eating disorders programme within Tier 4 CAMHS. She was a founding member of the Quality Network for Inpatient CAMHS (QNIC) and sits on the accreditation committee. Since becoming a nurse consultant in 2003, Angela has spent 50 per cent of her time in direct clinical practice as the responsible clinician for eating disorder cases including young people under the Mental Health Act. This is alongside delivering on other core domains of her role. She has been the RC for 130 inpatient cases and conducted over 200 assessments. As an approved clinician, Angela has the power to renew detention, make a Community Treatment Order and recall or discharge someone on a Supervised Community Treatment Order.

The following are extracts from the testimonial of a young person and parent submitted as part of the AC portfolio application:

> I am delighted in every way to support Angela's desire to be appointed as an approved clinician. Angela always took into account my views. Throughout my time under her care, she always knew what she was talking about and she never made me worry that I had someone who was not professional or fair. She made an effort to make me feel like a person, not just another annoying patient.
>
> Angela may not have been the responsible clinician (this was prior to approved clinician status approval) for my daughter's case, but she completely managed my daughter's case in the most professional way possible. Her style was inclusive, ensuring that all the members of the team including parents were informed and included in the decisions around treatment.

ACs take several years to achieve the level of expertise required, and this includes lots of extra studying. Those that make the grade are all senior clinicians. They have all added higher levels of competency to their skills, particularly in relation to the application of the Mental Health Act.

An AC has to be a registered medical practitioner, a registered psychologist, a mental health or learning disability nurse, a registered occupational therapist or a registered social worker and have undergone specific training relating to the application of the Mental Health Act. ACs have various responsibilities under the Act. These include acting as the RC for detained and Supervised Community Treatment patients, having overall responsibility for a patient's case.

So what does the future hold for extended and advanced nursing roles?

When NHS England recently published the *Five Year Forward View* (2014), it set out the challenges faced by the NHS and the steps needed to address these. It challenges everyone to think differently about new care models by focusing on prevention and working across cultural and organisational divisions with patients, communities and other healthcare professionals. The *Five Year Forward View* was developed in partnership with a number of organisations at local and national levels, placing greater emphasis on building health around populations rather than professionals and buildings.

This is in keeping with the approach that Health Education England (HEE) is taking in their workforce planning. They are moving away from a process of essentially planning numbers through the lens of registered professionals towards a system that identifies the 'numbers, skills, values and behaviours' that patients and their families need both today and tomorrow (Willis 2015). As the planning for 2015/16 education commissioning unfolds, HEE will develop more specific guidance notes covering medical workforce planning and other groups. This may indicate the need for even more specialist advanced nursing roles. The planning process for new care models to integrate acute and community care may transform the workforce further and provide new opportunities for advanced and extended nursing roles.

Conclusion

Nurses in the new and extended practice roles are expected to lead services with confidence and competence and to champion care quality with a powerful voice and positive impact. It is the task of those already in leadership positions to inspire and nurture the next generation of nurse leaders through a wide range of development programmes, such as the Consultant Practitioner Trainee programme. Many of them will already be qualified at master's degree and doctorate levels, but may need clinical development opportunities.

References

Begley, C., Elliott, N., Lalor, J., Coyne, I., Higgins, A. and Comiskey, C. M. (2013) Differences between clinical specialist and advanced practitioner clinical practice, leadership, and research roles, responsibilities, and perceived outcomes (the SCAPE study). *Journal of Advanced Nursing*, 69(6): 1323–37.

Commission on the Future of Nursing and Midwifery in England (2010) *Front Line Care: The Future of Nursing and Midwifery in England*. London: Department of Health.

Department of Health (2015) *Future in Mind: Promoting, Protecting and Improving Our Children and Young People's Mental Health and Wellbeing*. London: Department of Health.

Department of Health (2011) *No Health Without Mental Health*. London: Department of Health.

Department of Health (2010) *Responsibility and Accountability Moving on for New Ways of Working to a Creative, Capable Workforce. Best Practice Guidance*. London: Department of Health.

Department of Health (2007) *Mental Health: New Ways of Working for Everyone: Developing and Sustaining a Capable and Flexible Workforce. Progress Report*. London: Department of Health.

Department of Health (2003) *Modern Matrons – Improving the Patient Experience*. London: Department of Health.

Department of Health (2001) *Implementing the NHS Plan: Modern Matrons: Strengthening the Role of Ward Sisters and Introducing Senior Sisters*. London: Department of Health.

Department of Health (2000) *The NHS Plan: A Plan for Investment, A Plan for Reform*. CM 4818-I. London: The Stationery Office.

Department of Health (1999) *Getting it Right for Children, Young People and Families. Maximising the Contribution of the School Nursing Team: Vision and Call to Action*. London: Department of Health.

Doherty, C., Gatenby, M. and Hales, C. (2010) Role of the ward sister: tensions, pressures and opportunities. *Nursing Standard*, 24(51): 35–40.

Giles, M., Parker, V. and Mitchell, R. (2014) Recognising the difference in the nurse consultant role across context: a study protocol. *BMC Nursing*, 13: 30.

Kennedy F., McDonnell, A., Gerrish, K., Howarth, A., Pollard, C. and Redmond, J. (2011) Evaluation of the impact of nurse consultant roles in the United Kingdom: a mixed method systematic literature review. *Journal of Advanced Nursing*, 68(4): 721–42.

Latter, S., Blenkinsopp, A., Smith, A., Chapman, S., Tinelli, M., Gerard, K., Little, P., Celino, N., Granby, T., Nicholls, P. and Dorer, G. (2011) *Evaluation of Nurse and Pharmacist Independent Prescribing*. University of Southampton and Keele University.

McDougall, T. (2016) Child and adolescent mental health nursing: a call for action. *British Journal of Mental Health Nursing*, 5(1): 10–14.

McDougall, T. (2003) *Nurse Consultants: Children's Champions. Mental Health Practice* 6(9): 34.

McDougall, T. (2000) Child and adolescent mental health nursing: the role of the nurse specialist. *Nursing Times*, 96(28): 37–8.

McDougall, T. and Ryan, N. (2016) Nurse prescribing in CAMHS: an evolving role. *British Journal of Mental Health Nursing*, 5(2): 62–7.

Mangle, L., Phillips, P., Pitts, M. and Laver-Bradbury, C. (2014). Implementation of independent nurse prescribing in UK mental health settings: focus on attention-deficit/hyperactivity disorder. *ADHD: Attention Deficit Hyperactive Disorder*, 6(4): 269–79.

Morris, T., Anderson, Y. and Nixon, B. (2009) New Ways of Working in child and adolescent mental health services: 'keep the baby but throw out the bathwater'. *Journal of Mental Health Training, Education and Practice*, 4(3): 10–14.

NHS England (2014) *Five Year Forward View*. London: NHS England.

NHS Executive (1999) *Nurse, Midwife and Health Visitor Consultants: Establishing Posts and Making Appointments*. London: NHS Executive.

Nursing and Midwifery Council (NMC) (2008) *The Code: Standards of Conduct, Performance and Ethics for Nurses and Midwives*. London: NMC.

Nursing and Midwifery Council (NMC) (2007) Advanced nursing practice – update, 19 June [online]. London: NMC. Available from: https://www.nmc.org.uk/standards/code/ (accessed 20 July 2016).

Nursing and Midwifery Council (NMC) (2006) *Standards of Profiency for Nurse and Midwife Prescribers*. London: NMC.

Rolfe, G. (2014a) Advanced nursing practice 1: understanding advanced nursing practice. *Nursing Times*, 110(27): 20–3.

Rolfe, G. (2014b) Advanced nursing practice 2: a new vision for advanced nursing practice. *Nursing Times*, 110(28): 18–21.

Royal College of Nursing (RCN) (2014) *Specialist and Advanced Children's and Young People's Nursing Practice in Contemporary Health Care: Guidance for Nurses and Commissioners*. London: RCN.

Royal College of Nursing (RCN) (2012) *RCN Fact Sheet: Nurse Prescribing in the UK*. London: RCN.

Royal College of Nursing (RCN) (2009) *Breaking Down Barriers, Driving Up Standards*. London: RCN.

United Kingdom Central Council for Nursing, Midwifery and Health Visiting (1994) *The Future of Professional Practice: The Council's Standards for Education and Practice following Registration*. London: United Kingdom Central Council for Nursing, Midwifery and Health Visiting.

Willis, P., Lord (Chair) (2015) *Raising the Bar. Shape of Caring: A Review of the Future Education and Training of Registered Nurses and Care Assistants*. London: Health Education England. Available at: https://www.hee.nhs.uk/sites/default/files/documents/2348-Shape-of-caring-review-FINAL_0.pdf (accessed 21 July 2016).

Woodward, V. A., Webb, C. and Prowse, M. (2005) Nurse consultants: their characteristics and achievements. *Journal of Clinical Nursing*, 14(7): 845–54.

Chapter 6

Working in partnership with children and young people to tackle mental health stigma

Together we can change minds

Fiona Warner-Gale, Leanne Walker and Amanda Tuffrey

Key points:

- Some people who have experienced stigma and discrimination because of their mental health problems say this can be as difficult as, if not worse than, the mental health problem itself.
- Stigmatising views about mental health problems are not just limited to the general population but can exist amongst well-trained professionals, including those from mental health disciplines.
- Stigma is a major concern for young people. It can impact on self-worth and leave them feeling so ashamed that they do not want to tell others or ask for help.
- Developing anti-stigma programmes that incorporate all of these elements has been found to be effective at achieving change not only in individuals but on a systems and organisational level, thus creating a bottom-up and top-down approach.
- The most effective programmes to tackle stigma are not one-off interventions but, rather, mainstream approaches. This is so that positive change can be sustained and embedded across all elements of society and at a cultural level.

Introduction

As evidence has shown us, emerging mental health problems are very common in children and young people, affecting at least one in every four each year. At any given time, one in ten children and young people have a diagnosable mental health problem (Green *et al.* 2005). However, only 40 per cent of these receive professional help (Murphy and Fonagy 2013). Evidence indicates that in general children and young people tend to show low levels of help-seeking in relation to their mental health (Time to Change 2012). In particular, this avoidance of help-seeking is more of an issue amongst boys and young men than it is for girls and young women. Time to Change (2012) reports that the stigma attached to being identified as having a mental health problem results in many young people avoiding asking for help to the point that their mental health problem becomes a very real crisis for them.

This chapter was written in partnership with two exceptional young people who have given their time to deliver positive messages about mental health and who both have lived experience of mental health problems and stigma. It includes their thoughts, ideas and testimonies about what we, as the professionals supporting them, can do to tackle stigma with children and young people.

Background

It is estimated that half of mental health problems in adulthood start around the age of 14 (Kessler *et al.* 2007), and three-quarters of adults who have mental health problems had some kind of diagnosis as a child (New Philanthropy Capital 2008). The extent of stigma is widespread, far-reaching and can affect people throughout their lifespan. In a study by Time to Change (2014a), nine out of ten people interviewed reported that they had experienced some form of stigma related to their mental health problems. It is described as having a severe impact on the confidence and ability of those needing help. In fact, some people who have experienced stigma and discrimination because of their mental health problems have described the experience as equal to if not worse than the mental health problem itself (Pescosolido *et al.* 2007).

The NHS Benchmarking Network (2013) found that nurses are the largest professional group within child and adolescent mental health services (CAMHS) at 73 per cent of the workforce. With this in mind, there is a great opportunity for nurses, in partnership with other professionals, to be the driving force behind the change that is needed in attitudes toward mental health. It is only through a hard-hitting and multidimensional approach that we can tackle stigma in its many different forms across the many levels of society in which it exists.

What is stigma?

In order to challenge the effects of stigma, it is necessary to understand its definitions, concepts and extent as well as its impact on the individual and within society. There are many definitions around that attempt to describe what is meant by stigma. The earliest usage of the term was in ancient Greece where stigma referred to the act of 'branding', which entailed cutting or burning signs into the body of people who were considered to be members of tainted groups; this was a way of exposing something unusual or bad about the moral status of the 'marked' person. These marks warned others that the bearers were blemished or polluted and so should be avoided, especially in public (Goffman 1963). The fact that the term has been around for such a long time indicates how embedded the process and the effects of stigma are in our society.

Erving Goffman stated in his classic work *Stigma: Notes on a Spoiled Identity* that stigma was socially discrediting, permanent and affected perceptions of the person as a whole. He defined stigma as 'the situation of the individual who is disqualified from full social acceptance' (1963: 9). He suggested that cues signalling sources of stigma are not always readily evident. With this in mind, it has been suggested that people with mental health needs can, to some extent, 'hide' the tarnish that identifies them with a stigmatised group. This can be seen to contribute to the fear of 'being found out' – being discredited by their condition – which can lead to withdrawal, isolation and secrecy and, ultimately, feelings of shame.

Nowadays, stigma is defined in terms of being categorised as different from the social norm, setting the person or group of people apart from others. The term 'stigma' is referred to as the negative effects of a label being placed on a group with the result that they are often shunned, pushed aside or devalued. The labelling associated with stigma can cover a wide range of experiences including mental illness, physical disability, race, culture or sexual identity, for example. Stigma has been shown to be pervasive and operating on a number of levels so that it doesn't just affect the individual, but also those around them, their community, culture and society as a whole.

The negative language surrounding how we talk about mental health is deeply embedded within society. Research into young people's understanding of mental health and illness has revealed at least 250 ways of talking about it, the large majority of which were negative or derogatory (Rose *et al.* 2007).

A complex and widespread phenomenon?

The stigma related to mental health has been described as a global concern (World Health Organization 2013), and it affects people with mental health problems worldwide in many different ways. It is said to be highly prevalent and has persisted over time. In fact, studies undertaken by the Indiana University Bloomington (Stigma in a Global Context; n.d.) have suggested that the disparity in outcomes for people with serious mental illness are, in part, due to cultural norms, attitudes and behaviours towards people with mental illness across societies. Some research has suggested that people with mental health problems, regardless of whether they have a diagnosis, are stigmatised to a greater degree that those with other health conditions (Kurzban and Leary 2001).

A very early study (Cumming and Cumming 1957) examining the attitudes of the general public in relation to mental illness concluded that most people feared and disliked the mentally ill and would avoid them at all costs. When we compare this to the revelations earlier that nine out of ten people with mental health problems experience stigma and discrimination, we can see that changing negative attitudes and beliefs can be a slow process.

Stigmatising views about mental health problems are not just limited to the general population. Some research on the attitudes of well-trained professionals, including those from mental health disciplines, has shown that they too can subscribe to prejudicial stereotypes about mental health problems and mental illness (Lyons and Ziviani 1995; Corrigan 2000). In a recent Australian study, GPs were found to have higher scores on personal stigma scales (Reavley *et al.* 2014), and whilst England's largest anti-stigma campaign, Time to Change, reported in 2013 that there had been notable improvement in scores on surveys across family and friends, no change was found in discrimination by mental health professionals. The Time to Change survey, which is conducted on an annual basis, has shown that people using mental health services report significant levels of discrimination coming from mental health professionals and that levels of discrimination from this group had not decreased during the lifespan of the Time to Change campaign, which began in 2007 (Brindle 2013; Time to Change 2014a).

The power of the mass media to influence public perception and the degree to which people are exposed to media representations of mental health make the mass media one of the most significant influencers in developed societies. It has contributed significantly to damaging depictions of mental health. Such depictions range from overt, negative reporting in the press and on the news to subtle stereotyping through insinuating remarks. Research has shown that many people obtain their information about mental health problems and mental illness through the media. In addition, poor portrayal of mental health can be seen as a subject in a wide range of media products, from horror films to children's comic books, computer games and soap operas.

One recent and memorable example of the pervasive effects of stigma was the newsworthy portrayal of a range of Halloween costumes in well-known supermarkets that were marketed as 'mental health patient' and 'psycho ward'. This was found to be staggeringly offensive to the digital community, forcing an outcry on Twitter that caused the products to be taken off the shelves. Another example concerns a popular Saturday night television show which, on Halloween, had dancers in strait jackets performing to a song called *Crazy*; this had the effect of sending a message that people with mental health problems are to be feared or humiliated.

However, working hand in hand with media can also challenge stigma and have a positive effect on the way that people see mental health issues. *Making a Drama out of a Crisis* (Time to Change 2014b) looked at how mental health depictions are becoming more authentic and how they can prompt people to seek help earlier. This report also found that over half of people said that seeing a well-known character on screen with mental health problems improved their understanding. Half said it helped to change their opinion about the kind of people who can develop such problems, and around a third said it actively inspired them to start a conversation about the storyline with friends, family or colleagues (Time to Change 2014b).

Although mass media can be a useful source of learning and information, it is important to recognise that the impact of negative attributions associated with mental health and illness can begin at a very early stage in development and can be sustained throughout the lifespan. Therefore, the focus of campaigns to combat stigma using media as a conduit must target children, as well as adults, if they are to elicit any change.

How does stigma happen?

The stigmatisation process has been found to be complex, and it has been said to have a severe impact on the individual and the way that they see themselves in relation to the rest of the community. However, it is not just the way that stigma itself affects a person with mental health problems but the discrimination and prejudice they experience from those around them that can have the greatest impact.

Stigma has specific dimensions. Three processes take place within the individual and across society: public stigma, self-stigma and courtesy stigma (Corrigan 2000; Ben-Zeev *et al.* 2010; see Box 6.1).

Box 6.1 Three processes of stigma

5 Public stigma – the negative reaction that the general population has towards people with mental health problems.

6 Self-stigma – the negative experiences of those people with mental health problems as a response to the stigmatisation process (i.e. the harm that occurs as a result of internalising or taking on board stigma). This may impact on self-esteem and self-worth, in turn affecting personal empowerment and personal pursuit of goals.

7 Courtesy stigma – social disapproval for people associated with a person with a mental health problem. Families, friends and even neighbours are possible recipients of the effects of courtesy stigma. In this respect, people who experience courtesy stigma as a result of their connection with an individual can experience varying levels of stigma, which they can regulate through their ability to distance themselves from the person with mental health problems.

Source: adapted from Corrigan (2000).

Recently, research undertaken by Warner-Gale (2008) found that the parents of children with mental health problems felt the severe effects of stigma much more than their children did. This has occurred because of their closeness and responsibility for their child (i.e. it is difficult to distance themselves). As a result, parents felt they were taking on the stigma themselves to try and protect their child – this additional dimension of the stigmatisation process was defined by Warner-Gale as 'stigma by proxy'. A similar phenomenon has been found in parents of children with autism or genetic disorders wherein the parent feels responsible for the effects of the stigma on their children. In this case, parents find it hard to dissociate from the child in order to avoid the effects of stigma, as they would in courtesy stigma.

The stigmatisation process incorporates three elements that happens within individuals, groups and society as a way of communicating the negative effects of stigma: problems of ignorance (knowledge), problems with attitudes (prejudice) and problems with behaviour (discrimination) (Thornicroft et al. 2009; see Box 6.2).

Box 6.2 Three elements of the stigmatisation process

1 Knowledge – relates to poor understanding and ignorance about mental health and wellbeing and how it can affect people and potentially themselves.

2 Prejudice – relates to negative, emotive prejudgements and attitudes about mental health.

3 Discrimination – can be defined as the poor or less favourable treatment of people, including a reduction in access to life chances, opportunities and resources, which can arise as a result of stigma. Discrimination may be applied to people with mental health problems on the basis of belief, perceptions and alleged or other attributed characteristics rather than actual ones. It can also be actual discrimination or intended discrimination.

Source: adapted from Thornicroft et al. (2009).

The effects of stigma can have a significant impact on the individual and result in diminished self-esteem, self-value and confidence. This is a cycle that is hard to break. The results can become so enduring that a person with a mental health problem can become secretive and will selectively avoid those people who know about it. This might cause them to reduce their participation in social life, work or education and potentially in all levels of society. In a survey by Time to Change (2008), more that 71 per cent of people with mental health problems said that they stopped doing the things that they wanted to because of mental health stigma.

Mental health stigma and children and young people

Developing beliefs and attitudes

Although we know that beliefs and perceptions surrounding mental health are formed in early childhood and are influenced by peer group, family, the community and the media, there has been little contemporary research to help understanding of children and young people about their own mental health.

Research shows that children as young as those in preschool can start to develop negative attitudes about mental health. Younger children have been shown to be aware of everyday terms about mental health and the language that is used to stigmatise those with mental health problems; much of this is proffered by the adults around them. These negative attitudes have been found to increase with age, although it has been found that at around 9 years old, children show more empathy with those with mental health difficulties (Warner-Gale 2006). However, research into the development of social cognition suggests that the development of mature attributional styles and personality traits is still in progress between the ages of 6 and 12, making the primary school years a key place to start to embed positive attitudes about mental health (Flavell *et al.* 1993).

Many studies on the process of stigmatisation in children have focused on physical disability, race, ethnicity and religious groups. In studies that examined racial attitudes, very young children were found to have developed some negative attitudes, and as they grew older, children were more likely to possess a negative attitude over a positive one (Goodman 1970). Indicators that relate to the negative acquisition of beliefs and the beginning of the process of stigmatisation at an early age suggest that children first display reactions to those who are physically or visually different. In fact, distinct attitudes towards people seen as 'different' can be seen as early as infant school. Some research suggests that children's reactions toward mentally ill people seem to receive the most negative association (Wahl 2002). Although there is no evidence to suggest why this might be, there appears to be an implication that the more negative attitudes toward mentally ill people were learned within the family and established before entry into the school system. Evidence from other research suggests that the process of stigmatisation can begin in preschool years and that children display a preference for those who are similar to themselves, as opposed to those who they identify as being dissimilar. Even infants, when attempting to make sense of their world and their identity, will categorise others as 'like me' or 'not like me', preferring the former to the latter. Theories around the acquisition of beliefs suggest that children acquire understanding about mental health in three ways: through socialisation, by contribution from significant others and through the mass media (Wahl 2003).

In more recent qualitative studies around perceptions of mental health stigma, children were clear about the difference between mental health and physical health problems and were able to articulate this. There was also evidence of empathy and help-seeking knowledge in relation to those with mental health problems. The children's level of understanding enabled them to contribute to discussions about service development and to make suggestions about how needs should be met (Warner-Gale 2008; Warner-Gale/Time to Change 2012). These contemporary findings are significantly different from earlier studies as they indicate an increase in children's positive perceptions about mental health and the potential for them to make valuable contributions about how to tackle issues around stigma.

Amongst young people, stigmatising attitudes are found to be more common during adolescence, and these can lead to negative attitudes, stereotyping and discriminatory behaviours towards people with mental health problems. Stigmatising attitudes can differ according to the type of mental health problem, and stigma can be multidimensional with attitudes varying according to age, gender, peer group and culture. Overall, young people are more likely to show stigmatising attitudes towards people with serious mental illness, thinking that they are dangerous and unpredictable and showing a desire for social distance (Hennessy *et al.* 2008). It is also suggested that when children reach their teenage years, they begin to understand that behaviours expressed externally could be a result of inner distress. This enables them to form more positive opinions about behaviours related to mental illness that they had previously deemed to be irrational (Wahl 2002).

Recognising the effects of stigma on children and young people

> The stigma associated with mental health leaves a person feeling ashamed and 'little' …
> they feel singled out and isolated.
>
> – Young person with mental health problems, aged 17

Although children and young people have been found to have variable degrees of understanding about 'mental health' as a concept, those with poor mental health have described the profound negative experiences that the associated stigma has on them. They are clear about how stigma impacts on them in their everyday lives and on their ability to seek help when it is needed. The effect of internalising stigma can cause them to believe that they are 'spoiled' and of less value than 'normal people'. This can result in feelings of guilt, shame, self-protective denial and reluctance to talk to others about their mental health problems.

Although often mistaken for symptoms of their mental health problem itself, young people have described feelings of being set apart from their peers, excluded and rejected in relation to stigma (Hinshaw 2005; Warner-Gale 2008; Warner-Gale/Time to Change 2012). Based on this, it is the responsibility of every health professional to recognise how stigma can impact on the individual and how they engage with the treatment process. More often than not, professionals can fail to consider how stigma associated with getting help can impact on young people's willingness to seek help. Often the journey that has led them to their first meeting with a mental health professional has been a long and difficult one, tainted by experiences of stigma.

Young people with mental health problems have been found to experience higher levels of stigma than adults, and as a result, through no fault of their own, many children and young people have found themselves denied help and respect, education, employment, social interaction, their families and their homes and other basic rights. Moreover, young people with mental health problems are likely to internalise stigma, leading to low self-esteem and sense of hopelessness. This can often go unnoticed by those around them, and is frequently attributed to their mental health need.

Mental health stigma has been found to be a major concern to young people who have mental health problems, and many studies show that stigmatising attitudes can interfere with getting help, treatment outcomes and quality of life as the feelings associated with it can contribute to feelings of being different, disconnecting with society and an increased dependency on others.

How do children and young people conceptualise mental health and stigma?

Qualitative research was undertaken by the author of this chapter with younger children aged 5–11 and their parents and with young people aged 14–25 around their understanding of mental health and experiences of stigma. These children had all been referred to specialist mental health services for help. Key themes emerged for each age group that can help us to understand what we need to do to effect positive change (Warner-Gale and Sedgewick 2012).

Younger children and their parents

In younger children and their parents, seven key elements around how they experience stigma were identified. These can help us to think about the areas we need to focus on as the professionals supporting a family and in helping to change the way we tackle stigma and shape services.

1   Struggling to understand mental health
     Younger children were able to recognise the term 'mental health' from an early age (5 years old). They described it as feeling happy or playing with friends, and defined it in a 'healthy' context rather than to do with ill health. They explained that they had learned about physical health in school and used this learning to try to understand mental health. As they got older, children increasingly defined mental health in negative terms and applied negative stereotypes. Their parents tended to define mental health as mental illness, seeing the associated terms as representing the more severe end of the mental health continuum. This explains why it can be helpful to bring children and parents together to learn about mental health, thus breaking the negative cycle of attitudes.

2   Experiences of self-stigma
     Both parents and children experienced profound effects of stigma and described an enhanced cycle of powerlessness and low self-worth. This resulted in them being unable to talk to others, including close family members or friends, and feeling unable to ask for help. Children as young as 6 communicated feelings of shame and difference, both directly and indirectly.

     I feel ashamed and I can't talk about it … I have a dark secret.
                                                                    – William, aged 10

3   Impact of public stigma
     Experiences of public stigma contributed to shame and low self-esteem. Parents often became anxious in a bid to protect their children, and the anxiety was communicated and exacerbated between parent and child.

     I'd just like him to be like other children … [the public] step back and walk the other way.
                                                                    – Angela, parent

4   Contributing to (unintentional) stigma
     Paradoxically, both children and their parents showed a desire to change perceptions about mental health stigma, but also contributed towards it inadvertently through use of negative language and attitudes. Therefore, the cycle of stigma continued.

     People who are mental are horrible.
                                                                    – Marc, aged 7

5   The legacy and language of mental illness
     Both children and their parents had some difficulty in talking about concepts of mental health. Language used included stigmatising words and descriptions of violent and disturbed imagery, which seemed entrenched in everyday language.

What you would call 'nutters' [describing a mental health unit]. I know I shouldn't be saying that.

– Vanessa, parent

6   Fear of developing mental illness
     Both parents and children, but especially children, feared they may develop severe mental illness. This was often due to a lack of knowledge. As a result, they had avoided asking for help.

     I am very scared … there is something wrong with me … I think I might be [mentally] ill.

– Robyn, aged 11

7   The negative impact of services
     Both parents and children expressed similar views on the contribution of children's services to the experience of seeking help for mental health problems. Deficit in professionals' knowledge about mental health, poor communication strategies (with families and across organisations) and lack of clarity about referral criteria were cited as issues that contributed to stigmatisation and deterred help-seeking.

Young people

In research with young people, they explained that the stigma associated with mental health was a major concern for them. They felt that it had a huge impact on them and on younger children. These experiences were coupled with descriptions of how stigma impacted on self-worth, how it had mainly come from peers, education staff, healthcare professionals, including nurses, doctors and strangers, and how it made them feel so ashamed that they didn't want to tell others or ask for help. Figure 6.1 outlines how young people describe 'stigma' and what it means to them.

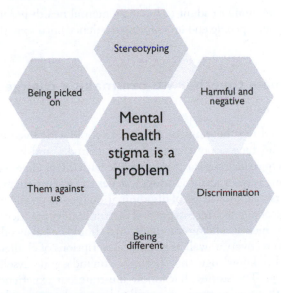

Figure 6.1 Young people's perceptions of stigma
Source: Warner-Gale and Sedgewick (2012).

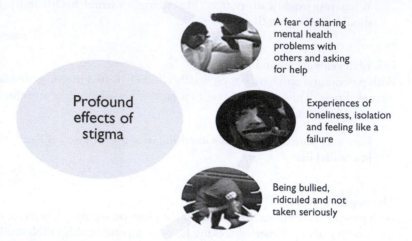

A fear of sharing mental health problems with others and asking for help

Experiences of loneliness, isolation and feeling like a failure

Being bullied, ridiculed and not taken seriously

Profound effects of stigma

Figure 6.2   Profound effects of stigma
Source: Warner-Gale and Sedgewick (2012).

Young people described mental health stigma as having profound effects on them and also on their family (Figure 6.2). They felt discredited, lonely and isolated. Many described scenarios where they were bullied by their peers and often ridiculed and made fun of. They explained that stigma scares young people and they don't seek help as a result. They also felt they would be treated badly by professionals if they did ask for support. Sometimes they felt their problems were not seen as serious and they 'suffered in silence' until a crisis happened. In addition, as a result of stigma, there could be an increase in family stress and worries about mental health; this was often compounded by not knowing how or where to get the help needed.

> Young people are afraid to admit to having a mental health problem through fear and shame. Many young people end up suffering in silence until something drastic happens.
> – Chloe, aged 18

Tackling stigma – together we can make a change

Hearing our stories

It is well documented that hearing the stories of people with lived experience of mental health difficulties can have a positive impact on attitudes and knowledge about mental health and services to reduce stigma. Young people with direct experience of mental health problems are in many ways crucial to the approaches to tackling stigma. As a result of their experiences and personal knowledge of discrimination, young people with lived experience are ideally placed to challenge stereotypes and discriminatory practices (Ministry of Health 2007). However, the messages being communicated should be balanced and include positive messages focused on recovery as well as personal descriptions of challenging experiences.

It is based on this knowledge that Leanne, Amanda and myself want to share our experiences with you. The stories that follow illustrate our experiences of mental health stigma in the hope that we can communicate the damage that stigma has on individuals, on families and on the recovery process. With this understanding, we hope that you can join us in making sure that the approach you choose is based on partnerships with people who have lived experience and on an understanding of the processes at play.

Leanne's story

As a young person with mental health difficulties, it was hard; but it was made even harder by the misconceptions people held of mental health, the lack of knowledge and the stigma surrounding me. This included my peers, friends and family.

I struggled a lot with anxiety and behaviours which came from these feelings. Things like getting buses, talking in front of the class at school and making choices such as deciding to go out to meet friends were all things I really struggled with. People called me names and said all kinds of unhelpful things such as: 'it's only a bus, just get on it'; 'stop being silly'; 'you just need to get over this'; 'just pick one, it's not difficult – I can do it!' Not only did this lead me to feel so misunderstood and different, but it also led me to feel so very alone; and loneliness leads people to very dark places.

When I finally opened up about the problems I had to a school teacher, I was relieved to be sharing my difficulties and the thoughts and feelings I was experiencing at last. However, as my family and friends learnt about these difficulties, my feelings about talking changed. Instead of warmth, care and understanding, I was faced with misconceptions, lack of knowledge and so much stigma. Sometimes I felt others thought I wanted to be the way I was, that struggling with my mental health was something I was choosing to do and, equally, that it was something I could choose not to do. It reached a point where I stopped talking to my friends and family about how I was feeling and my difficulties.

The stigma was too much for me to process and stunned me into literal silence. My family especially didn't understand much about mental health and saw mental health in stigmatising terms. My problems became the unspoken elephant in the room, no one would ask and I wouldn't say anything, although the difficulties I had were clear. It is sad to think because of this stigma, it was easier to keep these things to myself and say nothing at all, hiding my problems and pretending they didn't exist being so much easier due to this fear of what others thought, what they would say or how they would treat me.

It reached a point where I was carefully guarding the fact that I was seeking help for my problems at CAMHS. I felt ashamed, not understood and largely alone in terms of support from family and friends. I went to great lengths to hide the support I was accessing, such as seeing my CAMHS worker during breaks within my school day so no one would question where I had been. Eventually, I chose not to tell anyone at all that I was accessing services. Going through things alone without the support of my family and friends was easier than facing the stigma and discrimination of having mental health difficulties.

Unfortunately, with those closest to me, my mental health problems remained unspoken about despite my obvious difficulties. Things escalated and reached a point where I thought taking my life would be better than feeling that alone with what I was experiencing. The saddest thing about this is that with support, care, understanding and knowledge, the place I reached with how I felt could have been prevented.

I have now learnt, just like physical health, mental health is something we all have; and also like physical health, we struggle with it sometimes in our life – some more than others. There is no shame.

Amanda's story

Not only did I have to face my own illnesses, but also the stigma and being ostracised by my family, my friends and my work colleagues. Personally, being diagnosed with severe depression, anorexia nervosa and adjustment disorder made me quite an introverted person. I didn't want to draw attention to myself or have to deal with any type of confrontation. No one fully understood what mental torment I was experiencing as sometimes my behaviours were so extreme. How can a 15-year-old explain to a family member why they hide food or visit 'pro-ana' websites without experiencing some kind of stigma associated with the misconceptions that are sensationalised in the media? I began to live by the thought process: 'if no one listens to what I'm saying, why should I speak?' This led me to become a mute towards my friends, family and some mental health professionals. I feared the stigma I would face would be so great that I thought it was better not to talk at all.

School was a really big help for me when experiencing mental health problems. I had several tutors in sixth form who would always ask me how things are going or whether I wanted to talk about anything that was worrying me. Without their support and open-door policy I would have never completed my A levels to the high standard I did. Just a small question like 'how has this week been?' made a huge difference towards my self-esteem and my ability to talk through the problems I was experiencing. For them to listen and appreciate how hard it must be to suffer from mental illnesses was all I needed to ensure that I felt supported and not alone in my battle.

As I have grown older and entered the workplace, I fear this can be one of the most stigmatising settings young people could find themselves in. Comments such as 'What have you got to be depressed about?' and 'Why is she off sick just for depression?' can really put shame onto sufferers. If someone were off sick because they had a cancer screening, I doubt people would be commenting on the reasons why they were off sick. Therefore, this highlights the absolute need for parity of esteem in the workplace.

Most importantly, the stigma I have witnessed that has been most surprising was amongst mental health professionals. Thinking of people as numbers or statistics increases the likelihood of 'do not attends'. The use of the words 'severe', 'entrenched' and 'not ill enough' create a negative self-fulfilling prophecy. I have had some shocking things said to me by mental health professionals – things that no one should have said to them. There is a need for awareness around vocabulary and the labelling of sufferers. People who are suffering from an illness are human beings; they are someone's daughter or son and they deserve to be treated with respect.

Fiona's story

When I experienced a severe bout of postnatal depression after the birth of my lovely daughter, I battled with stigma and in admitting that 'mental health' was actually my problem. I also battled with the healthcare professionals who tried to pass it off as something physical. As a mental health professional, I found it extremely difficult to get people to listen to me and to hear that I might be struggling with my own issues. The difficulty in getting healthcare practitioners to recognise that my anguish, my weight loss, my sleeplessness and my inability to cope with the tiniest of challenges, which could be attributed to depression, was a long and drawn-out process. I was in a tricky place.

Although in my case I did ask my healthcare providers directly for help (admittedly after several visits when I plucked up the courage to say 'I have depression'), I was often pushed towards trying to explain my sheer exhaustion and physical decline through physical health investigations. Unlike some mums with postnatal depression, I didn't experience problems with attachment to my child; I became hypervigilant instead, constantly worrying and having severe anxiety about my daughter's wellbeing. I went to the GP practice and to Accident and Emergency on a number of occasions with my daughter, although for genuine reasons (she suffered quite severe reflux for the first year of her life).

Not once did anyone ask me how I was feeling; in fact, one doctor suggested I was neurotic. If I hadn't stumbled upon a GP who was willing to listen, I don't know what my prognosis would have been. Consequently, my postnatal depression lasted around two and a half years, much longer than it needed to. I'm only just able to talk about my experiences (my daughter was 5 when I wrote this); some of this is down to the stigma surrounding mental health – a stigma that I have been trying to fight for the last 12 years to help others. If we are to help others in similar situations, then we need to understand mental health and the stigma that surrounds it, not only in the GP practices or through other healthcare providers but in places that mothers who haven't plucked up the courage to access services might present.

The road to feeling back to 'me' was long, but I'm here, and I'm me. We must fight against the stigma – we all have a right to mental health.

Why bother to tackle stigma?

So as we can see, mental health stigma is fairly commonplace in society, yet stigma processes have a dramatic effect on the distribution of life chances – the need to create flourishing communities where everyone has a positive start in life, where everyone can contribute to tackling stigma and promoting mental health, and where everyone has access to interventions as early as possible has never been so apparent. It has been suggested that developing an understanding of the meanings that mental health and stigma have for children and young people will prompt us to develop creative and sustainable approaches to changing attitudes that last throughout the lifespan. Young people have said that tackling stigma really matters to them. Leanne and Amanda certainly give us some food for thought in their testimonies that follow.

Leanne's testimony for change

The power of our minds means we can ask ourselves 'what if' questions and reflect on what if things were different. My mind asks me: What if the people around me understood mental health and mental health problems? What if I was able to be open about my mental health problems to the people around me? What if I knew I wasn't alone? What if stigma did not exist?

Making a change individually is so important, not just because of my personal experience but because my personal experience is not a one-off example. Making a change, such as seeking understanding of mental health, can make a massive difference to someone who is struggling.

We can do this through approaches such as talking about mental health, not using stigmatising terms and seeking to understand mental health. This will help to give other people the courage they need to speak out about problems they are experiencing, and it will also reduce stigma on a wider level. The more we talk, the more we learn, the more we share, the more 'normal' mental health will become. Making a change and holding this in mind as a goal to work towards is important because it will help people to feel less alone, it will help more people feel able to access the support they need and, ultimately, this will help people lead better, healthier lives, creating a better future for us all – and there is nothing greater than that. To do this, we all have to believe that our voice is important, that we can change things – because if we don't believe this, then who will?

Box 6.3 *Together we can make a change: a poem by Leanne Walker*

Leanne has been involved in many events to raise mental health awareness and tackle stigma in schools. She wrote this poem to get her message across at a mental health conference for Year 9s.

When I was younger, someone said to me
Leanne, you're crazy.
And they meant it,
And it spread,
This word they said, this word they attached to me stuck in my head,
And sometimes when I was in bed,
I really thought who I was, was something that was wrong,
I felt this strongly, it made me feel I didn't belong.
When inside I was already struggling,
This stigma and discrimination, the names and the labels,
Created more misery until I felt like nobody cared and I was unable
To change
And people began to ignore me, wouldn't even look me in the face,
Like they'd catch my problems right there in that place,
They looked at me like I was a disgrace.

And I was sad, and it made me feel sadder.
And I felt mad and it made me feel madder.
And I was alone and it made me feel even more on my own.
But most of all I could feel it deeply, this stigma that hung in the air,
This perception that ill mental health meant I was crazy,
And it made me feel so sad, that my world became hazy.

This isn't just the reason we should make a change because
Of this stigma that I felt on an individual level.
Because the fact is, this is felt more widely by so many others,
Such as people's sisters, their brothers, or mothers.
But let me tell you about the facts that exist.
For ill mental health has no set list,
Mental health problems have no race, no gender, religion or culture,
There is no set example shaped like a sculpture.
Their boundaries are blurry like looking under water, they are not restricted,
So why are these Individuals being treated like they are convicted?
What I'm trying to say is, ill mental health cannot be clearly predicted.

The statistics show that mental health problems affect one in four,
But I want to question that and state, mental health affects us all.
Even if not directly,
So let's support mental health correctly,
Tackling stigma isn't the problem of individuals but all of us together.

And this is why it's important for us all to make a change,
Change our own ways,
Stand up and make that change today.
And I'm reaching out to all of you here,
Whose voices can sing out,
Together, they can sing so clear.
And together who can unite on dispelling this stigma,
Getting rid of this enigma.
Together we can learn to understand mental health,
Develop this wealth
In knowledge
And generate this shift in our culture,
Let's together unite
To break this fear and this dread,
Turn it into a united front instead

I hope these words have given you a small amount of contemplation,
And I hope together
We can work on ending this discrimination.
I hope together we can create a movement of supporting wellbeing which spreads across the
whole population.

Create an atmosphere of inclusion and help stop this spreading confusion.
And I hope you will stand with me and pledge to make a change,
I hope you will stand with me and help to change our ways.

Amanda's testimony for change

One of the most unhelpful phrases anyone in the healthcare provision could say is 'we've always done it this way'. Change is a necessity for progression; keeping the same attitudes and stigma towards mental health means we will never end stigma and discrimination for sufferers of mental illness. Changing attitudes will alleviate the shame and secrecy surrounding talking about mental illnesses. Many people fear they will not be believed or will become an outcast to society if they talk about their mental illness. If attitudes changed, we could see parity of esteem and fewer young people presenting mental health crisis, and we could ensure sufferers get the respect and care they deserve when accessing treatment.

How to make a change – what works for children and young people in tackling stigma?

Several approaches for challenging public views and behaviours towards people with mental health problems have emerged, and these broadly reflect the issues discussed in this chapter. They do not need to be implemented in isolation, and often a combination of approaches can have the greatest reach. Three examples follow of different models of stigma.

- The biomedical model – this tends to promote the view that mental ill health is an illness like any other. When implementing a biomedical model, stigma and discrimination can be reduced because people understand that there are underlying physiological causes behind mental health problems, as there are with physical illnesses, and that the individual is not to blame.

- The social model – this locates stigma not only in the individual but also in the social setting. Stigma is seen as a social process that results in the labelling of certain individuals. When implementing a social model, stigma and discrimination can be reduced because the distance between 'them' and 'us', people with mental health problems and those without, is reduced. Such approaches would include hearing the stories of people with lived experiences first-hand, which can significantly improve issues to do with social distance.

- The systems model – the systems model locates the stigma processes in the social, health and care, education, justice, community and political systems that surround us, with the power to make changes in attitudes being out of reach for the individual. Using a systems change approach, which places citizenship and participation at the highest level in the centre of the process, enables empowerment of individuals from within the system while working to change attitudes and behaviour across all elements and levels of the system (Warner-Gale 2006, 2008; Warner-Gale/National CAMHS Support Service n.d.).

When considering what approach to take, there are some key elements that need careful thought. Evaluation of a range of anti-stigma approaches has found that some anti-stigma programmes do more harm than good by confirming negative stereotypes and negative messages about very severe presentations of mental health, especially where people with lived experience are part of the approach. Therefore it is really important to ensure that any personal stories that are told are balanced and give positive messages, especially about hope and recovery.

Furthermore, the person telling their story needs to feel comfortable to answer questions and be supported through training in facing an audience, speaking and presenting and answering difficult questions. Having pre-briefs and debriefs are very useful in ensuring that people with lived experience feel supported and empowered and that they have a true partnership with all involved in delivering the key messages of the programme. Ideally, they should be matched to the age group they are talking to, although this is not entirely necessary; they should, however, be able to relate to the key issues and concerns of their audience.

The most effective programmes are also not one-off interventions. Although short-term campaigns can raise awareness, it is really important to mainstream approaches, so that positive change can be sustained and embedded across all elements of society and at a cultural level. When considering approaches that work with school-age children and young people, whole school approaches are seen to be most effective and should include booster sessions and student-led activities that involve partnerships with staff, families and the community.

Before embarking on the development of an anti-stigma programme, there are a few fundamental aspects to consider – getting these right will ensure that strong foundations are built that provide a locus for positive attitudes going forward.

Building social capital and empowering children and young people

As a result of experiencing stigma, it is likely that young people's social capital will be affected. Young people's social capital has been associated with a certain level of quality in their social networks, youth bonding, engagement in leisure time and trust in others

(Odegard and Berglund 2008). However, there are a number of definitions of social capital in respect of children and young people; in order to show how mental health stigma can impact on them, the key elements that are important to consider for young people are brought together (Green *et al.* 2005). On this basis, we see good social capital relies on:

- Social support and social networks and their quality – this includes supports from family and other peers or adults outside of the family from whom young people may benefit (e.g. leaders, role models and mentors).
- Active participation in social and community life and the extent and quality of engagement within these domains – this may include participation in the school extracurricular community or youth groups, for example.
- Resourcefulness – this refers to the ability to engage with the community in order to access opportunities and solve problems (how the young person links in with others to gain access to social activities, learning opportunities, employment, practical help, etc.).
- Reciprocity – this is the level to which young people identify the need to give help to others and to receive help themselves.
- Trust – this is the level of trust and confidence young people have in others, those they know and those they don't know, as well as trust in institutions such as the police, health services, education, etc.

Anti-stigma approaches should be designed with these elements in mind so that the programme can have a dual benefit, changing negative attitudes and enhancing social capital at the same time. Involving young people is important as they can understand how to enhance their own mental wellbeing whilst learning to be responsible for the mental health of others – giving the key message that everyone has mental health.

Changing the way we think and talk about mental health

Moving from a continuum-based model to a 'wellness-based model' can serve to ensure that children and young people with a diagnosed mental health disorder or mental illness are never excluded from their ability to achieve optimum wellbeing. Being able to view mental health as a 'wellness continuum' means that we must add an extra axis, which takes into account the wellbeing of the individual according to their own abilities and whether or not they are subject to distress. For example, a young person could have a diagnosed mental health disorder or illness, yet be achieving good mental health – i.e. accessing help, enjoying a good quality of life and being free from distress (Jorm *et al.* 1997). This approach gives children and young people hope and shows that there can be positive outcomes for recovery and wellness.

Thus, the mental health wellness continuum can be viewed as a four quadrant model wherein a young person can move from one quadrant to another depending on their current life situation and state of wellbeing. It enables the development of positive knowledge, attitudes and behaviour about mental illness and in relation to recovery for those who may have a diagnosis; it also supports mental health promotion, positive mental health behaviours, identification of mental health problems and help-seeking for mental health problems. It therefore reaches across all children and young people to include everyone, both with and without mental health problems (see Figure 6.3).

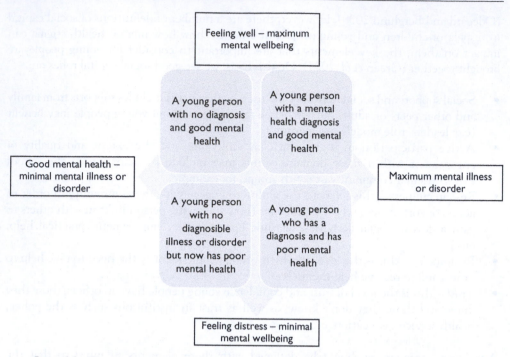

Figure 6.3   The 'wellness continuum' of mental health in children and young people

Involving children and young people at the centre of ways to tackle stigma

Amanda's thoughts on why involving young people is paramount

It is vital to involve young people in tackling stigma, especially as one in ten young people will experience a mental health problem. It would be irresponsible to exclude the next generation from opportunities to promote change and to create a more positive understanding towards mental health. We should be encouraging young people to support their peers if they are worried about their mental health and to really normalise talking about how they are feeling. I have participated in various mental health awareness programmes, which has really boosted my confidence as I can now speak in front of over a hundred people both nationally and internationally. Young people are very passionate and it only takes a spark to ignite a fire of passion within a young person. This is what I experienced, all I needed was the opportunity to be given a voice and an opportunity to change my negative experiences into positive ones. This could be so true for many young people who haven't been given the opportunity yet.

Leanne's perspective

Involving young people is important so they can learn that we all have mental health. When I was at school and first started having problems with anxiety, I didn't even know the word anxiety existed. I didn't know about mental health or symptoms of poor mental health, and consequently I didn't know how to help myself.

Involving young people in programmes to reduce stigma will help them to understand and recognise problems they may have early on, and it will help them to support their peers and to be compassionate and understanding to the people around them experiencing poor mental health.

In effect, this will not only create a more accepting society but it will also support and encourage people to seek help when they need it and to not be afraid or hide their problems right from the start. It's important to create an empowering atmosphere where talking about mental health is as natural as speaking about physical health. This can be achieved by taking small active steps in researching understanding of mental health, talking more about mental health and being more open about your own mental health.

Taking a systems approach for whole systems change

Developing meaningful and effective interventions nearer to home in partnership with children and young people will ensure that they feel listened to and connected. Whole systems change approaches coupled with education and training programmes for nurses and other professionals as well as parents and children and young people can have good long-term effects on childhood mental health problems and on reducing the effect of stigma (Warner-Gale/Time to Change 2012). Working in partnership with children, young people, families, schools and communities can create a vision of wellbeing, improve wider sustainability and help to provide services that are inclusive and reduce stigma (Pinfold *et al.* 2003; Right Here 2010). Engaging the public and professionals who work with children and young people at all levels in a collaborative approach that develops a strong partnership with children and their families will ensure that we are able to tackle stigma across a number of domains and across generations to guarantee sustainable change.

Developing anti-stigma programmes that incorporate all of these elements has been found to be effective in achieving change not only in individuals but at a systems and organisational level, therefore creating bottom-up and top-down approaches. It has been suggested that systems around us can contribute to our beliefs and attributions about mental health and that stigma change is most effective when it includes all the power groups and stakeholders and looks at the social and systems contexts within which people live (Corrigan and Gelb 2006).

The Tackling Stigma Framework was developed by Warner-Gale to be implemented as part of wider children and young people's mental health services improvement strategy in England, addressing mental health stigma and building on early support and targeted intervention work (Warner-Gale/National CAMHS Support Service 2010). The framework is based on the research undertaken with children and their families described earlier, examining their experiences of the stigma associated with mental health (see 'How do children and young people conceptualise mental health and stigma?'). It is a whole systems change initiative that aims to help children, young people, their families and professionals to work together to think about tackling stigma and improving mental health awareness. It also helps children's organisations to assess where the key places are to reduce stigma and to involve the right people in order to have the greatest impact.

The Tackling Stigma Framework has eight domains that, when applied simultaneously, should minimise the stigma linked to children and young people's mental health (see Figure 6.4). The domains can be applied in a range of settings and at a number of levels. An evaluation of the framework found that two domains are pivotal to the success of the rest of the approach: 'citizenship and participation' – ensuring that children and young people are at the centre of the programme to tackle stigma; and 'mainstreaming' – embedding the framework and associated activities in the ethos of organisations that work with children (Barham and Smith 2010).

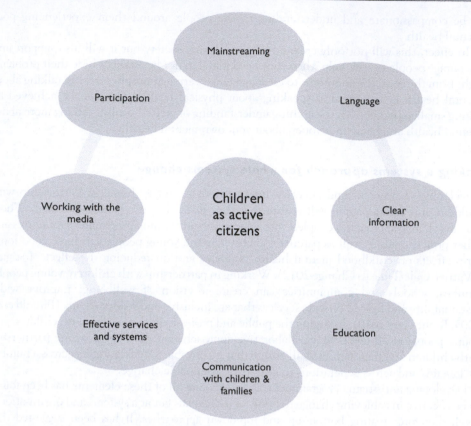

Figure 6.4   The Tackling Stigma Framework
Source: Warner-Gale (2006).

1   Participation
Involving children and parents/carers as citizens, partners and decision-makers requires a coordinated and practical approach at a local level. It requires professionals at all levels to identify opportunities for participation. In order to develop a participatory approach, professionals need to understand techniques to promote it and ensure that these are embedded within their service ethos.

The benefits of participation are that it gives children and young people a voice and influences significant changes for them and in the wider community. As a result, their services will be less stigmatising, more effective and better targeted and received. The involvement of children and young people is also key to sustaining developments and positive attitudes about mental health through the life course.

2   Mainstreaming
The mainstreaming and integration of tackling stigma programmes, stigma awareness and education about children's mental health is the business of all commissioners and service providers across the spectrum of services, and this works most effectively when it is integral to each individual professional's value base.

Mainstreaming approaches to tackling stigma involves embedding the framework and associated actions as a philosophy that underpins all structures and related actions, ensuring that they are continually considered in planning and developments. At a service level, mainstreaming action to tackle stigma is about a multifaceted process of ensuring that children and their families are key partners in the tackling stigma process.

Obtaining the commitment of key professionals, including the nursing workforce, and changing policies, procedures, strategies and action plans so that they are consistent with the Tackling Stigma Framework is also very important. Similarly, at strategic or multi-agency partnership level, it is also about the active involvement of children, young people and families as well as embedding activity to tackle stigma within strategic documents and getting formal support from relevant local strategic partnerships and commissioners at the highest level.

3   Agree a definition and work towards a common language of mental health
Collaboratively, all services should develop and work with an agreed definition of mental health and related terminology. It is often the confusion about the language used in talking about mental health that alienates children and their families and makes them wary of accessing services.

Developing age-appropriate explanations of mental health and mental health problems will go a long way to encouraging people to talk about mental health freely and will, as a consequence, assist in the development of non-stigmatising services. Children and families' involvement in developing a shared understanding of mental health terminology will provide a sound base from which to launch programmes to promote mental health awareness and challenge stigma. It will also ensure that children and their families are engaged in the journey to tackle stigma from the very start.

It is not challenging to find definitions of mental health as there are a number of good examples that can be used. The challenge lies in agreeing the terminology to be used across an area, especially around the words and terms used to talk about emotional wellbeing, mental health and mental health services.

The best way to do this is to work with young people and their families, professionals and stakeholders. Everybody should sign up to the agreed definitions and they should be publicised and used consistently across all partners.

4   Developing information for children and families
Children and young people have highlighted their concerns about seeking help and attending mental health services. Many were uncertain about what might happen when they attended their first appointment and they have explained that they were not sure where to go or which was the right service for their mental health needs. These issues contribute to the mystique and fear which surrounds mental health and the adverse effects of stigma.

Useful interventions to combat these concerns include the development and dissemination of age-appropriate and user-friendly information about children's mental health and mental health services, developed in partnership with children and families. Methods for successfully developing information to tackle stigma include producing leaflets, pamphlets and websites about services and having good-quality information about mental health problems that is accessible in a number of mediums to both children and their families.

5   Educating children, families and professionals

As the reform of children's services has indicated the need for the early recognition of child mental health problems and for increased capacity and knowledge about children's mental health across services, it is necessary to develop robust local education programmes. Such education programmes should be delivered in multiple contexts, across agencies and levels of provision, and they must include a curriculum on children's mental health and stigma. In addition, the inclusion of knowledge about child mental health and the stigmatisation process could be included in training courses, at a pre-registration and postgraduate level, for nurses and other professionals that work with children.

Local services would also need to consider how children and their families can best contribute to education programmes and how they might benefit from them. Such involvement would be beneficial in empowering children to promote their own mental health, to recognise their mental health needs and to challenge the negative impact of stigma. This approach could be specifically targeted within schools so that learning about mental health becomes part of the curriculum.

6   Communicating with children and families

Poor communication with children and their families/carers and between agencies can result in loss of faith in the systems and leave children and families feeling unsupported. Children often perceive that they are not listened to and have indicated that they wish to be part of the decision-making process about their problems. Such concerns would suggest that services need to consider their relationship with users. Inclusive models of working should be developed to ensure that children and parents/carers are active partners in determining the care process and in measuring and understanding their own outcomes and progress.

Ways of achieving this include putting children and families at the centre of their treatment and care process. Keeping them well informed about treatment options and choices as well as dates and times of appointments will enable them to have a very active part in their care. This can be done through their involvement in the care planning process or by agreeing goals and outcomes so they can have a role in and responsibility for their own care.

7   Developing effective organisation systems and accessible services

Policy recommendations for more accessible, responsive, timely and comprehensive mental health provision point to the requirement for revision of some local organisational structures. Lack of clarity in referral routes and criteria for services for children across levels of provision, uncertainty about their remit, lack of knowledge about community and specialist or targeted services, and ambiguity about joint agency working can contribute to experiences of self-stigma, shame and powerlessness.

The priority here is having clearly defined and well-communicated care pathways and referral criteria that children, families and professionals can understand and act upon. This is not just about making it easy to access services but also about making the process of moving through and then out of services effortless and seamless.

The provision of timely services is key so that children and families do not feel marginalised by having to wait. Effective service provision is also about having flexible services for young people that are integrated into school provision or in 'one-stop shops' where accessing emotional wellbeing and mental health services are normalised.

8   Partnerships with the local media – engaging them as allies
Involving the communications departments of the local organisations right from the start of the programme or campaign is a good idea. In this way, the positive stories of tackling stigma strategies and actions can be reported in the local press, providing accurate information about mental health issues and raising awareness of the devastating effects of stigma.

Ultimately, the aim is for journalists to develop awareness of the harm that negative stereotypes can provide. Training young journalists would also be a key goal, but working with journalists and improving their awareness of mental health problems is also likely to have an impact on their practices.

There may be other ways of targeting media organisations locally, such as speaking to radio stations who may be willing to do interviews or play recordings about mental health issues. Also, some cinemas have been able to help by playing excerpts from videos during pre-film advertising.

Practical approaches to tackling stigma for nurses and other professionals

Leanne shares a message with us about how to tackle stigma:

It's up to us, the people that make up society, to share our experiences. By doing this, we let other people see that they are not alone. The more we talk, the more we share, the more people will see that it is ok to do this and the more 'normal' mental health with become. It's like a Mexican wave – it cannot be done on its own, but it takes one person to start it.

In a consultation with young people in an online survey and consultation groups, several key themes were revealed by young people as important in terms of how they would like to be involved in tackling stigma (Warner-Gale and Sedgewick 2012). These included young people leading approaches to challenge and reduce stigma, using peer mentoring and peer networking. They also talked about standing up for mental health by creating champions amongst young people. As well as developing their leadership skills and ensuring activities are fun, this would also give young people something back that helps to build their futures (e.g. certificates and award schemes or testimonials for their portfolio). Young people also talked about the importance of starting conversations. They pointed out that challenging and reducing stigma is not just about education and awareness but learning how to support friends and peers. One young person said:

No sitting and listening 'cos we don't take it in – action stuff is better. It needs to be fun and engaging activities.

Figure 6.5 illustrates how young people want to tackle stigma.

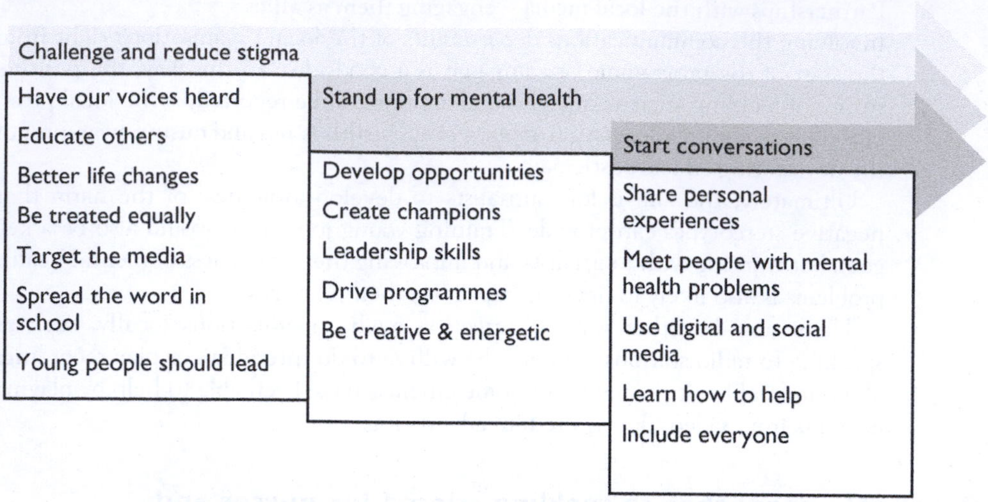

Challenge and reduce stigma

Have our voices heard	Stand up for mental health	
Educate others		
Better life changes		Start conversations
Be treated equally	Develop opportunities	Share personal experiences
Target the media	Create champions	Meet people with mental health problems
Spread the word in school	Leadership skills	Use digital and social media
Young people should lead	Drive programmes	Learn how to help
	Be creative & energetic	Include everyone

Figure 6.5   Challenging and reducing stigma, standing up for mental health and starting conversations
Source: Warner-Gale (2013).

Amanda and Leanne have identified some helpful practical approaches to help tackle stigma that they have been involved in:

1   Small steps
    Creating posters, badges, postcards, key chains or leaflets with information such as top tips of what helps when feeling down, supportive quotes, symptoms of mental health problems, where to get support or statistics. This will get people thinking about mental health, open up conversations and put mental health on the agenda.

2   Education in schools, colleges and universities
    Education about stigma in schools, colleges and universities can be very wide-reaching but it can be very uncomfortable to sit through a lesson plan on different mental illnesses. The best way to engage young people is to be interactive. Mental health awareness is very important but it doesn't have to be boring. Posters about the myths and facts of mental illnesses can be placed in corridors and in classrooms to promote positive attitudes. Getting involved in mental health awareness week or identifying a school mental health awareness day/week is also a great opportunity to put mental health as a top priority.

3   Making films
    Creating videos of young people's personal accounts can really break down the barriers of stigma – they are hard-hitting and will be memorable. Stop-motion animation is an alternative solution to personal accounts, and it can also be used as a tool to decide 'what to do next' in different mental health-related scenarios.
    A useful example could be to have a discussion on how young people would like to be treated if they were struggling with their mental health or that of a close friend or family member. Talk about what they would like people to say or how they'd like people to treat them. This naturally draws out what isn't so helpful. Filming this voice can be powerful to look back on and to share with others.

4   Young people-led mental health conferences
Having recently attended one of these events within a school, we can tell you what an active approach this is. Ten people from each of ten local schools attended, and the day was filled with information about mental health, including addressing stigma. The idea was that the messages from the day will spread out across all ten schools and they will develop their own plans to tackle mental health stigma. From an early age, this educates young people in knowing that everyone has mental health, encouraging a more supportive environment.

5   Empowering young people and sharing personal experiences
We believe this to be one of the most powerful shapers and influences in creating action. Be it talking in schools, universities or with smaller groups, sharing real-life experiences (although not always easy) not only opens up conversation but also allows others to feel your emotions. I have found this encourages others to take a more active approach such as talking about their own experiences, talking to friends and family, being careful about words they use when talking about mental health, or simply posting supportive messages about mental health on social media.

6   Getting out into the community
Getting out into the community is a great way of spreading the work about mental health. A new approach is 'pop-up villages' – mini tented villages where you can have conversations about mental health. One that we got involved with was an arts and crafts village that had activities like: sewing patchwork onto a quilt, creating badges, a movie theatre with popcorn dispenser showing mental health films, a news stand with different promotion materials and freebies, a five-minute drama piece where everyone stopped and passers-by were asked to interact with the performance and also a pledge wall.

Other anti-stigma key strategies and approaches can include:

- Face-to-face approaches led by young people
  Examples include:
  o   teaching sessions and approaches to learning about mental health and stigma in personal, social, health and economic (PSHE) education within the school curriculum;
  o   live drama in the school setting, including role play and theatre group productions – one approach is to use Forum Theatre as a medium for engaging the audience, where they can become involved in deciding a range of outcomes;
  o   social contact and conversations with young people with mental health problems;
  o   groups of young people aiming to change behaviours through activities and campaigning using peer-to-peer approaches – these can be via social media or in person;
  o   public events, such as organised events that focus on mental health in the community, or attendance at major events to raise awareness about mental health in young people.
- Multimedia campaigns
  It can be challenging to captivate the attention of young people by using leaflets and booklets as they may be bombarded by similar materials on a daily basis. As traditional reading material has started to be replaced by ever more intensive

engagement with media (e.g. TV, Internet, social media), campaigns too need to follow this trend.

Social media approaches are said to play a key role in helping anti-stigma campaigns reach out to target audiences. There are Internet sites, Facebook and Twitter groups and blogs dedicated to young people's mental health. There is huge potential for the use of social media to change knowledge and attitudes as it has the ability to stimulate the involvement of young people in local issues and, therefore, to make the messages more meaningful to them. Convenience, speed and cost are all important factors influencing this. If successful, the potential for the use of social media in increasing capacity to engage young people and enabling them to have their say is endless. A variety of approaches can be adopted to convey messages, using a range of media. These might include:

○ distribution of dedicated DVDs through schools, youth organisations and mental health trusts;

○ dedicated newspapers such as a mental health and wellbeing magazine for young people that can be accessed online;

○ films and multimedia presentations about mental health problems on Internet channels, such as YouTube, or blogs and posts on social media.

• Social marketing programmes

Social marketing approaches have generally been successful in challenging stigma where they combine more than one method of engaging with their target audience. The programmes that focus solely on advertising space (posters and logos) have reported less success. One effective multi-method social marketing programme put young people in the driving seat and created a rich mix of multimedia resources that included:

○ a short film about how stigma can affect young people and how mental health problems can make them feel;

○ a website that contained a wealth of information and support for young people on mental health issues and stigma;

○ a leaflet about mental health and stigma for young people to be distributed through schools and youth organisations;

○ a theatre production about mental health and stigma;

○ a PSHE education pack to be delivered in schools to 14- to 18-year-olds that included four sessions to teach young people about mental health and challenged them to take responsibility for tackling stigma and discrimination – it had young people with lived experience as part of the delivery team;

○ numerous radio interviews and presentations at events and conferences.

Youth groups who don't specifically have a focus on mental health, such as the Girl Guides, have also been key to getting the message about young people's mental health to a wider audience.

The involvement of the public is generally seen as a positive mechanism in anti-stigma programmes, but it has been found to be counterproductive when the messages were general in nature and aimed at the public without any particular focus. Key messages of anti-stigma campaigns can be understood differently by different age groups and genders and by different communities and cultures so there is also a need to develop a focused message. It must be emphasised that there is a need for piloting messages before they appear in advertising materials.

Working with key stakeholders and partners

There are generally three operating levels for this particular strategy. The key stakeholder levels are the individual, a group of people who form a 'community' (people who work together, who live in the same neighbourhood or who go to the same school or youth organisation) and the general public. On all three levels, successful programmes will draw on the principles of social marketing and campaigning in general to effectively identify audience characteristics and develop appropriate methods to reach them.

The need to clearly set out the target audiences for anti-stigma programmes has been emphasised in many papers and studies. The target audiences will be the key stakeholder groups who can benefit from the message. When taking this approach there are a set of key 'rules' to follow:

- All participants need to have equal status.
- There needs to be an opportunity to get to know each other.
- Information to challenge negative stereotypes ought to be available.
- There is active cooperation between participants.
- Participants share a mutual goal.

Young people's top tips for tackling stigma

Whatever approach is chosen, children and young people suggest some top tips for ensuring a successful programme to tackle stigma in Box 6.4.

Box 6.4 *Young people's top tips for tackling stigma*

- Be inclusive – include all young people, including those who are disabled and those from other potentially excluded or vulnerable groups.

- Use a multi-method approach.

- Be creative – use arts, crafts, drama, role play, photography, video work. Creative approaches offer the opportunity to express ideas visually as well as verbally or in written form.

- Support young people to think beyond their lived experiences – ensure young people are supported to stretch their imaginations beyond their existing knowledge.

- Invest time and commitment – meaningful involvement cannot be a 'tick box' exercise, rushed or in addition to existing work. Genuine involvement takes time and commitment.

- Form partnerships and work with others – make sure everyone is involved and working together, and make links with the key professionals who have the expertise that you need.

- Use the resources and networks out there – ask for advice and support when needed. Make contact with those who have already tried it out.

Summary

Young people have shared their experiences, thoughts and ideas about stigma and how to change for the better the way that people view mental health. They feel that stigma should be tackled early on and across generations and organisations. They can see that the key places to talk about mental health are in schools and colleges and that messages can be communicated through digital methods including social media and by hearing real stories about mental health and recovery.

Children, young people and their families want to be at the centre of approaches to tackling stigma and they want to learn new skills and gain confidence in talking about mental health. They want programmes to tackle stigma to be innovative and creative. Above all, they want to target those who wouldn't ordinarily show an interest in mental health and for them to see that it is something that matters to them. They say it is the responsibility of us all to make a change.

References

Barham, J. and Smith, N. (2010) *Tackling Stigma Framework Pilot: Evaluation Update Report. A Report to the National CAMHS Support Service*. Birmingham: ECORYS. Available at: www.chimat.org.uk/default.aspx?RID=97132 (accessed 21 July 2016).

Ben-Zeev, D., Young, M. and Corrigan, P. (2010) DSM-V and the stigma of mental health. *Journal of Mental Health*, 19(4): 318–27.

Brindle, D. (2013) Mental health campaign fails to shift health professionals' attitudes. *The Guardian*, 3 April. Available at: www.theguardian.com/healthcare-network/2013/apr/03/mental-health-anti-stigma-campaign (accessed 21 July 2016).

Corrigan, P. (2000) Mental health stigma as social attribution: implications for research methods and attitude change. *American Psychological Association*, 7(1): 48–67.

Corrigan, P. and Gelb, B. (2006) Three programs that use mass approaches to challenge the stigma of mental illness. *Psychiatric Services*, 57(3): 393–8.

Cumming, E. and Cumming, J. (1957) *Closed Ranks: An Experiment in Mental Health Education*. Cambridge, MA: Harvard University Press.

Flavell, J., Miller, P. and Miller, S. (1993) *Cognitive Development* (third edition). Englewood, NJ: Prentice Hall.

Goffman, E. (1963) *Stigma: Notes on the Management of a Spoiled Identity*. Middlesex: Pelican Publishing.

Goodman, M. (1970) *Race Awareness in Young Children*. New York: Collier Books.

Green, H., McGinnity, Á., Meltzer, H., Ford, T. and Goodman, R. (2005) *Mental Health of Children and Young People in Great Britain, 2004*. London: Office for National Statistics.

Hennessy, E., Swords, L. and Heary, C. (2008) Children's understanding of psychological problems displayed by their peers: a review of literature. *Child Health Development*, 34(1): 4–9.

Hinshaw, S. (2005) The stigmatization of mental illness in children and parents. *Journal of Child Psychology and Psychiatry*, 46(7): 714–34.

Indiana University Bloomington (n.d.) Stigma in a Global Context – Mental Health Study [online]. Available at: www.indiana.edu/~sgcmhs/index.html (accessed 16 May 2016).

Jorm, A., Korten, A., Jacomb, P., Christensen, H., Rodgers, B. and Pollitt, P. (1997) Mental health literacy: a survey of the public's ability to recognise mental disorders and their beliefs about the effectiveness of treatment. *Medical Journal of Australia*, 166(4): 182–6.

Kessler, R., Angermeyer, M., Anthony, J. C., De Graaf, R., Demyttenaere, K., Gasquet, I., De Girolamo, G., Gluzman, S., Gureje, O., Haro, J. M., Kawakami, N., Karam, A., Levinson, D., Medina Mora, M. E., Oakley Browne, M. A., Posada-Villa, J., Stein, D. J., Adley Tsang, C. H., Aguilar-Gaxiola, S., Alonso, J., Lee, S., Heeringa, S., Pennell, B. E., Berglund, P., Gruber, M. J., Petukhova, M., Chatterji, S. and Üstün, T. B. (2007) Lifetime prevalence and age-of-onset distributions of mental disorders in the WHO World Mental Health Survey Initiative. *World Psychiatry*, 6(3): 168–76.

Kurzban, R. and Leary, M. R. (2001) Evolutionary origins of stigmatization: the functions of social exclusion. *Psychological Bulletin*, 127(2): 187–208.

Lyons, M. and Ziviani, J. (1995) Stereotypes, stigma and mental illness: learning from fieldwork experiences. *American Journal of Occupational Therapy*, 49(10): 1002–8.

Ministry of Health (2007) *Like Minds, Like Mine. National Plan 2007–2013.* New Zealand: Ministry of Health.

Murphy, M. and Fonagy, P. (2013) Mental health problems in children and young people. Chapter 10 in *Chief Medical Officer's Annual Report 2012: Our Children Deserve Better: Prevention Pays.* London: Department of Health.

New Philanthropy Capital (2008) *Heads Up: Mental Health of Children and Young People. A Guide for Donors and Charities.* London: New Philanthropy Capital.

NHS Benchmarking Network (2013) *CAMHS Benchmarking Report.* London: NHS Benchmarking Network. Available at: www.rcpsych.ac.uk/pdf/CAMHS%20Report%20Dec%202013%20v1(1).pdf (accessed 21 July 2016).

Odegard, G. and Berglund, F. (2008) Opposition and integration in Norwegian youth networks: the significance of social and political resources 1992–2002. *Acta Soociologica*, 51(4): 275–91.

Pescosolido, B., Perry, B., Martin, J., McLeod, J. and Jensen, P. (2007) Stigmatising attitudes and beliefs about treatment and psychiatric medications for children with mental illness. *Psychiatric Services*, 58(5): 613–18.

Pinfold, V., Toulmin, H., Thornicroft, G., Huxley, P., Farmer, P. and Graham, T. (2003) Reducing psychiatric stigma and discrimination: evaluation of educational interventions in UK secondary schools. *British Journal of Psychiatry*, 182(4): 342–6.

Reavley, N., Mackinnon, A., Morgan, A. and Jorm, A. (2014) Stigmatising attitudes towards people with mental disorders: a comparison of Australian health professionals with the general community. *Australian and New Zealand Journal of Psychiatry*, 48(95): 433–41.

Right Here (2010) *Not So Trivial a Pursuit.* Sheffield: Right Here.

Rose, D., Thornicroft, G., Pinfold, V. and Kassam, A. (2007) 250 labels to stigmatise people with mental illness. *BMC Health Services Research*, 7: 97.

Thornicroft, G., Rose, D., Law, A., Evans-Lacko, S., Leese, M., Lewis-Holmes, E., Little, K., McCrone, P., Rhydderch, D., Flach, C., Henderson, C., London, J., Corker, E. and Genziani, M. (2009) *Moving People Evaluation Protocols: Evaluation of the National Anti-Stigma Programme in England 2008–2011.* Institute of Psychiatry [unpublished report].

Time to Change (2014a) *National Attitudes Report 2013.* London: Time to Change.

Time to Change (2014b) *Making a Drama out of a Crisis.* London: Time to Change. Available at: www.time-to-change.org.uk/sites/default/files/Making_a_drama_out_of_a_crisis.pdf (accessed 21 July 2016).

Time to Change (2012) *Children and Young People's Programme Development: Summary of Research and Insights.* London: Time to Change. Available at: www.time-to-change.org.uk/sites/default/files/TTC%20CYP%20Report%20FINAL.pdf (accessed 21 July 2016).

Time to Change (2008) *Stigma Shout: Service User and Carer Experiences of Stigma and Discrimination.* London: Time to Change.

Wahl, O. (2003) Depictions of mental illnesses in children's media. *Journal of Mental Health*, 12(3): 249–58.

Wahl, O. (2002) Children's views of mental illness: a review of the literature. *Psychiatric Rehabilitation Skills*, 6(2): 134–58.

Warner-Gale, F. (2013) *Qualitative Evaluation of the Time to Change in Schools Competition: Birmingham and the West Midlands Pilot.* Time to Change [unpublished report].

Warner-Gale, F. (2008) Tacking the stigma of mental health in vulnerable children and young people. In P. Vostanis (ed.) *Mental Health Interventions and Services for Vulnerable Children.* London: Jessica Kingsley Publishers, pp. 58–81.

Warner-Gale, F. (2006) *Children and Parents'/Carers' Perceptions of Mental Health and Stigma.* PhD thesis, University of Leicester.

Warner-Gale, F. and Sedgewick, J. (2012) Parlez! Key messages from children, young people and parents about mental health, stigma and help-seeking. Poster presentation at the *International Stigma Conference*, Ottowa, Canada, 4–6 June 2012.

Warner-Gale, F./Time to Change (2012) *Learning from Approaches to Tackle Stigma.* Time to Change [unpublished report].

Warner-Gale, F./National CAMHS Support Service (2010) Tackling Stigma Toolkit [online]. Available at: www.chimat.org.uk/tacklingstigma (accessed 21 July 2016).

World Health Organization (2013) *Mental Health Action Plan 2013–2020.* Geneva: World Health Organization.

Chapter 7

Education, training and workforce development for CAMHS nurses

Rachel Hadland and Fred Ehresmann

Key points:

- It could be argued that the child and adolescent mental health service (CAMHS) nursing identity is stronger within specialist inpatient settings where the traditional nurse's caring role and its associated activities are more clearly defined, delineated and observed. Within community CAMHS teams where the therapeutic task and associated interventions are organised differently, it can sometimes be more challenging for nurses to articulate clearly what skills, knowledge, qualities and values they contribute to the multidisciplinary team.

- It is vital that education, training and workforce development is shaped by the needs of children, young people and families rather than just those responsible for delivering them. An attempt to design and deliver education and training that does not take account of the voices of young people and families is unlikely to meet their needs and creates practitioners who consider themselves 'experts' and are less able to work in a meaningful and collaborative way with families.

- A great deal of work has been done in recent years to try to address the emotional wellbeing and mental health needs of children and young people, and there has been a particular focus on prevention and early intervention. Subsequently, it has been important not to separate completely the workforce development issues related to CAMHS from those which are more broadly associated with the children's workforce agenda.

- Not all staff working in CAMHS require different levels of training. Getting this personalisation right is fundamental to achieving the optimum skill mix within the workforce and managing resources. Not everyone needs to be an expert in all areas, and the skill mix within the CAMHS nursing workforce should be tailored to local service requirements.

- There has been a serious lack of attention paid to workforce development in mental health and more specifically in CAMHS. A research programme centred on the therapeutic impact and contribution of CAMHS nursing is much needed in order to explore helpful and effective interventions delivered by nursing staff. This should include safe staffing in CAMHS inpatient areas, development of specialist and expanding roles, and exploration of the experiences of unregistered staff working in CAMHS who generally assist nursing staff.

Introduction

The national vision for the education, training and workforce development of child and adolescent mental health services (CAMHS) nurses is ambitious. Therefore, practitioners must demonstrate excellent practice, use evidence-based care and work in partnership with children, young people, families and their fellow professionals. In clarifying definitions and terms of reference for this chapter, it is important to acknowledge that there are several groups of nurses working as autonomous practitioners across the full range of comprehensive CAMHS. While the majority are mental health nurses, there are also a growing number of registered children's nurses, learning disability nurses and health visitors working to support the emotional needs of children and young people.

Nevertheless, it is probably only nurses working within specialist community and inpatient settings that might identify themselves as CAMHS nurses. This picture is further complicated by the fact that within this group, there are nurses who have undergone additional training who no longer identify themselves by profession but, rather, by therapeutic modality (e.g. family therapist or child psychotherapist) and are employed as such. Alongside this, there are those who are employed as primary mental health workers (PMHWs) or specialist practitioners under a generic set of competencies rather than as part of a profession.

This chapter is written within the spirit of the RCN guidance *Children and Young People's Mental Health – Every Nurse's Business* (Royal College of Nursing [RCN] 2014) and aims to describe and critically reflect on factors influencing the knowledge, skills, competencies and capabilities of the existing and future CAMHS nursing workforce in its broadest sense. This is in keeping with other developments in the field, including the latest review of CAMHS, *Future in Mind* (Department of Health 2015), which stipulates that the entire children's workforce should be appropriately trained and supported to meet the emotional and mental health needs of children and young people. It is vital that education, training and workforce development is shaped by the needs of children, young people and families rather than those responsible for delivering them. An attempt to design and deliver education and training that does not take account of the voices of young people and families is unlikely to meet their needs and creates practitioners who consider themselves 'experts' and are less able to work in a meaningful and collaborative way with families.

Box 7.1 illustrates children and young people's views about the workforce qualities and behaviour they would like to see, based on the latest review of CAMHS (Department of Health 2015).

Box 7.1   Children and young people's views about the CAMHS workforce and what they would like to see

- A workforce which is equipped with the skills, training and experience to best support children and young people's emotional and mental wellbeing.

- Staff who are positive, have a young outlook, are relaxed, open-minded, unprejudiced and trustworthy.

- Behaviour that is characterised by fairness, and a willingness to listen to, trust and believe in the child or young person.

- Everybody should work from a basis of asking and listening, being prepared to be helpful in creating understanding among other members of the workforce.

- Their processes should be transparent, honest and open to being both inspected and clearly explained. Visible actions should result from such scrutiny, enabling children to voice their opinions.

- The workforce should provide real choice of interventions supported by enough resources to follow through, whilst remaining honest and realistic.

Source: Department of Health (2015: 63).

The organisational context of CAMHS

Nurses working with child and adolescent mental health find themselves doing so within a complex set of systems that, for the purposes of clarity, might be divided under two broad headings – CAMHS subsystems and nursing subsystems. The structure and operation of CAMHS can appear complex at first as the organisation differs from both traditional secondary mental health services for adults and the majority of general services for children and young people (specifically in relation to multi-agency relationships and interdependencies). The structure of CAMHS is often best explained in terms of how a child or young person accesses the service within the current four 'tiers' of service provision. Alongside this, there are differences in the levels of support and types of intervention offered in the different tiers and also in how each of the tiers is commissioned.

The range of professionals involved and the different services this encompasses provides challenges for the way in which the CAMHS workforce is trained and developed. This is due to the range of different professionals working across different sectors, organisations, services and age groups. Nurses, health visitors and midwives work across a range of settings and are one of the largest groups of healthcare professionals coming into contact with children and young people (RCN 2014).

Within Tier 1, nurses are in key positions to promote the psychological and emotional wellbeing of children and young people, and they have the potential to identify those who are at risk and to intervene early (Department of Health 2004a; Department for Education and Skills 2003). This is highly significant within the current policy climate that focuses on the importance of early intervention and appropriate referral and support, which can substantially reduce the likelihood of long-term psychological difficulties (Early Intervention Foundation 2014).

Beyond Tier 1, there are several groups of nurses working as autonomous CAMHS practitioners across Tiers 2, 3 and 4. Therefore it is likely that the education and training needs of the CAMHS workforce will differ depending on where they work and the stage of career they are at. This in turn poses challenges around effective curriculum design and continuing professional development (CPD) provision. The education and training available to staff needs to be suitable as not all staff working in CAMHS require the same level of training. Getting this personalisation right is fundamental to achieving the optimum skill mix within the workforce and managing resources. Not everyone needs to be an expert in all areas, and the skill mix within the CAMHS nursing workforce should be tailored to local service requirements.

Whilst there is no evidence that having all staff as higher qualified and more expert practitioners equals better care or better outcomes (Morris *et al.* 2009), the majority of children with difficulties either go undetected or are cared for in primary care settings (Kramer and Gerralda 2000) by nurses who do not always have appropriate training. It is therefore vital to develop the capabilities of all nurses in identifying and addressing child and adolescent mental health issues (RCN 2014).

The publication of *Together We Stand* (NHS Health Advisory Service 1995) and *A Handbook on Child and Adolescent Mental Health* (Department of Health 1995) paved the way for moving from a traditional child guidance model of service delivery and towards developing CAMHS within a four-tiered framework. Within this framework, everyone working with children and young people was envisaged as having a contribution to make to the mental health of this group. The impact of this and several years of subsequent policy and guidance has been that nurses working with the mental health needs of children and young people have been practising in a complex and constantly evolving multi-professional and inter-agency environment. The plethora of reviews, reports and guidance to improve the mental health outcomes for children and young people, including looked-after children and young people in youth offending institutions, has been accompanied by the advent of Sure Start and the National Healthy Schools Programme.

A great deal of the work done in recent years to try to address the emotional wellbeing and mental health needs of children and young people has had a particular focus on prevention and early intervention (Early Intervention Foundation 2014). Subsequently, it has been important not to separate the workforce development issues related to CAMHS completely from those that are more broadly associated with the children's workforce agenda.

There is a wealth of evidence and good practice to build on including key strategies, reports and initiatives such as the National Service Framework (Department of Health 2004a, 2004b) and *Every Child Matters* (Department of Education and Skills 2003). More recently, *Making Children's Mental Health Everyone's Responsibility* (National Advisory Council 2011), the *Report of the Children and Young People's Health Outcomes Forum* (Department of Health 2012) and *Improving Children and Young People's Health Outcomes* (Department of Health 2013a) emphasised the need to develop a workforce with the right mix of skills competencies to support children and young people with mental health needs at a national level. However, despite a regular flow of policy reports, reviews, initiatives and guidance from central government, a recent report from the Chief Medical Officer (Department of Health 2013b) led to the Health Select Committee launching an inquiry into CAMHS. Following this inquiry, a taskforce was put together and *Future In Mind* was published (Department of Health 2015).

These findings highlight the need to bring together education, health and social care more closely in order to develop a model of services that focuses on the whole child and family. Whilst *Future in Mind* echoes themes prevalent in earlier reviews and publications, it is the first to state explicitly that the four-tiered service system around which CAMHS services have been organised for the past decade should be replaced in its entirety. Furthermore, there is the added suggestion of a move away from specialist community CAMHS services to a model of specialist liaison and consultation based within other services. Nevertheless, the report is clear in reiterating that all those working with children and young people have a role in supporting their social, emotional and mental wellbeing.

Whilst *Future in Mind* is critical of current service design and provision, it does not fully acknowledge the current competing and demanding pressures that exist within the CAMHS workforce. This was previously noted in the New Ways of Working in CAMHS initiative, which highlighted that clinical capacity cannot be expanded simply by increasing workforce numbers or streamlining processes (Morris and Nixon 2008). The need to train and develop new and enhanced roles alone will not address some of the broader systemic challenges facing CAMHS services, and this issue to date has not been debated widely enough within the literature. Therefore, in order to achieve the vision set out in policy, change is needed at a strategic level; and within the current climate of reduced service provision, this is considerably challenging.

At present, there has been a serious lack of attention paid to workforce development in relation to mental health and, more specifically, CAMHS. A research programme centred on the therapeutic impact and contribution of CAMHS nursing is much needed in order to explore helpful and effective interventions delivered by nursing staff. This should include safe staffing in CAMHS inpatient areas, the development of specialist and expanding roles and an exploration of the experiences of unregistered staff working in CAMHS who generally assist nursing staff.

The political context of nursing

There have been profound changes in the wider context of mental health nursing, which have added to the complexity facing CAMHS nurses. The focus of policy recently has emphasised that mental health is a priority for society, communities and, in particular, health professionals. Whilst in the past, much of policy has focused on adult mental health services (AMHS), more recently, the publication of *No Health Without Mental Health – A Cross-government Mental Health Outcomes Strategy for People of All Ages* (HM Government/Department of Health 2011) reflects a more integrated lifespan approach to thinking about the mental health of people of all ages.

This is alongside reports such as *Starting Today – The Future of Mental Health Services* (Mental Health Foundation 2013), which, whilst being focused largely on AMHS, also contains a theme on lifespan issues, linking poor mental health in childhood to the mental health problems in adult life. It refers in detail to child and adolescent mental health, discussing issues related to CAMHS service design and delivery. Therefore, it is possible that these developments might have profound implications for mental health nurses whose education and training have largely equipped them for working with adults, viewing children and young people's mental health as an optional speciality.

Together with these changes, the landscape within nurse education has also been transforming. Over the last several years, media coverage, both positive and negative, has placed nurses and nursing in the public arena. The Francis inquiry (2013) highlighted issues associated with the quality of nursing care and called for better education and training. Following this, *The Cavendish Review* was published, highlighting the need for formal training for healthcare assistants and support workers who make up the majority of the nursing workforce, particularly in inpatient CAMHS (Department of Health 2013c).

Against the backdrop of these and other recent high-profile national reports, the need for care to be person-centred, compassionate and well informed has been emphasised in the recently published *Shape of Caring Review* (Health Education England 2015). This highlights the need for more flexible provision of education and training across nurse education. The recommendations include better access to quality training for unregistered staff with flexible pathways into nurse education. This is alongside pre-registration nurse education becoming less rigid across the four fields in order to develop parity between mental health and physical health. The importance of access to CPD for registered nurses is further discussed as well as the development of career pathways that allow nurses to transition across clinical, managerial, research and education posts.

The role of CAMHS nurses

The problem of clear role-identity for mental health nurses in general has received no small amount of attention, and this problem is no less an issue for nurses who work in CAMHS settings. The issue of blurred roles and lack of clarity around occupational boundaries in relation to multidisciplinary working in community mental health settings has been debated in the literature for many years (Brown *et al.* 2000). This is largely because aspects of mental health nursing and its subspecialties are hard to define (Rasmussen *et al.* 2014). Baldwin found that although nurses in the UK have worked in community CAMHS settings for almost 20 years, 'they are frequently unclear about what their nursing contribution is to the multidisciplinary team' (2002: 520). This may be because many of the characteristics that nurses have developed within specialist areas are tacit or intuitive. However, Baldwin warns that there is a risk that if nurses cannot develop a clearer rationale for their role or be better able to articulate what they do in these teams, their roles might be lost.

Specialist CAMHS services are organised around a mix of modality-specific professional identities (e.g. family therapists) and profession-specific identities (e.g. clinical psychologists). It could be argued that the CAMHS nursing identity is stronger within specialist inpatient settings where the traditional nurse's caring role and its associated activities are more clearly defined, delineated and observed. Within community CAMHS teams where the therapeutic task and associated interventions are organised in a different way, it can sometimes be more challenging for nurses to articulate clearly what skills, knowledge, qualities and values they contribute to the multidisciplinary team. This may be brought about by or reflected in the lack of a clear specific training and development pathway for nurses who wish to work in this field. This is particularly pertinent since professional training and professional confidence and identity appear to go hand in hand. Furthermore, many CAMHS nurses seem to address this lack of a clear developmental pathway by retraining and rebranding themselves as therapists providing cognitive behaviour therapy (CBT) or dialectical behaviour therapy (DBT). Alternatively, they might use their professional qualification to gain access to newer roles such as the PMHW. The question is: are they still nurses? A further question might be: does it matter?

The advent of the Choice and Partnership Approach (CAPA) (York and Kingsbury 2009) with its emphasis on the core assessment, behavioural, cognitive, dynamic and systemic CAMHS skills required to meet the bulk of the clinical demand might have been an opportunity to reassert the value of CAMHS nursing with its non-specialist and eclectic approach to delivering interventions. However professional leadership in CAMHS nursing locally and nationally has not yet evolved consistently to the point where it can take up and run with these sorts of opportunities. New and expanded roles within CAMHS nursing are not as well established as in other specialisms, such as children's cardiac care or children's cancer care (RCN 2011, 2012a), and there are noticeably only a handful of CAMHS nurse consultants, whose roles remain poorly defined and whose potential is not yet fully realised despite guidance from the RCN (2012b). This further reflects a continued lack of UK-wide leadership in CAMHS nursing, and the RCN (2014) has made some important recommendations in order to ensure that there is effective nurse leadership within CAMHS (see Box 7.2). Strong leadership both in clinical and managerial nursing positions is fundamental to advocating for the role and contribution of nursing within CAMHS settings.

Box 7.2 Recommendations for effective nurse leadership in CAMHS

- the continued development of specialist nurses to influence practice and strategic level service developments

- the continued development of specialist nurses to promote integrated working and succession planning across all professional groups

- CAMHS nursing representation in the local service planning and delivery of mental health services for children and young people

- CAMHS representation to ensure that accessible and appropriate education provision is contracted during pre-registration and post-registration to meet the current and future needs of local service providers

- areas of excellence identified and processes put in place to share and disseminate good practice

- further investment made in the research field of child and adolescent mental health.

Source: RCN (2014: 8).

In the context of this complicated picture of CAMHS nursing, there has been a move in community CAMHS teams across the country towards new posts being offered as generic competency-based positions. These include the introduction of the position of CAMHS practitioner, replacing what were once nursing posts. Although nurses make up a significant proportion of clinicians working within CAMHS, within the latest review, there is a focus on skill mix and capabilities. This is reflected in a growing preoccupation in mental health education and service delivery with concepts of competence and professionalism. Competence itself is complex and hard to define. Within caring, it encompasses knowledge, performance, skills and attitudes, which in themselves are hard to articulate. This move towards a competency-driven workforce has seen the decline of some professional groups, and the difficulties in recruiting to profession-specific posts in some areas has further added to this.

The case for a shift away from a workforce that is defined and restricted by professional qualifications and roles to one that is defined by skills, competencies and capability was first outlined in the New Ways of Working in CAMHS programme (Care Services Improvement Partnership/National Institute for Mental Health [England] 2007). So far, it appears to have impacted most strongly on nursing roles for reasons that currently do not appear clear. The resulting deficit is all the more significant during a time when strategic change and leadership is essential and may leave the role of the CAMHS nurse vulnerable to other specialisms or open to the development of more generic roles. The skills of CAMHS nurses working with CAMHS need to be better articulated by nurses themselves and better advocated for by nurses working in senior and leadership positions. Research is further needed to support nurses in taking a strong and valid stance on this. This may help to redefine and focus the CAMHS nursing role in order to protect these roles and avoid further role blurring. Box 7.3 is an attempt to highlight some of the key capabilities required of CAMHS nurses.

The National Service Framework (Department of Health 2004a, 2004b) and *Every Child Matters* initiative (Department for Education and Skills 2003) indicated for the first time that there were to be clear standards for the delivery of services for working with the health

---

Box 7.3   Key capabilities required of CAMHS nurses

- Ability to work in a recovery-oriented way, focusing on the strengths of the individuals and family and working towards shared goals collaboratively

- Ability to work flexibly and in an integrative way, drawing on a range of theory and therapeutic skills

- Ability to build meaningful relationships with young people, families and professionals alike

- Ability to deliver care that is individualised, tailored and focused as part of the nursing process

- Ability to discuss and manage risk effectively in collaboration with young people and their families

- Ability to use clear, plain and jargon-free language

- Ability to work collaboratively in multi-professional and inter-agency contexts

- Ability to engage in and utilise reflective practice.

---

and emotional wellbeing of children and young people, with the expectation that all child healthcare professionals should have education and training to meet these needs. Although *Future In Mind* (Department of Health 2015) appears to signal a major strategic and operational change for the way in which CAMHS services are delivered, there is still a need to make an important distinction. This is between practitioners for whom the mental health and emotional wellbeing of children is a part of their work but not their core business, and specialist practitioners for whom this is their main role.

A review of the post-registration training needs of nurses working with children and young people with mental health problems (RCN 2004) came to the conclusion that pre-registration nurse training did not prepare nurses with the adequate knowledge, skills or experience to work with child and adolescent mental health and made key recommendations in relation to the importance of relevant post-registration education. Although around this time, nurses were able to access a range of multidisciplinary post-registration and postgraduate CAMHS training offered by a range of higher education institutions, the formal articulation of specific competencies in working with children and young people with complex and severe mental health problems and systems of appraisal and CPD for nurses practising in specialist CAMHS settings remain undeveloped. This is despite the fact that nurses working in specialist CAMHS are required to have highly advanced practice knowledge and skills.

Whilst profession-specific education and training for nurses working in CAMHS seems to have been elusive, the National Service Framework (Department of Health 2004a) signalled the beginning of much thinking and work around the development of the CAMHS workforce as a whole. It recommended that arrangements be put in place to ensure that specialist multidisciplinary teams were of sufficient size and had appropriate skill mix, training and support to function effectively (Department of Health 2004a). Between 2003 and 2006, the CAMHS mapping exercise sought to provide information about, amongst other things, the make-up of specialist CAMHS (Wistow 2007). Interestingly, this data showed nursing to be the largest professional group, forming a third of this workforce in 2006.

However, as Nixon (2007) points out, the issue of sufficient size is not adequate to satisfy demand for services. Additionally, practitioners must be appropriately trained and supervised. New Ways of Working for CAMHS served to underline the need for a change in organisation of services and working practices to be more aligned with demonstrated need and not rooted in historical precedent. This would have to include education and training for practitioners. This again highlights the need for further skills analysis of the current nursing workforce in order to identify how we can further develop the skills and competencies of those supporting children and young people with emotional and mental health needs.

Workforce development initiatives in specialist CAMHS were also to take into account the wider children's workforce development initiatives signalled by *Every Child Matters* (Department for Education and Skills 2003). A number of government documents, including the *Children's Workforce Strategy* (Department for Education and Skills 2005), stated that government departments would work closely together to ensure a coherent strategic approach to workforce development across all children's services of which specialist CAMHS were a part. Following this, we have seen the development of expanded roles such as the PMHW and specialist practitioner role introduced to CAMHS with their associated competency and capability frameworks (Gale *et al.* 2005).

This is a prime example of innovative thinking and creative new role developments that seem to point the way forwards and which also reflect a move away from the medical model towards a more holistic and systemic way of working. These roles are based not on a profession-centric or modality-centric view of practice, but on a clearly articulated set of competencies and capabilities that are open to any children's practitioner who can demonstrate an ability to meet them. Additionally, it can be argued that they play a central part in providing training and consultation for practitioners working in universal and targeted children's services.

Existing competency frameworks

Competencies are descriptors of the performance criteria, knowledge and understanding that are required to undertake work activity. They describe what staff members in CAMHS need to do and to know in order to carry out relevant activities, regardless of who it is that performs the task (Sergeant 2009). University College London in partnership with Health Education Scotland developed a full competence framework for CAMHS services that seeks to encompass the full range of comprehensive CAMHS from universal to specialist inpatient provision (NHS Education for Scotland 2011). This competency framework uses the main principles of evidence-based practice and is focused on clinical work as opposed to leadership and management. Whilst the CAMHS framework is most relevant to those working in Tiers 2, 3 and 4, it may also be valuable for professionals working in broader universal services at Tier 1. It helpfully differentiates between core skills that all workers in CAMHS should have and specialist skills for those working in more specific settings. This further illustrates the need for appropriate and tailored training in order to develop competencies across services rather than a 'one size fits all' approach. Alongside this competency framework, Skills For Health (2007) has produced core functions for CAMHS practitioners working in specialist CAMHS services, and these are summarised in Box 7.4.

Box 7.4 Core functions of CAMHS practitioners

- Effective communication and engagement with children, young people, families and carers

- Comprehensive assessment taking account of all aspects of a young person's development

- Safeguarding and promotion of the welfare of children

- Support for all aspects of care coordination

- Promoting health and helping young people understand the importance of wellbeing

- Supporting transitions and identifying the likely impact of different types of transition on individual children and young people

- Multi-agency working, establishing and maintaining effective joint working with other agencies and services

- Information sharing with colleagues and other agencies following agreed procedures for confidentiality and disclosure

- Professional development and learning, supporting others to understand young people's mental health needs and how these can be addressed in their work.

Source: adapted from Skills for Health (2007).

Exposure to CAMHS in pre-registration nurse education

Pre-registration nurses receive comprehensive training within a variety of settings with a diverse range of needs including mental health. The Nursing and Midwifery Council (NMC) sets out learning outcome standards that should be obtained by every entry-level nurse. The Council specifically requires nurses to be able to identify risks and needs in relation to psychological health and to be able to implement a plan of care in partnership with clients. It states that theory and practice learning outcomes must take account of the essential physical and mental health needs of all people, including babies, children and young people, pregnant and postnatal women, adults and older people. This includes people with acute and long-term conditions, people requiring end of life care, people with learning disabilities and people with mental health problems (Nursing and Midwifery Council 2010).

Whilst the NMC standards are clear and complete, there are differences in the way in which they are interpreted and embedded across pre-registration programmes. The amount that is taught in relation to child and adolescent mental health in pre-registration nurse education is limited at best and absent at worst. Furthermore, the quality and content of this taught content is disparate across university programmes and tends to be determined by the skill mix of the particular programme team. Additionally, there is a lack of placements in specialist CAMHS settings, meaning that many students do not get exposed to this area of practice during their training. This is despite there being clear evidence regarding the benefits of this – particularly in relation to attitudes towards working with young people with mental health problems (Richardson 2011) – and the anecdotal experiences of students who happen to get placed in CAMHS.

Within the majority of children's nursing and mental health nursing programmes, there is an emphasis in the former with working with 'sick children' and in the latter with working with 'disordered adults'. The rigidity of pre-registration programmes in relation to the four fields of nursing was heavily criticised within the *Shape of Caring Review* (Health Education England 2015), which highlights the marginalisation of mental health and a need to achieve parity across all four fields of nursing practice; this is generally consistent with the notion of holistic nursing. In order to achieve this, there is a need to understand the importance of good mental health and the impact of poor mental health on broader health and social outcomes. This will require a fundamental move away from programmes that focus disproportionally on illness and acute care towards those that are better aligned to promoting wellness and working collaboratively in care and community nursing.

Given that it is now well known and understood that half of all mental illness occurs during childhood, there is a need for nurse education to take a lifespan approach in the way in which learning is structured. This is so that the complexity of the problems people present with are appreciated and so that students engage in consideration of broader systemic issues. Therefore, in order to achieve this, there are some core aspects of learning that need to be addressed more specifically than those set out by the NMC, taking into account the current policy drivers (see Box 7.5).

Box 7.5 *Key aspects of learning for nurses*

Pre-registration programmes should address:

- the historical perspectives and the development of current CAMHS provision;
- developmental theories and their relationship to the mental health of children and young people;
- the relationship within and between agencies that promote children and young people's health, education and wellbeing;
- the legal and policy frameworks for working with children, young people and their families;
- how to engage with children and young people;
- frameworks for assessment and referral processes;
- evidence-based interventions.

Current policy drivers

Infancy and young children

- Perinatal mental health
- Attachment and relationship formation in vulnerable children
- Promoting infant mental health
- Developmental theories and normal child development
- Parenting
- Parental mental illness
- Eating and sleep patterns.

5- to 11-year-olds

- Self-esteem and self-concept
- Parenting.

Young people

- Developing a sense of self and identity formation
- Importance of social identity and role of peers/peer pressure
- Impact of loss and bereavement on young people
- Assessment of need and referral pathways in CAMHS services
- Caring for children from hard-to-reach communities
- Vulnerable children, including looked-after children.

The development of newly qualified and existing CAMHS nurses

It is important to acknowledge that for nursing staff that are new to the field of CAMHS, there will be gaps in knowledge, skills and competencies (Morris *et al.* 2009). Newly qualified nurses joining the CAMHS workforce cannot be considered the finished product; they will require a focused period of induction alongside a more defined career pathway that supports ongoing education that is part of a CAMHS workforce strategy. Alongside addressing the needs of newly qualified staff, attention needs to be paid to developing a future workforce that is fit for purpose, which means that there needs to be adequate support for and investment in current nursing staff working in CAMHS.

Nurses continue to make up the largest part of the CAMHS workforce; therefore, its potential must be maximised in order to meet the needs of young people and their families. Over a decade on since the RCN (2004) report on the post-registration education and training needs of nurses working with children and young people with mental health problems, the vast majority of the current nursing workforce has had limited opportunity to engage in post-registration education. There has been significant variation in the level and degree of investment in the qualified workforce, leading to differences in the level of post-qualification attainment (Health Education England 2015). This illustrates the need to develop broad CPD programmes that are relevant and address common themes for nurses and other professionals working across CAMHS services. As part of this, there is a continued need for targeted education and training in order to achieve the outcomes in Box 7.6 as defined by the RCN (2014).

Adequate CPD programmes for nurses working within CAMHS are fundamental to the provision of safe nursing care and quality services as well as the ongoing development of knowledge, skills and personal reflection. The current system of CPD provision has evolved in complexity and with inconsistencies; as a result, though several local and regional programmes have been developed, these have been difficult to deliver and sustain due to the cuts to funding and pressures on staff time. This is further complicated by the distinct lack of a presiding and overarching CAMHS nursing competency framework alongside the absence of clear national guidance and curricula to support the education and training of CAMHS nurses working in England.

Box 7.6 *Key outcomes of targeted education and training*

- ensure evidence-based best practice

- continue to promote mental health pre-registration placements

- develop the skills and knowledge of non-specialist child and adolescent workers

- enable post-registration nurses working at tier 1 and 2 the opportunity for reflective practice and clinical supervision

- enhance the knowledge and skills of specialist child and adolescent mental health workers

- ensure that all nurses working within specialist child and adolescent mental health services have access to clinical supervision

- provide both general and specialist child and adolescent mental health workers with a flexible framework of learning for progression and professional development.

Source: RCN (2014: 7).

This lack of organisation around the development and provision of post-registration education in nursing is reflected in the absence of qualifications that are recognised by all employers and the unavailability of a clear career pathway. This ultimately leads to a disparity in knowledge, skills and competence at varying levels in nursing across services and organisations, which further affects the existing inequities within the provision of CAMHS. Furthermore, it is important to state the obvious in that if training programmes that led to a recognised qualification were to be designed, there would need to be support from managers and organisation to enable staff to engage in this.

Considerable funding has been invested by the Department of Health and NHS England into the Children and Young People's Improving Access to Psychological Therapies (CYP IAPT) programme, which is a service transformation programme delivered by NHS England that aims to improve existing community CAMHS teams. This has gradually supported the transformation of local services. However, there remain significant and unacceptable gaps and variations in consistency and coherence within and across services and how they are commissioned.

The programme has several core principles which include participation, accessibility, evidence-based practice and routine outcome monitoring. It differs from the provision of Adult IAPT training as it does not create stand-alone services. The purpose of the training is to equip professionals working within specialist community settings with the necessary knowledge, skills and competence to work in partnership with young people and families in a way that is therapeutic, evidence-based and outcome driven. The curriculum has been designed to focus on psychological therapies that have been approved by the National Institute for Health and Care Excellence, with a clear focus on evidence-based practice and core therapeutic skills.

Future in Mind (Department of Health 2015) made recommendations to extend the roll-out of the CYP IAPT programme and to consider developing the curricula and training programmes to train staff to meet the needs of children and young people who are currently not supported by the existing programmes. Thus CYP IAPT ceased in 2015 when a broader CAMHS transformation programme replaced it. This was to extend and adapt the approach to meet the needs of professionals working within schools. Furthermore, skills and training programmes need to be made available to all staff working in inpatient CAMHS settings, which support the most vulnerable young people who often have the most complex sets of problems. At the time of writing this chapter, aspects of the CYP IAPT programme were being piloted in inpatient settings.

This would help assist the development of core competencies that are specific to inpatient CAMHS settings and linked to career progression for unregistered and registered staff. It is essential that staff on inpatient units have the adequate level of competence, to ensure that they are delivering evidence-based, integrative care, alongside the necessary knowledge and understanding of the theory which underpins this. However crucial to the success of inpatient units will be the consideration of wider issues to do with recruitment and retention of staff due to the high level of staff turnover that these services tend to experience, particularly in relation to their nursing staff. This continual attrition of nursing staff within inpatient settings means that there is an ongoing skills deficit and, in some units, a lack of senior nursing staff to lead care delivery and provide role models for more junior members of staff – in particular, unregistered staff who make up a significant proportion of the inpatient staffing. Within the CAMHS workforce, there is a need to recognise and better support the training needs of unregistered staff who work as part of the nursing teams and deliver a significant proportion of care to vulnerable young people and who often feel undervalued within their clinical roles.

Conclusion

Nurses, and in particular mental health nurses, who wish to work within children and young people's mental health could potentially find themselves caught between a lack of sufficient pre- and post-registration profession-specific training on the one hand and a move away from traditional professional demarcations towards generic roles on the other. However, amongst the current policy drivers, service transformation projects and potential role confusion, there is perhaps an opportunity for nurses in the field to better articulate their purpose and value.

CAMHS nurses are resilient and used to working under pressure and in uncertain circumstances; however, there is an important need to advocate for and protect important nursing roles within CAMHS across all tiers. It is particularly important for nurses to highlight the skills that they bring to multidisciplinary teams through their eclectic use of models, risk management, communication and team work. This is particularly important at a time where competency over profession is desired and preferred amongst service managers.

Alongside this, there is a need to develop the existing nursing workforce within CAMHS and not rely solely on those who currently hold the expertise and experience to take care of the future workforce. Whilst it would be timely for nurse educators to reconsider the way in which the mental health and wellbeing of children and young people is addressed in pre-registration nurse education, this needs to be alongside the development of CPD modules and programmes aimed at existing CAMHS nurses. Furthermore, at a time where significant and strategic change is signalled in relation to the way in which CAMHS services are delivered and how they relate to the wider systems that support children and young people, it is timely to revisit the role of the CAMHS nurse who, amidst this change, may be required to take on new roles and challenges.

Particular attention needs to be paid to the development and sustainability of clinical nurse specialists, nurse consultants and modern matrons and their roles in relation to education and training, bridging of community/inpatient services and leading the strategic development of CAMHS services in order to deliver the vision laid out in policy.

References

Baldwin, L. (2002) The nursing role in outpatient child and adolescent mental health services. *Journal of Clinical Nursing*, 11(4): 520–5.

Brown, B., Crawford, P. and Darongkamas, J. (2000) Blurred roles and permeable boundaries: the experience of multidisciplinary working in community mental health. *Health and Social Care in the Community*, 8(6): 425–35.

Care Services Improvement Partnership/National Institute for Mental Health (England) (2007) *New Ways of Working for Everyone: Developing and Sustaining a Capable and Flexible Workforce*. London: Department of Health.

Department for Education and Skills (2005) *Children's Workforce Strategy. A Strategy to Build a World-class Workforce for Children and Young People*. London: Department for Education and Skills.

Department for Education and Skills (2003) *Every Child Matters*. London: Department for Education and Skills.

Department of Health (2015) *Future in Mind: Promoting, Protecting and Improving Our Children and Young People's Mental Health and Wellbeing*. London: Department of Health.

Department of Health (2013a) *Improving Children and Young People's Health Outcomes: A System Wide Response*. London: Department of Health.

Department of Health (2013b) *Chief Medical Officer's Annual Report 2012: Our Children Deserve Better: Prevention Pays*. London: Department of Health.

Department of Health (2013c) *The Cavendish Review: Review of Health Care Assistants and Support Workers in NHS and Social Care*. London: Department of Health.

Department of Health (2012) *Report of the Children and Young People's Health Outcomes Forum*. London: Department of Health.

Department of Health (2004a) *National Service Framework for Children, Young People and Maternity Services*. London: Department of Health.

Department of Health (2004b) *National Service Framework for Mental Health Services*. London: Department of Health.

Department of Health (1995) *A Handbook on Child and Adolescent Mental Health*. London: Department of Health.

Early Intervention Foundation (2014) *Getting It Right for Families*. London: Early Intervention Foundation.

Francis, R., QC (Chair) (2013) *Report of the Mid Staffordshire NHS Foundation Trust Public Inquiry*. London: The Stationary Office.

Gale, F., Hassett, A. and Sebuliba, D. (2005) *The Competency and Capability Framework for Primary Mental Health Workers in Child and Adolescent Mental Health Services (CAMHS)*. London: National CAMHS Support Service.

NHS Health Advisory Service (1995) *Together We Stand: Thematic Review of the Commissioning, Role and Management of Child and Adolescent Mental Health Services*. London: HMSO.

Health Education England (2015) *Shape of Caring Review*. London: Health Education England.

NHS Education for Scotland (2011) *A Competence Framework for Child and Adolescent Mental Health Services*. Edinburgh: NHS Education for Scotland.

Department of Health (2011) *No Health Without Mental Health: A Cross-government Mental Health Outcomes Strategy for People of All Ages*. London: Department of Health.

Kramer, T. and Gerralda, E. (2000) Child and adolescent mental health problems in primary care. *Advances in Psychiatric Treatment*, 6(4): 287–94.

Mental Health Foundation (2013) *Starting Today – The Future of Mental Health Services*. London: Mental Health Foundation.

Morris, T. and Nixon, B. (2008) New Ways of Working in CAMHS. *The Journal of Mental Health Training, Education and Practice*, 3(1) 22–7.

Morris, T., Anderson, Y. and Nixon, B. (2009) New Ways of Working in child and adolescent mental health services – 'keep the baby but throw out the bathwater'. *The Journal of Mental Health Training, Education and Practice*, 4(3): 10–14.

National Advisory Council (2011) *Making Children's Mental Health Everyone's Responsibility*. London: National Advisory Council.

Nixon, B. (2007) Understanding the key workforce issues facing child and adolescent mental health services. *The Journal of Mental Health Training, Education and Practice*, 2(4): 40–7.

Nursing and Midwifery Council (2010) *Standards for Pre-registration Nurse Education*. London: Nursing and Midwifery Council.

Rasmussen, P., Henderson, A. and Muir-Cochrane, E. (2014) Conceptualizing the clinical and professional development of child and adolescent mental health nurses. *International Journal of Mental Health Nursing*, 23(3) 265–72.

Richardson, B. P. (2011) Child and Adolescent Mental Health Service (CAMHS) placements for pre-registration child branch nursing students: potential benefits. *Nurse Education Today*, 31(5): 494–8.

Royal College of Nursing (RCN) (2014) *Children and Young People's Mental Health – Every Nurse's Business*. London: RCN.

Royal College of Nursing (RCN) (2012a) *Advanced Nurse Practitioners: An RCN Guide to Advanced Nursing Practice, Advanced Nurse Practitioners and Programme Accreditation*. London: RCN.

Royal College of Nursing (RCN) (2012b) *Becoming a Nurse Consultant: Towards Greater Effectiveness Through a Programme of Support*. London: RCN.

Royal College of Nursing (RCN) (2011) *Children and Young People's Cardiac Nursing: RCN Guidance on Roles, Career Pathways and Competence Development*. London: RCN.

Royal College of Nursing (RCN) (2004) *The Post-registration Education and Training Needs of Nurses Working with Children and Young People with Mental Health Problems in the UK: A Survey Conducted by the RCN Mental Health Programme in Collaboration with the RCN Children and Young People's Mental Health Forum*. London: RCN.

Sergeant, A. (2009) *Working Within Child and Adolescent Inpatient Services: A Practitioner's Handbook*. Wigan: National CAMHS Support Service.

Skills for Health (2007) *Core Functions: Child and Adolescent Mental Health Services, Tier 3, 4 (Specialist Targeted)*. Bristol: Skills for Health.

Wistow, R. (2007) Mapping the CAMHS workforce: 2003–2006. *The Journal of Mental Health Training, Education and Practice*, 2(4) 30–9.

York, A. and Kingsbury, S. (2009) *The Choice and Partnership Approach: A Guide to CAPA*. Surrey: CAMHS Network.

Part 2

Common mental health and psychosocial disorders

Chapter 8

Nursing children and young people who self-harm

Marie Armstrong

Key points:

- The number of young people admitted to hospital for self-harm has been increasing in recent years. Despite figures being alarmingly high, reported figures are far from representative since most young people who self-harm do not attend hospital for assessment or treatment.
- Nurses in child and adolescent mental health services (CAMHS) take a holistic stance, seeing the young person as a whole and recognising that child and family needs are broad and varied. This insight is enabled by nurses' well-developed communication skills and ability to engage with the young person and their family.
- As well as understanding the significance of self-harm in the context of adolescent development, it is also important to be aware of the social context in which young people harm themselves. For some young people, self-harm may be symptomatic of a serious mental health disorder such as depression, whilst for others, it may be the result of experimentation as part of adolescent identity and self-image.
- Guidelines in England and Wales provide health professionals with evidence and standards for the assessment of young people who self-harm. These can be applied by nurses across a range of paediatric, school, mental health, community and forensic settings.
- In order to help young people who self-harm, the nurse must understand, communicate this understanding and create a therapeutic alliance, which is the bedrock for positive change.
- It is important that nurses who work with young people who self-harm have regular clinical supervision. This is essential to ensure practice is safe and effective and so that the nurse remains supported, up to date and professionally accountable for their work.

Introduction

Nurses in schools, hospitals, prisons and community settings come into contact with children and young people who harm themselves. This chapter explores some of the myths and realities about self-harm and uses an evidence-based framework to guide nurses and other professionals who are required to assess, treat and support children in both front-line services and residential settings. Self-harm is heterogeneous, which means that it signifies different things in different people. Current evidence for the assessment of self-harm and clinical interventions are discussed. The development of mental health nursing in relation to self-harm is also described. Case vignettes are used to illustrate the different ways in which self-harm is understood and how a variety of nursing interventions can be used to meet young people's needs.

Terminology, distinctions and definitions

A range of terms are used to describe self-harm, self-injury, parasuicide and attempted suicide. In order to clarify what is meant by self-harm, Kerfoot (2000) suggests some distinctions (see Box 8.1).

Box 8.1 Terminology, distinctions and definitions

- Suicide – those who intentionally kill themselves

- Attempted suicide – those who self-harm with the intention of suicide but survive

- Parasuicide or self-harm – those who self-harm with little or no intention of killing themselves.

Source: adapted from Kerfoot (2000: 111–2).

However, it is important to recognise that definitions are far from straightforward. Categories often overlap, and the suicidal intent of young people may be changeable or unclear. The term self-harm is therefore often used to describe a young person's behaviour rather than their intent. Nurses and other professionals often use the term 'deliberate self-harm'. This can be misleading since the term 'deliberate' implies premeditation and wilfulness (Pembroke 1994). Indeed, self-harm is atypical, often spontaneous and not obviously preceded by awareness and conscious thought. The following definition of self-harm – which is now commonly accepted and which is used in this chapter – is from the National Institute for Health and Care Excellence (NICE) guidelines for the short-term physical and psychological management of self-harm in primary and secondary care (2004: 6):

Self-harm – 'self-poisoning or injury, irrespective of the apparent purpose of the act'.

How common is self-harm?

Ten years ago, there was concern that rates of self-harm in the UK had increased and were amongst the highest in Europe (NICE 2004). As many as 25,000 young people were presenting to general hospitals in England and Wales with problems involving self-harm, most having taken an overdose or cut themselves (Samaritans and Centre for Suicide Research 2002). This represented an increase of almost 30 per cent since the 1980s and repetition rates had doubled (Hawton *et al.* 2000). Though alarmingly high, these figures were far from representative. A large school survey of young people who self-harmed (Hawton *et al.* 2002) indicated that 1 in 15 self-harmed with most incidents not reaching the attention of services or professionals; only 12 per cent of episodes resulted in attending hospital. Ten years on, it is reported that the number of young people admitted to hospital for self-harm has increased by 68 per cent (Cello 2012).

The trend in suicide rates in the general population decreased in England between 1999 and 2008 from 10.1 per 100,000 to 8.2 per 100,000. However, since 2008, we have seen a gradual increase with the 2013 rate being 8.8 per 100,000 (see www.samaritans.org.uk for statistics on suicide). Childline report that 65 per cent of their referrals in 2013 were about suicide and that referrals about suicide from children aged 11 or younger had doubled from the previous year (NSPCC 2014). There are also significant differences in suicide rates according to race and cultural background. For example, the rate of suicide for young Asian women in England and Wales has been reported as three times that for women of white British origin (Raleigh and Balarajan 1992). These trends clearly demonstrate the urgent need to find effective ways to help distressed young people.

Why is self-harm common in young people?

Adolescence

Adolescence marks the transition from childhood to adulthood. It is a period when young people experiment, question and try to make sense of physical, emotional and social changes in their lives. Adolescence is a developmental phase during which time a number of significant tasks are usually on the way to being achieved. These include the attainment of independence, establishment of sexual orientation, self-control of aggressive and oppositional impulses and formation of identity. Peer groups often become more intense and are important in terms of influencing interests and behaviour. The age range that spans adolescence and the timing of specific developmental changes varies from one young person to the next.

Social context

As well as understanding the significance of self-harm in the context of adolescent development, it is also important to be aware of the social context in which young people harm themselves. For some young people, self-harm may be symptomatic of a serious mental health disorder such as depression (Pfeffer *et al.* 1991). For others, it may be the result of experimentation as part of adolescent identity and self-image (Anderson *et al.* 2004). A significant proportion of young people who self-harm experience difficulty in solving problems in non-destructive ways and may struggle to cope with difficult and intolerable feelings (McLaughlin *et al.* 1996). Such feelings may be generated by current or previous abuse or trauma, or they may be linked to problems with family, friends or school. Factors such as unwanted pregnancy, bullying, parents who argue, abuse, rape and bereavement have all been associated with self-harm (National Children's Home 2002). Self-harm by young people often occurs impulsively and with little thought about consequences. At other times, self-harm may be preceded by varying degrees of planning. It has been suggested that the media is responsible for perpetuating self-harm in young people. Various soap operas, artists and musicians have been criticised for increasing self-harm and suicide in young people.

A growing influence is that of social media, young people having 24/7 access to each other and the wider world being an integral part of their life. The negatives of this are the greater risk of bullying (i.e. cyberbullying) and sexual exploitation as well as sites advocating self-harm/suicide including posting of photos of injuries which can 'trigger' other young people to self-harm and social contagion. Social contagion occurs by means of social modelling/learning – young people with certain individual and/or psychiatric characteristics imitating self-harm through identification with others. Positives of social media include the many websites offering helpful advice and support, such as coping strategies and ideas to increase skills to manage emotions. Young people can also communicate their distress to friends/family immediately and access urgent help. The development of new technology such as BuddyApp (www.buddyapp.co.uk) offers resources that nurses can use to engage and help young people.

Whilst these issues may help increase our understanding about why young people self-harm, the thought that a child may want to die or harm themselves may be difficult for nurses to cope with. Until 1961 in the UK and 1993 in the Republic of Ireland, suicide was a criminal offence (Hill 1995). Some communities may therefore regard suicide as shameful and treat relatives of those who have killed themselves or who have attempted suicide accordingly. It is important for nurses to be aware that cultural issues may influence the young person's willingness to seek help.

National policy and guidelines

The Royal College of Psychiatrists (RCP) has produced council reports related to managing self-harm in young people (1982, 1998, 2014). These reports recommend that young people who self-harm with an acute presentation should be admitted to general hospital since the annual rate of repetition is higher for adolescents that are not admitted (Hawton and Fagg 1992). Despite the existence of national guidelines, a review of protocols for the management of self-harm by young people revealed that many services fail to implement the recommendations (Dorer 1998). These findings are consistent with the findings of Armstrong (1995), who explored the management of young people who self-harm. In this study, nine hospital departments and six GP practices were asked about their referral and treatment guidelines. The study found that only four services had formal guidelines. Although, more recently, NICE (2004, 2011) guidelines for the short-term and longer-term management of self-harm have been produced, there continues to be the same inconsistency and variation in practice that has been described previously (Department of Health 2014).

The prevention of suicide has also been the subject of national guidelines (NHS Health Advisory Service 1994; Department of Health 2002). These guidelines were followed by the current outcomes strategy *Preventing Suicide in England* (Department of Health 2012a), accompanied by an annual progress report (Department of Health 2014). These reports identify the need to reduce access to means of suicide, promote the responsible representation of suicidal behaviour by the media and provide better information and support to those bereaved and affected by suicide. From this, every local authority has a responsibility to produce a multi-agency strategy and framework for action to address local needs. Standard 9 of the *National Service Framework for Children, Young People and Maternity Services* (Department of Health 2004) also identified good practice applicable to self-harm. This included mental health promotion, early intervention, partnership working and easy access to local services. *No Health Without Mental Health* (Department of Health 2011) supports these practices and also includes an expectation of parity of service provision between physical and mental health.

Assessing young people who self-harm

National guidance provides nurses with evidence and standards for the assessment of all young people who self-harm (RCP 1998, 2014; NICE 2004, 2011). This can be applied across a range of settings by different professionals who work with young people. The development of MindEd, an e-learning portal that includes modules on assessing and managing risk in self-harm and suicidality (https://www.minded.org.uk/), allows easy access to much-needed training.

Nurses in primary care settings

School nurses, practice nurses in GP practices and youth workers as well as other primary care professionals come into contact with many young people who self-harm (Hawton *et al.* 2002). NICE (2004) guidelines recommend that primary care workers should assess the urgent physical and mental health needs of young people who have self-harmed during the previous 48-hour period. In the case of self-poisoning, primary care workers should refer the young person to the emergency department and also consider referral for other forms of self-harm such as cutting. If dealing with an acute presentation, referral of a young person to the emergency department will depend on the severity, intention and frequency of the self-harm. The need to inform parents or carers will need to be discussed with the young person. Sometimes referral to the emergency department is not made as the primary care worker's assessment is that risk is low and chronic and that the needs of the young person can be met more appropriately elsewhere. Where school nurses or other primary care workers suspect that a young person is harming themselves, they should consider discussing this with a colleague in a targeted/specialist child and adolescent mental health services (CAMHS) team. This may result in a formal consultation and the referral of the young person for a specialist CAMHS assessment.

Nurses in emergency departments

Overarching principles of the NICE (2004) guidelines for emergency departments include those shown in Box 8.2.

Box 8.2 NICE guidelines for self-harm in emergency departments

- Professionals should be respectful and understanding.

- Paediatric staff should undertake physical and mental health triage in a specific area for children and young people.

- Young people should normally be admitted to a general paediatric or adolescent hospital ward.

- Once admitted, a referral should be made to the specialist child and adolescent mental health service for a comprehensive psychosocial assessment in accordance with national (NICE) and locally agreed guidelines.

Source: adapted from NICE (2004).

Nurses in specialist CAMHS

Specialist CAMHS provide a comprehensive psychosocial risk assessment that involves talking with the young person individually, meeting with the parents or carers and then making a collaborative management plan. Specialist CAMHS professionals will consult with the paediatric team and, as necessary, social services, education and other agencies. The primary aim of the assessment is to engage the young person and family in a therapeutic process while also considering knowledge of risk factors, child protection issues and the needs of the young person. Information should be sought about the factors listed in Box 8.3.

> **Box 8.3 Important areas to cover in a self-harm assessment**
>
> - Family tree, including family physical/mental health problems
> - Peers, school and hobbies
> - Other agencies/professionals involved
> - Developmental history and sexual orientation
> - Physical health, mental wellbeing and history of abuse or neglect
> - Alcohol or substance misuse
> - Relationships, support systems, protective factors/resources
> - History of previous self-harm, including their knowledge of others who self-harm
> - Detailed account of presenting episode of self-harm, including precipitating factors, their intentions, how they feel now and if they think they are likely to do it again
> - Hopefulness and hopelessness
> - What the young person thinks needs to change to improve their situation.

Standardised risk assessment tools can be used to aid clinical assessment. However, risk assessment measures should not be used to decide whether a person is offered treatment or to predict future risk of self-harm (NICE 2004; RCP 2014). Details of the assessment and management plan should be clearly documented in the young person's case record. With appropriate consent, this plan should be communicated to all professionals and other workers involved in the young person's care, welfare and education. It is considered good practice to copy such letters to young people and their parents unless there are good defensible reasons why this would not be in their best interests (Department of Health 2000).

What does the research tell us about young people who self-harm?

A major systematic review of the efficacy of psychosocial and pharmacological treatments for the prevention of repetitive self-harm has been reported elsewhere (Hawton 1998). This meta-analysis evaluated a series of 20 randomised controlled trials (RCTs). However, only one study specifically involved adolescents (Cotgrove et al. 1995). This study assessed the value of readmission to hospital on demand and found that the intervention failed to have a positive effect. Since this systematic review took place, further studies have been published.

A RCT of home-based family intervention for young people who had self-poisoned did not result in better outcomes than the 'routine care' provided to the control group, though a moderate decrease in suicidal ideation was identified in the subgroup without major depression (Harrington et al. 1998). In this study, the term routine care was used to describe a diverse range of interventions provided in the hospital setting. Harrington et al. (2000) set out to explore why a brief family intervention worked well with some young people and not with others. Their follow-up results showed that improvements in the group of young people who were not depressed were not related to changes in family functioning. A nursing service in Glasgow has implemented an adapted version of this home-based intervention model (Fyfe and Dale 2002).

There have now been three RCTs measuring effectiveness of group therapy for adolescents who repeatedly harm themselves. The first (Wood *et al.* 2001) showed no reductions in levels of depression or suicidal thinking but did report reduced rates of self-harm. However, the sample size of this study was small and the confidence intervals were wide, which means up to 14 young people may need the group intervention before one is prevented from repeating. In contrast when this study was then repeated in Australia, more people repeated self-harm in the group treatment (Hazell *et al.* 2009). The third and largest RCT measured frequency of repeat self-harm and showed no added benefit of group work (Green *et al.* 2011).

Depression and measures of depressive behaviour are often core elements of quantitative research. This is because major depression is a strong predictor of outcome in relation to young people who harm themselves (Pfeffer *et al.* 1991). Hopelessness has been found to be another significant factor reported by young people who self-harm, even after the effects of depression have been taken into account (McLaughlin *et al.* 1996). This study also identified problem-solving difficulties in young people who harm themselves and suggested that this should be a focus for intervention.

Research on the use of cognitive behaviour therapy (CBT) with young adults has suggested that this intervention is no more effective than 'routine care' in reducing depression, hopelessness and suicidal ideation (Linehan *et al.* 1991). Dialectical behaviour therapy (DBT) is used to help adults and, more recently, adolescents who engage in repetitive self-harm and is associated with helping people who have borderline (and emerging) personality characteristics (Linehan 1993; Miller *et al.* 2007). DBT is designed to help people learn skills to cope with life stresses and to understand and resist their urges to self-harm.

Impulsiveness also seems to be a key factor. In a follow-up study of 48 young people who had attempted suicide, Keinhorst *et al.* (1995) suggested that suicidal behaviour in young people was commonly a 'phasic' desire for relief rather than a reasoned and long-standing decision. Hence the importance in follow-up of trying to reduce impulsive behaviour since delaying self-harm by half an hour may be sufficient to implement an alternative safer strategy and therefore prevent a potential suicide attempt. During this crucial (impulsive) period, the reduction of access to tablets through the safe storage of medicines is also known to assist in the prevention of overdoses by young people (Hawton *et al.* 2004).

Mentalisation is a promising new treatment; a 12-month programme rooted in attachment theory has currently been shown to reduce self-harm and depression in adolescents (Rossouw and Fonagy 2012). Other intervention studies are currently underway (e.g. in relation to remote CBT; see the UK Clinical Trials Gateway, www.ukctg.nihr.ac.uk). It is also recognised that a high-quality mental health risk and needs assessment is an important intervention that can reduce repetition and aid recovery in itself (Kapur *et al.* 2013). Additionally, a recent multicentre trial concluded that cutting conveyed a greater risk of future suicide than poisoning/overdose, though different methods are usually used for suicide (Hawton *et al.* 2012).

What do young people tell us about self-harm?

Various consultation exercises have been undertaken to elicit young people's views about the services they receive. A project for young people aged between 13 and 25 in Leeds sought to understand the factors that make services for self-harm effective (Neill 2003). Confidentiality, having choice and being respected were identified as important factors. In a further study with young people aged between 15 and 25 that looked at their views of self-harm services (Spandler 1996), a key theme was the need for control, both of the self-harm and of the meaning this had for the young person. Young people explained that when control was taken away from them, this often felt like abuse. This had the paradoxical effect of the young person harming themselves more.

A qualitative study by Le Surf and Lynch (1999) set out to understand the perceptions and attitudes of young people towards counselling. The need for confidentiality, as highlighted by Neill (2003), was a consistent theme. This was often associated with stigma and the effects of having counselling as well as a deeper experience of shamefulness. This implies that young people often may not want others to know they are having counselling for their self-harm.

Overall, the evidence of what works for young people who self-harm suggests that a good service should involve a number of factors, and these are presented in Box 8.4.

Box 8.4 Good practice in working with young people who self-harm

- Removal of easy access and safe storage of medication
- Identifying and treating depression
- Identifying and responding to hopelessness and impulsivity
- Strategies to enhance problem-solving
- Developing skills and alternative coping strategies
- Maintaining confidentiality
- Enabling choice
- Respect and a non-judgemental approach
- Collaboration in safety planning rather than over-control
- Addressing stigma and shame.

Young people continue to feel that professionals, including teachers and GPs, either overreact to self-harm or trivialise it; and professionals often feel they lack the skill and confidence in dealing with self-harm (Cello 2012). Since problems surrounding self-harm are diverse, it is important that nurses adapt the above markers of good practice according to the needs of the young person at any one time.

Child and adolescent mental health nursing

The role and function of mental health nurses has generated much debate with mental health nursing going through a significant period of change (Jackson and Stevenson 2000). Schon (1987) observed a move away from a practical, task-orientated role towards reflexive involvement with patients. Michael (1994) suggests that this shift has made it more difficult for nurses to recognise and define their role. This is because working alongside patients means their skills have become less visible. A focus group study facilitated by Jackson and Stevenson (2000) asked nearly 100 participants to explore what people need mental health nurses for. Their results indicated that service users valued nurses who were able to move across domains and dimensions in response to need. The focus groups reported that nurses were experienced by service users as both a friend and a professional.

Mental health training requires nurses to spend significant periods of time with patients and fosters closeness and an approach to mental health care that is different to that of other professionals such as psychiatrists (Baldwin 2002). The role of nurses in CAMHS is not well defined in the literature, despite concerns that such a lack of clarity may lead to the loss of the role (McMorrow 1995). The unique contribution that nurses make remains undefined but implicitly accepted. Indeed, they are considered to be core members of the CAMHS multidisciplinary team (NHS Health Advisory Service 1995). Nurses in CAMHS take a holistic stance, seeing the young person as a whole and recognising that the child and family needs are broad and varied. This insight is enabled by nurses' well-developed communication skills and ability to engage with young people and their families. Like all areas of nursing, implementing standards set out in *Compassion in Practice* (Department of Health 2012b) is fundamental for CAMHS nursing.

Vignettes

So how does this translate into nursing young people who self-harm? The case vignettes in this section illustrate how self-harm can represent a range of meanings. Each vignette focuses on different nursing interventions that are used to help young people and their families or carers. It is intended that these descriptions of practice go some way to depicting part of the essence of child and adolescent mental health nursing.

Ann

Ann, aged 15, is a dual-heritage white/black Caribbean British girl who has taken an overdose of 28 paracetamol tablets. Ann was assessed by a CAMHS nurse on a general paediatric ward in accordance with national and local guidelines. The overdose had been precipitated by a recent disclosure of sexual abuse and a family bereavement. Ann reported that she had been feeling down for a couple of weeks and believed that she did not have much to live for.

Nursing is in part about 'being' with a person. A fundamental component of all interventions with young people is to establish a good therapeutic relationship. In order to understand Ann's self-harming behaviour, the nurse sought first to understand what it was like to be Ann. The nurse aimed to make Ann feel at ease by listening to her thoughts and feelings and encouraged her to share her distress and fears. The better the knowledge about a young person is, the better the risk assessment becomes.

Prior to asking detailed questions about self-harm, the nurse collected some background information about family and friends, school and other professionals who were involved. Brief assessments of mood and mental state were also undertaken. In order to understand Ann's self-harming behaviour, a series of questions were used to explore the overdose, assess risk and inform the intervention strategy:

- How much medication was accessible/available/taken?
- Were drugs or alcohol involved? If so, which drugs or alcohol and how much?
- Was the overdose planned or impulsive?
- Was the overdose taken whilst the young person was alone? If not, who was present?
- How much does the young person know about the lethality/harmful effects of the overdose?
- Was a suicide note written or were there texts/messages left on social media?

- Did the young person tell anyone before or after the overdose?
- Is the young person regretful or disappointed to be alive?
- Would the young person take another overdose?
- Is the young person planning to take another overdose?
- How hopeful/hopeless does the young person feel about the future?

Involving the parents or carers of young people who self-harm

Parents sometimes have a different understanding than their child about why the self-harm has occurred. Ann's mother strongly believed that her daughter's disclosure of sexual abuse explained the self-harm. Ann herself thought that recent changes in family relationships were more significant. The disclosure of sexual abuse can generate many strong emotions in parents such as anger, guilt and shame (Jones 2003). After meeting her, the nurse became aware that Ann's mother also needed support and arranged this with a local voluntary organisation. Ann was clear that she wanted her session work to remain confidential. Whilst she did not want anyone at school to know about her overdose, Ann gave permission for the nurse to inform the GP about the overdose and ongoing support. Ann accepted that her mother had a duty to ensure she was safe. The nurse explained to Ann's mother that most overdoses by young people are impulsive, and the importance of safe storage of medicines was discussed.

The importance of follow-up

By asking Ann a series of questions about her intentions and thoughts and feelings before, during and after the overdose, it is possible to form an opinion about risk. After interviewing Ann, the nurse assessed the risk of further self-harm as medium and the risk of suicide as low. One of the aims of the assessment was to enable Ann to feel more hopeful about the future than she was at the time of the overdose. During the interview, it became apparent that Ann had high expectations of herself and rarely allowed herself to feel sad, upset or angry. Giving a young person permission to cry and acknowledging their feelings in a safe and supportive environment can be both validating and liberating for them. All young people who self-harm should be given at least one follow-up appointment in which to review their risks and needs. Ann has fortnightly sessions to discuss her thoughts, feelings and fears and has not harmed herself further.

Sue

Sue, aged 16, is a white British girl who took five diazepam tablets to sleep for a prolonged period. She had no intention of killing herself. Sue has a two-year history of cutting her arms and legs, and she described feeling unloved by her family who have multiple social problems. Her attendance at school was poor, and Sue left school with no qualifications. After briefly attending college, Sue dropped out and was told to leave the family home. At this time, she began to regularly get drunk and engaged in petty crime. The Police and Youth Offending Team became involved.

When Sue was assessed by the nurse specialist, it became apparent that many of Sue's peer group were involved in self-harming behaviour. She has previously cut herself at the same time as her friends; she believes they are supportive and understand how she feels. This was in contrast to some of the adults and professionals who Sue had encountered who had 'disapproved' of her cutting. One of the biggest challenges faced by young people who self-harm is the stigma and negative attitudes they can encounter. This is addressed in the NICE (2004) guidelines on self-harm, which state that people who self-harm should be treated with the same care, respect and privacy as any patient whilst taking into account the likelihood of their additional distress.

Reducing self-harm through alternative coping strategies

After the nurse had completed an initial assessment of mental state and risk, Sue reported that she wanted help to stop cutting herself. Cutting can be compared to other behaviours, such as smoking, eating or exercising, in that a person has to want to change their behaviour or they will continue as before. Even if a young person wants to change their self-harming behaviour, it is important to remember that this may be difficult. When cutting has developed as a coping strategy over a long period of time, young people may need help to identify and use different coping strategies. In the meantime, young people are likely to continue to self-harm. Whilst the nurse would never condone or encourage self-harm, it is important to be non-judgemental and understanding. Sue and the nurse met again for several sessions. This was to help Sue better understand the situations and triggers that precipitated her cutting. Sue used a diary to help her remember the circumstances that had led her to cut. This assisted the nurse in recognising patterns and identifiable triggers for self-harm.

Working as part of a specialist CAMHS team can bring a wealth of experience and knowledge about young people who self-harm. Whilst maintaining confidentiality, this breath of experience can often be shared to benefit young people who self-harm. Sue appeared to gain hope and confidence from knowing that other young people had been able to reduce or stop cutting. This was a belief that was shared by Sue and the nurse throughout their sessions. As well as identifying risk situations that appeared to trigger cutting, a range of alternative coping strategies were discussed and explored by Sue. These included distraction techniques, ventilating emotions and the use of alternative or safer pain, which are methods described as helpful by people who self-harm (The Crisis Recovery Unit 1998). Sue decided to combine several components of these strategies, which involved her leaving the house, having a freezing shower and blasting her music when faced with a situation which made her want to cut. Some young people who self-harm report that snapping an elastic band on the wrist, tightly holding ice cubes and snapping wood are ways of inflicting less severe pain or discomfort on themselves. Some young people also draw on themselves with a red marker pen or use ketchup or red food colouring to replicate self-harm in a way that is less destructive and permanent than cutting.

The cutting continued while Sue was being supported to use alternative coping strategies, though it did become less frequent. As recommended by the NICE guidance on self-harm, the nurse provided advice about harm minimisation. Sue was advised against cutting using broken glass to reduce the risk of infection and scarring. Education about first aid was provided, and the need to have access to clean wound care supplies was recommended. A harm minimisation approach needs to be used in conjunction with understanding the underlying issues and meaning of self-harm. During the course of treatment, it became apparent that the social and family factors that made Sue feel sad were unlikely to change. The focus of therapeutic sessions was therefore to enable Sue to identify a positive future and support her in achieving independence. The nurse supported Sue in making a housing application, made links with Connexions in order for her to return to college and arranged transport for appointments. Noticing positive changes and rewarding these with praise and encouragement made notable differences to Sue's self-esteem.

Jackie

Jackie, aged 13, is a British black Caribbean girl. Although this is her first admission to hospital after an overdose of codeine, the assessment reveals that Jackie has taken several small overdoses and has cut herself on numerous occasions. Jackie is unclear about why she took the six tablets. She reports feeling unhappy, hates herself and does not want to live any more. Jackie feels that life is a struggle but cannot think of any particular reason why. She describes a need to punish herself and reports that self-harm helps her release tension. She does not like being at home or school and has recently begun to truant. Jackie is offered individual sessions to explore the reasons why she is unhappy and self-harming. It soon becomes apparent that there are family relationship problems and that Jackie often gets angry, refuses to talk or runs away for short periods.

In terms of adolescent development, it is important to remember that adolescents do not have the breadth of life experiences to draw on. Their personalities are developing and they do not put things into perspective the way adults might be able to do. Jackie, like many young people her age, was struggling with the developmental task of controlling her emotions and constructing her self-identity (Hoare 1993; Anderson et al. 2004).

Family therapy

Although Jackie did not initially want her parents involved in her follow-up care, the nurse enabled her to recognise that their involvement was crucial to therapeutic change. Had Jackie continued to refuse to share her self-harm with her parents, the nurse would have weighted up her rights to confidentiality and risks of significant harm and, if needed, overridden confidentiality and informed her parents.

Jackie did not initially want to engage in family therapy, and working with young people in a collaborative way is a key function of the nursing role. This involves supporting them in decision-making and in planning and evaluating the care programme. Inevitably, there may be different views about the usefulness of family therapy between the young person, their parents and the nurse. This was addressed by explaining the process in advance, visiting the room in which family therapy takes place and talking about the one-way screen and observation suite.

In the first session, Jackie said nothing at all. However, she heard other family members say things she had never heard before and managed to stay in the room. As the sessions progressed, family members developed a growing understanding of each other. Where rigid beliefs had become entrenched, these were replaced with new meanings and explanations. Jackie's 'bad' behaviour, previously met with hostility and criticism, became understood as a sign of distress and was met with care and compassion. One positive change led to another and as well as a general improvement in family relationships, Jackie's self-esteem and confidence increased. Self-harm rarely featured during the family therapy; instead, the focus was on improving relationships and enhancing communication.

Ben

Ben, aged 14, is a white British boy who took an overdose of 80 paracetamol tablets with the clear intention of dying. The overdose was discovered when Ben was heard vomiting by his younger brother. It was two weeks before he was medically fit to be assessed by the nurse specialist from the CAMHS team. This was because the possibility of a liver transplant was being discussed by the paediatric team. When Ben recovered sufficiently, his story was clear. He was intimidated by a local gang and feared for his life. Ben made a decision to kill himself before the bullies killed him. Ben's family were distraught but shared Ben's fears as their house had been vandalised and a window had recently been smashed.

Therapeutic relationships

Fear often features in young people's accounts of their self-harming behaviour. This can be generated by a number of factors including bullying, exam stress or abuse. It was fundamentally important to Ben that the nurse created a plan where Ben felt safe, protected and supported. In order to help him feel safe, Ben was initially encouraged to bring one of his parents to the sessions. After just a few sessions, he felt more relaxed and reassured that the nurse understood his fears and was there to help him.

Part of establishing a therapeutic relationship involves decisions by the nurse about how much self-disclosure is appropriate. Ben asked the nurse whether she had children and if they had been bullied. In keeping with the theory of practice where nurses move across domains of intimate friend and knowledgeable professional (Jackson and Stevenson 2000), the sharing of personal information can sometimes be appropriate and helpful. Initially, Ben did not feel safe to leave his house, so sessions with the nurse took place in the family home. Flexibility about where to see young people can increase their control and responsibility and is an important part of the collaborative therapeutic process. After initially meeting at Ben's house, his confidence improved and he utilised and valued the support of his family and friends. Ben became more socially included and joined clubs outside of his immediate neighbourhood. In time, Ben was able to reflect on his overdose and felt confident that he could keep himself safe when faced with difficult situations.

The importance of clinical supervision

Clinical supervision is essential for the provision of safe and accountable nursing practice and the governance of CAMHS. It is important that nurses who work with young people who self-harm have regular clinical supervision. This is to ensure their practice is safe and effective and so that the nurse remains up to date and professionally accountable for their work. Supervision can take many forms and can take place across a range of settings. Nurses can receive supervision individually, in groups and from nurses or other colleagues with understanding of the key issues in relation to young people and self-harm. Ben's nurse discussed his case with the CAMHS multi-disciplinary team. This provided evidence-based reflection on practice, helped to develop a case management plan and supported the nurse in the individual work he was doing with Ben.

Conclusion

Self-harm by young people is increasing. The vignettes illustrate that self-harm is heterogeneous and means different things to different people. The chapter provides an overview of national strategy and research evidence in relation to the assessment and management of self-harm, and describes a range of interventions to support young people, their families or carers. Whilst notoriously difficult to articulate, the chapter attempts to capture some of the essence of nursing care. Theoretical concepts such as care and compassion are defined in terms of practical interventions and psychological approaches that nurses can undertake in order to engage, help and support young people who self-harm. Of fundamental importance is the message that to help any young person who self-harms, the nurse must understand, communicate this understanding and create a therapeutic alliance, which is the bedrock for change. A range of nursing skills such as the ability to listen, to be accepting and to appropriately use self-disclosure are identified as crucial in terms of helping young people who self-harm.

References

Anderson, M., Woodward, L. and Armstrong, M. (2004) Self-harm in young people: a perspective for mental health nursing. *International Nursing Review*, 51(4): 222–8.

Armstrong, M. (1995) *The Management of Self-harm in Children and Adolescents*. University of Lancaster [unpublished thesis].

Baldwin, L. (2002) The nursing role in out-patient child and adolescent mental health services. *Journal of Clinical Nursing*, 11(4): 520–5.

Cello (2012) *Talking Self-harm: Talking Taboos*. London: Cello and YoungMinds.

Crisis Recovery Unit, The (1998) *Working with the Work: Our Approach to Working with Individuals who Self Harm, Based on Our Experience* [unpublished]. South London and Maudsley NHS Trust.

Cotgrove, A., Zirinsky, L., Black, D. and Weston, D. (1995) Secondary prevention of attempted suicide in adolescents. *Journal of Adolescence*, 18(5): 569–77.

Department of Health (2014) *Preventing Suicide in England: One Year On. First Annual Report on the Cross-government Outcomes Strategy to Save Lives*. London: Department of Health.

Department of Health (2012a) *Preventing Suicide in England: A Cross-government Outcomes Strategy to Save Lives*. London: Department of Health.

Department of Health (2012b) *Compassion in Practice. Nursing, Midwifery and Care Staff: Our Vision and Strategy*. London: Department of Health.

Department of Health (2011) *No Health Without Mental Health: A Cross-government Mental Health Outcomes Strategy across All Ages*. London: Department of Health.

Department of Health (2004) *National Service Framework for Children, Young People and Maternity Services*. London: Department of Health.

Department of Health (2002) *National Suicide Prevention Strategy for England*. London: Department of Health.

Department of Health (2000) *The NHS Plan: A Plan for Investment: A Plan for Reform*. Cm 4818-I. London: The Stationery Office.

Dorer, C. (1998) An evaluation of protocols for child and adolescent deliberate self harm. *Child Psychology and Psychiatry Review*, 3(4): 156–60.

Fyfe, M. and Dale, M. (2002) Hope in the city. *Mental Health Practice*, 5(6): 18–21.

Green, J., Wood, A., Kerfoot, M., Trainor, G., Roberts, C., Rothwell, J., Woodham, A., Ayodeji, E., Barrett, B., Byford, S. and Harrington, R. (2011) Group therapy for adolescents with repeated self-harm: randomised control trial with economic evaluation. *British Medical Journal*, 342: d682.

Harrington, R., Kerfoot, M., Dyer, E., McNiven, F., Gill, J., Harrington, V. and Woodham, A. (2000) Deliberate self-poisoning in adolescence: why does a brief family intervention work in some cases and not others? *Journal of Adolescence*, 23(1): 13–20.

Harrington, R., Kerfoot, M., Dyer, R., McNiven, F., Gill, J., Harrington, V., Woodham, A. and Byford, S. (1998) Randomised trial of home-based family intervention for children who have deliberately poisoned themselves. *Journal of American Academy of Child and Adolescent Psychiatry*, 37(5): 512–18.

Hawton, K. (1998) Deliberate self-harm: systematic review of efficacy of psychosocial and pharmacological treatments in preventing repetition. *British Medical Journal*, 317 (15 August): 441–7.

Hawton, K. and Fagg, J. (1992) Deliberate self-poisoning and injury in adolescents: a study of characteristics and trends in Oxford 1976–1989. *British Journal of Psychiatry*, 161(6): 816–23.

Hawton, K., Bergen, H., Kapur, N., Cooper, J., Steeg, S., Ness, J. and Waters, K. (2012) Repetition of self-harm and suicide following self-harm in children and adolescents: findings from the Multicentre Study of Self-harm in England. *Journal of Child Psychology and Psychiatry*, 53(12): 1212–19.

Hawton, K., Simkin, S., Deeks, J., Cooper, J., Johnston, A., Waters, K., Arundel, M., Bernal, W., Gunson, B., Hudson, M., Suri, D. and Simpson, K. (2004) UK Legislation on analgesic packs: before and after study of long term effect on poisonings. *British Medical Journal*, 329(7474): 1076–9.

Hawton, K., Rodham, K., Evans, E. and Weatherall, R. (2002) Deliberate self harm in adolescents: self report survey in schools in England. *British Medical Journal*, 325(7374): 1207–11.

Hawton, K., Fagg, J., Simkin, S., Bale, E. and Bond, A. (2000) Deliberate self-harm in adolescents in Oxford: 1985–1995. *Journal of Adolescence*, 23(1): 47–55.

Hazell, P., Martin, G., McGill, K., Kay, T., Wood, A., Trainor, G. and Harrington, R. (2009) Group therapy for repeated self-harm in adolescents: failure of replication of a randomised trial. *Journal of the American Academy of Child and Adolescent Psychiatry*, 48(6): 662–70.

Hill, K. (1995) *The Long Sleep: Young People and Suicide*. London: Virago.

Hoare, P. (1993) *Essential Child Psychiatry*. New York: Churchill Livingstone.

Jackson, S. and Stevenson, C. (2000) What do people need psychiatric and mental health nurses for? *Journal of Advanced Nursing*, 31(2): 378–88.

Jones, D. (2003) *Communicating with Vulnerable Children: A Guide for Practitioners*. London: Gaskell.

Kapur, N., Steeg, S., Webb, R., Haigh, M., Bergen, H., Hawton, K., Ness, J., Waters, K. and Cooper, J. (2013) Does clinical management improve outcomes following self-harm? Results from the Multicentre Study of Self-harm in England. *PLOS ONE*, 8(8): e70434.

Kerfoot, M. (2000) Youth suicide and deliberate self-harm. In P. Aggleton, J., Hurry and I. Warwick (eds) *Young People and Mental Health*. Chichester: John Wiley and Sons Ltd, pp. 111–29.

Kienhorst, I., De Wilde, E., Diekstra, R. and Wolters, W. (1995) Adolescents' image of their suicide attempt. *Journal of the American Academy of Child and Adolescent Psychiatry*, 34(3): 623–8.

Le Surf, A. and Lynch, G. (1999) Exploring young people's perceptions relevant to counselling: a qualitative study. *British Journal of Guidance and Counselling*, 27(2): 231–43.

Linehan, M. (1993) *Cognitive-behavioural Treatment of Borderline Personality Disorder*. New York: Guilford.

Linehan, M., Armstrong, H., Suarez, A., Allmon, D. and Heard, H. (1991) Cognitive behavioural treatment of chronically parasuicidal borderline patients. *Archives of General Psychiatry*, 48(12): 1060–4.

McLaughlin, J., Miller, P. and Warwick, H. (1996) Deliberate self-harm in adolescents: hopelessness, depression, problems and problem-solving. *Journal of Adolescence*, 19(6): 523–32.

McMorrow, R. (1995) An eclectic model of care: the role of the community psychiatric nurse in child psychiatry. *Child Health*, 3(3): 95–8.

Michael, S. (1994) Invisible skills. *Journal of Psychiatry and Mental Health Nursing*, 1(5): 56.

Miller, A. L., Rathus J. H. and Linehan, M. M. (2007) *Dialectic Behaviour Therapy with Suicidal Adolescents*. New York: The Guilford Press.

National Children's Home (2002) *Look Beyond the Scars: Understanding and Responding to Self-harm*. London: National Children's Home.

National Institute for Health and Care Excellence (NICE) (2011) *Self-harm: Longer-term Management (CG133)*. Manchester: NICE.

National Institute for Health and Care Excellence (NICE) (2004) *Self-harm in Over 8s: Short-term Management and Prevention of Recurrence (CG16)*. Manchester: NICE.

Neill, L. (2003) Market forces: listening to what young people want. *YoungMinds Magazine*, 62: 20–2.

NHS Health Advisory Service (1995) *Child and Adolescent Mental Health Services. Together We Stand: The Commissioning, Role and Management of Child and Adolescent Mental Health Services*. London: HMSO.

NHS Health Advisory Service (1994) *The Challenge Confronted: Suicide Prevention*. London: HMSO.

NSPCC (2014) *On the Edge. ChildLine Spotlight: Suicide*. London: NSPCC.

Pembroke, L. (ed.) (1994) *Self-harm: Perspectives from Personal Experience*. London: Survivors Speak Out.

Pfeffer, C., Klerman, G., Hunt, S., Lesser, M., Peskin, J. and Siefker, A. (1991) Suicidal children grown up: demographic and clinical risk factors for adolescent suicide attempts. *Journal of the American Academy of Child Psychiatry*, 30(4): 609–16.

Raleigh, V. and Balajaran, R. (1992) Suicide and self-burning among Indians and West Indians in England and Wales. *British Journal of Psychiatry*, 161(3): 365–8.

Rossouw, T. I. and Fonagy, P. (2012) Mentalization-based treatment for self-harm in adolescents: a randomised control trial. *Journal of the American Academy of Child and Adolescent Psychiatry*, 51(12): 1304–13.

Royal College of Psychiatrists (RCP) (2014) *Managing Self-harm in Young People (CR192)*. London: RCP.

Royal College of Psychiatrists RCP (1998) *Managing Deliberate Self-harm in Young People (CR64)*. London: RCP.

Royal College of Psychiatrists RCP (1982) The management of parasuicide in young people under sixteen. *Psychiatric Bulletin*, 6(10): 182–5.

Samaritans and Centre for Suicide Research (2002) *Youth and Self-harm: Perspectives*. Oxford: University of Oxford.

Schon, D. (1987) *Educating the Reflexive Practitioner*. San Francisco: Jossey-Bass.

Spandler, H. (1996) *Who's Hurting Who? Young People, Self-harm and Suicide*. Manchester: 42nd Street.

Wood, A., Trainor, G., Rothwell, J., Moore, A. and Harrington, R. (2001) Randomised trial of group therapy for repeated deliberate self-harm in adolescents. *Journal of American Academy of Child and Adolescent Psychiatry*, 40(11): 1246–53.

Chapter 9

Nursing children and young people with eating disorders

Tim McDougall

Key points:

- Eating disorders tend to get worse if they are not treated; without help, children and young people place both their physical and mental health at risk. The sooner a young person starts evidence-based treatment for an eating disorder, the better the outcome. Evidence-based interventions can reduce the need for inpatient admission, improve the process of recovery and reduce relapse rates.
- Anorexia nervosa is a serious, life-threatening illness with one of the highest mortality rates of any psychiatric disorder. Children and young people with this condition have an extreme fear of being fat and suffer from distorted body perception and a range of related psychological difficulties.
- Bulimia nervosa is characterised by a cycle of starving and bingeing. Unlike the obvious weight loss that occurs in anorexia nervosa, young people with bulimia nervosa may not look overweight or underweight. As the bingeing and purging associated with bulimia nervosa is often a private activity, it can often go unnoticed by nurses and other professionals.
- Eating disorders can negatively affect families and carers, both intra-personally and socio-economically. Parents or carers may be required to make changes to work or family life in order to care for their child or young person. Eating disorders can also disrupt family functioning and activities, and they may have a significant effect on siblings. It is therefore essential that nurses understand the potential dynamics and dilemmas involved and that they take a family-based approach to care and treatment.
- Nurses and other professionals need to be able to respond to the broader needs of families and carers as well as to the child or young person with an eating disorder. This may include supporting parents with strategies to help manage their child's eating or providing information about eating disorders and access to specialist services.
- A number of evidence-based resources exist to guide nursing practice. These include National Institute for Health and Care Excellence guidelines, quality standards and the MARSIPAN guidance on the management of children and young people with anorexia nervosa.

Introduction

In her chapter on eating disorders, Lewer (2006) suggests that nursing young people with these conditions is a challenging experience that demands incredible curiosity, patience, persistence, resilience and humour. Ramjan (2004) concurs, pointing out that nurses caring for adolescents with eating disorders face a particular set of problems in seeking to establish therapeutic relationships and in navigating such issues as power and control struggles and overcoming despair and hopelessness.

Nurses and other professionals work with children and adolescents with eating disorders in a variety of practice settings. Whether this is in hospital, at home or in the community, they encounter young people with anorexia nervosa, bulimia nervosa and other difficulties with eating. This chapter explores the two most common eating disorders and discusses the role of nurses in recognising and supporting young people to recover. The role of clinical guidelines and quality standards in guiding best practice is also discussed.

Background

Eating is influenced by a combination of individual, social and cultural factors. As well as how we are feeling, our appetite, the views of friends and family, religious beliefs and customs all affect eating. Eating occurs in a social context where young people are high users of social media. This has been linked to appearance comparison and internalisation of body image ideals (Bell and Dittmar 2011; Gallagher et al. 2015). The impact of the media on adolescent eating disorders is closely associated with body image, self-esteem and weight reduction behaviours (Ahern et al. 2008). It is in the popular media where young people are likely to form their views about the 'ideal' image and how they should be, and it is social media where responses to those who do not fit the ideal image or happen to be different are played out – sometimes with serious or devastating consequences. The fashion industry is regularly criticised for portraying ultra-thin young women as models for clothes and make-up. However, it is the values, attitudes and beliefs that lie behind such campaigns that are the most difficult to tackle.

Children in hospital who are living away from family and friends may go off food, be selective about what they eat or simply refuse to eat at all. Nurses who work with children and young people in hospital will have experienced those who struggle with eating, and this is not unusual. Feeling ill causes a loss of appetite, and the unfamiliar hospital surroundings bring uncertainty and a change of routine. Food may be strange and eaten at different times to what the child or young person is used to. Some children eat more or less than usual if they are worried, anxious or depressed. Temporary changes in eating behaviour are not in themselves part of an eating disorder. Rather, they are likely to occur as part of a change of routine or trauma and will usually resolve without intervention. It is also common for children to go through food fads and for adolescents to go on diets. These transient episodes are not usually cause for concern.

What are eating disorders?

Eating disorders are involuntary, complex and sometimes life-threatening illnesses involving an unhealthy and unconventional view of and relationship with food, weight and shape. The most common eating disorders are anorexia nervosa and bulimia nervosa, and this chapter explores both. Obesity is also an eating disorder, but this is not usually regarded as a specific mental health problem. Studies have found anorexia nervosa to be the third most common chronic illness of adolescence, affecting 0.5 per cent of adolescent girls. Bulimia nervosa is slightly more common with a prevalence rate of 1 per cent, but the secretive nature of the disorder and young people's ambivalence about seeking help means that rates are likely to be higher (Nicholls and Viner 2005).

Eating disorders usually emerge during adolescence and often persist into adulthood, particularly in the absence of help and support for the sufferer. Eating disorders such as anorexia nervosa and bulimia nervosa are much more common in girls (Gowers *et al.* 2000), but boys also suffer (Kjelsas *et al.* 2004). In the UK in 2009, the highest incidence of both anorexia nervosa and bulimia nervosa was for girls aged 15–19 (Micali *et al.* 2013).

Eating disorders are often complex, and there is often variation in signs and symptoms. Indeed, it is not uncommon for young people to have a mixture of anorexia nervosa, bulimia nervosa and binge eating difficulties. Despite the high incidence of eating disorders in children and young people, very little has been written about nursing practice and care for this group (Halek 1997).

Anorexia nervosa

Whilst often used interchangeably, 'anorexia' and 'anorexia nervosa' are not the same thing, which can cause confusion. Whilst anorexia literally means loss of appetite, anorexia nervosa is a serious, life-threatening illness with one of the highest mortality rates of any psychiatric disorder (Gowers *et al.* 2000). Children and young people with this disorder have an extreme fear of being fat and an overwhelming drive to starve themselves in a relentless pursuit of thinness. Reporting on the phenomenon of self-starvation, O'Hara (2013) comments that admiration for the ascetic control of one's body and using food restriction to withdraw from an 'evil material world' has been observed and documented throughout history and across cultures.

Anorexia nervosa is characterised by a number of physical, behavioural and psychological changes. Severe weight loss, amenorrhoea (periods stopping), abdominal pain and dizziness are all physical signs that a young person may be anorexic. Their behaviour may also change. Wearing baggy clothes to disguise weight loss and being secretive about eating behaviour may indicate that the child is unhappy about their body image and may be seeking control. Over-exercising and using laxatives to induce fat and water loss are other ways in which young people attempt to control their weight.

Most of the physical complications associated with anorexia nervosa are directly caused by starvation, malnutrition and dehydration. Other physical changes may be less immediately obvious but are nonetheless concerning. Calorie restriction over a prolonged period can lead to widespread physiological disturbance. Hormonal and endocrinal changes are associated with a range of cardiovascular, gastrointestinal and gynaecological problems.

When a young person experiences severe weight loss, their body introduces a range of survival mechanisms. Young people with anorexia nervosa may complain of feeling cold and experience numbness in their feet and hands. This is caused by low body temperature, poor circulation and a lack of body fat to act as insulation. In extreme cases, this weight loss can lead to hypothermia or death (Lewer 2006). There are a number of cardiovascular complications associated with extreme low weight. These include bradycardia, T-wave inversions and ST segment depression. Additionally, arrhythmias and tachycardia can occur, which is why physical monitoring is essential.

Onset of anorexia nervosa before puberty can result in delayed growth. In older children, damage to internal organs and the risk of infertility increases into adult life. Young people with anorexia nervosa are particularly prone to develop osteoporosis (brittle bones). This is because peak bone density and strength develop during the period of adolescence, when bones are growing most. Disruption to nutritional and mineral metabolism before puberty and during the teenage years can lead to a range of other problems in adult life.

Table 9.1 Signs and symptoms of anorexia nervosa

Physical	Behavioural	Psychological
Extreme weight loss	Wearing baggy or oversized clothes	Mood swings and depression
Malnutrition		Impaired concentration
Dry or rough skin	Over-exercising	Preoccupation with body shape and size
Hormonal changes	Self-induced vomiting	
Delay in onset of puberty	Use of laxatives or diuretics	Intense feeling of being fat
Amenorrhoea	Water loading	Difficulty discerning hunger from satiety
Stomach ache or constipation	Social isolation	
Tiredness and lethargy	Decreased sexual interest	Heightened senses
Feeling cold	Self-harm	
Cyanosis	Suicidal behaviour	
Osteoporosis		
Lanugo (an increase in fine hair on the body)		
Cardiovascular abnormalities		
Hypotension		

Lewer (2006) reminds us that psychological signs and symptoms of anorexia nervosa can be difficult to detect. Young people often go to great lengths to mask their feelings and weight loss behaviours in an attempt to hide their eating disorder. Since the majority of interpersonal communication is non-verbal, it is important that nurses use their range of interpersonal skills to observe how young people behave.

Anorexia nervosa is characterised by a number of physical, behavioural and psychological changes, which nurses should watch out for and monitor if they are concerned (see Table 9.1).

Bulimia nervosa

The average age of onset for bulimia nervosa is 18, and the prevalence in adolescent girls has been estimated at 1 in 200. Bulimia nervosa is rare in children aged under 12 (Lask and Bryant-Waugh 2000). As with all eating disorders, children with bulimia nervosa use food in an attempt to cope with problems they may be struggling with. Bulimia nervosa is characterised by a cycle of starving and bingeing.

As with anorexia nervosa, young people who are bulimic may deny there is a problem or be evasive about their eating behaviour. Unlike the evident weight loss in anorexia nervosa, however, young people with bulimia nervosa may not look overweight or underweight. This makes the disorder even harder for nurses and other professionals to recognise. House and colleagues (2012) recommend that additional proactive measures are needed to improve case identification and early intervention for young people with bulimia nervosa so that they can be supported to access help.

One of the most obvious behaviours that indicate a young person may be bulimic is bingeing. This involves them eating large quantities of food in a short period of time, after which they may go to the toilet to make themselves sick. As this is a private activity, it can often go unnoticed by nurses and other professionals. Young people who eat compulsively may be depressed, feel out of control or seek comfort through eating. Weight

Table 9.2 Signs and symptoms of bulimia nervosa

Physical	Behavioural	Psychological
Frequent weight changes	Bingeing	Depression
Calluses on fingers	Vomiting	Anxiety
Dehydration	Excessive exercise	Low self-esteem
Tiredness	Use of laxatives and/or diuretics	Hopelessness
Headaches		Preoccupation with food, diet and weight
Chest pain	Solitary or secretive eating	
Electrolyte imbalance	Impulsivity	Denial
Gastro-oesophageal reflux	Self-harm	
Swelling of hands and feet	Suicidal behaviour	
Gum disease and tooth decay		
Hypertrophy of the parotid glands		
Electrolyte disturbance		
Arrhythmias		
Reverse peristalsis		
Hiatal hernias		

gain through excessive eating is a sign that the child may be unhappy, depressed and having trouble coping.

There are several physical signs that a young person may be bulimic. Some of these are a result of purging (self-induced vomiting). Young people may complain of having a sore throat, swollen glands or mouth infections. Their teeth may be decayed as a result of acid erosion, and skin may be dry or in poor condition due to the regular loss of nutrients (see Table 9.2).

The recommended treatment for bulimia nervosa is cognitive behaviour therapy (CBT) (National Institute for Health and Care Excellence [NICE] 2004) and enhanced CBT (Fairburn 2008), and some nurses in specialist CAMHS have been trained to use these approaches. Young people are helped to focus on and address negative cognitions and beliefs about weight and body image. Nurses using CBT for children and young people with bulimia nervosa will need to adapt their approach to suit the age, circumstances and developmental needs of the child. Contemporary training courses such as those governed through Children and Young People's Improving Access to Psychological Therapies (CYP IAPT) ensure that the approach taken is developmentally appropriate.

The importance of a thorough assessment

Talking with the young person about their eating may reveal an overwhelming fear of gaining weight and a distorted perception of their body image. They may claim to be fat even if they are seriously underweight. Their mood may also be labile (up and down) or depressed. It can sometimes be difficult for nurses to tell the difference between ordinary teenage dieting and a more serious problem that may require intervention, and they should always seek advice from an eating disorders specialist if they are uncertain. Specialists are usually located in community or inpatient CAMHS teams and can offer advice about whether the issues of concern are likely to be transient and manageable without specialist help or whether there is a more serious problem that requires assessment or treatment by a community eating disorders service for children and young people, which may include hospital admission.

Nurses who are worried about a child or young person's eating should always maintain a record of what they are eating and drinking. This is vital in terms of establishing whether the child is temporarily off food or 'dieting' or whether there is an underlying problem that requires further investigation. It is also essential to monitor elimination as use of diuretics and laxatives is not unusual among young people with eating disorders. Lewer (2006) suggests that nurses may find it helpful to consider some guidelines as part of the physical assessment process (see Box 9.1).

Box 9.1 *Guidelines for physical assessments*

- Observe the young person's general appearance. Are they wearing clothing to hide their body? Are they looking after themselves and attending to appearance? What is the condition of hair, skin and nails?

- Measure height and weight to work out the young person's body mass index (BMI).

- Record blood pressure, pulse and temperature.

- Examine the body for muscle wastage, signs of dehydration or evidence of self-harm.

- Examine head, eyes ears and throat (for swollen saliva glands, dental corrosion or tiny haemorrhages in back of throat).

- What is the young person's complaint about weight? When did they first become concerned? Have they used vomiting, laxatives or diuretics to control weight?

- What have been the young person's highest and lowest weights? What were the circumstances?

- What does the young person typically eat in a day?

- What is the young person's experience of hunger? Do they have urges to eat? Do they binge? If so, what on? How does it start and end and what is felt afterwards?

- What is a young person's typical day like in terms of eating? Is it ritualised? Does the young person eat alone or in company?

- Does the young person use excessive exercise to control weight? If so, what kind, how often and for how long?

Source: Lewer (2006: 101).

For a diagnosis of anorexia nervosa to be made, body weight must be at least 15 per cent below that which is normal for the child's expected age and height (see Box 9.2).

However, it is important not to rely on weight and BMI scores alone, and these should never be used to delay treatment decisions. NICE (2004) is clear in stating that although weight and BMI are important, they are unreliable and should not be used as the sole indicators of physical risk.

Box 9.2 *How to work out a child or young person's body mass index (BMI)*

BMI is a measure of weight-to-height relationship. It is not an exact science due to developmental variations and differences in body shape.

To work out a child's BMI, you must carefully measure their height and weight. The BMI score is calculated by dividing weight in kilogrammes by height in metres squared ($BMI = kg/m^2$).

For example, if a child weighs 35 kilogrammes and is 1.5 metres in height, their BMI equals 15.6.

There are minor sex differences in BMI calculations. Individual BMI scores should be plotted on BMI reference curves. These are population norms for boys and girls. Like height and weight charts, ranges are set in centiles. A child's BMI score can then be plotted according to their age.

A healthy BMI is in-between 20 and 25. Children with a BMI of less than 20 are underweight.

What services are available for children and young people with eating disorders?

Service provision for children and young people with eating disorders is variable across England (National Collaborating Centre for Mental Health [NCCMH] 2015). Services that are generally regarded as comprehensive offer a 'stepped care' model of treatment, more intensive support being offered to those who are more severely unwell. While most children and young people receive treatment in community services, some receive treatment as day patients or inpatients.

Generic community CAMHS

These will usually, but not always, be commissioned to provide eating disorder services. However, the availability and level of expertise in assessing and managing children and young people varies across the UK.

Eating disorder 'mini-teams' or 'special interest groups' within generic CAMHS

These have often evolved around the skills base of individuals rather than in response to a specific commissioning function. Such teams offer a limited level of specialist assessment and treatment provision and are usually only able to manage small caseloads. Mini-teams tend to serve a smaller geographical area than generic community CAMHS and require close links with these 'parent' services.

Highly specialised child and adolescent eating disorder services that are commissioned to only assess children and young people with eating disorders

These services should consist of multidisciplinary teams of medical and non-medical professionals including nurses. They have significant training and experience in the assessment, risk management and treatment of children and young people with anorexia nervosa, bulimia nervosa and other related conditions. These teams require a high level of expertise to be able to manage the levels of medical risk safely and to provide continuous high-quality supervision for the psychological treatments (NCCMH 2015).

Inpatient mental health and paediatric settings

Treatment in hospital takes place most often in general psychiatric child or adolescent inpatient units, some of which have developed expertise in eating disorders. As many as a quarter of all inpatient admissions are of young people with eating disorders (O'Herlihy *et al.* 2007). Day services are sometimes available as a step down from inpatient care (James and Worrall-Davies 2015). Alternatively, children and young people can be discharged to the care of their local generic or specialist community CAMHS team. Shorter acute admissions to paediatric wards may be required for children and young people who are physically unwell. In some areas of the UK, well-established and effective care protocols exist between local paediatric and mental health services in relation to treatment of eating disorders, but in other areas, arrangements are more sporadic.

Sometimes young people with severe anorexia nervosa require refeeding in a hospital environment. Where physical wellbeing is at serious risk such as through dehydration, circulatory failure or significant growth delay, a programme of nasogastric feeding may be necessary. Refeeding should only be performed under medical supervision and the nasogastric tube usually remains in place until the young person can manage without its support (Lewer 2006). Small feeds in bolus form are given throughout the day so as to mimic normal eating patterns, and the content should be reviewed regularly. NICE (2004) recommends that total parenteral nutrition should not be used for young people with anorexia nervosa unless there is significant gastrointestinal dysfunction.

Physical monitoring during refeeding is crucially important because a young person who has starved themselves for a prolonged period is at risk of developing refeeding syndrome. This occurs when a young person who has been previously malnourished is fed with high-carbohydrate meals (Lewer 2006). A range of medical complications can occur due to changes in magnesium, potassium and phosphate levels. A young person who is receiving nasogastric refeeding should still be encouraged to attend mealtimes and have a small meal placed in front of them. This is so that the expectation that eating normally will happen is consistent and reinforced.

In some situations, young people with severe eating disorders who require mental health hospital admission are not being placed in inpatient CAMHS because of limited or variable local bed availability. Instead, they are admitted to paediatric or adult mental health wards, which are usually unsuitable care settings. Indeed, the number of young people being admitted to hospital for inpatient care has been increasing steadily in recent years (Health and Social Care Information Centre 2014).

What is available to guide nursing practice?

A number of evidence-based resources exist to guide nursing practice in relation to supporting children and young people with eating disorders.

National Institute for Health and Care Excellence

Guidelines published by NICE set standards for the assessment, treatment and management of eating disorders in children and adults. This includes recommendations about assessment, treatment and care. However, there is no reference to specific nursing interventions, which is an oversight given nurses provide the bulk of direct care. The NICE guidance was primarily focused on working age adults. However, a number of important treatment principles apply to the care and treatment of children and young people (see Box 9.3).

Box 9.3 Recommendations for the care and treatment of children and young people

- Children and young people should be offered evidence-based family interventions that directly address the eating disorder.

- Family members, including siblings, should normally be included in treatment.

- Interventions should include sharing of information, advice on behavioural management and facilitating communication.

- Services should offer care that is age-appropriate, accessible to females and males and culturally appropriate.

- Most children and young people should be treated in the community.

- Inpatient admission should be considered where there is high or moderate physical risk.

- Admission should be to appropriate facilities with access to educational provision and related activities.

- When inpatient admission is required, this should be within reasonable travelling distance.

Source: adapted from NICE (2004).

The sooner a young person starts NICE concordant treatment for an eating disorder, the better the outcome. Evidence-based interventions can improve recovery, reduce relapse rates and reduce the need for inpatient admission.

MARSIPAN

The Royal College of Psychiatrists (2012) published the *Junior MARSIPAN: Management of Really Sick Patients Under 18 with Anorexia Nervosa* guidelines for the management of children and young people under 18 with anorexia nervosa. These refer to the need for adequately trained and suitably resourced paediatric, nursing and dietetic staff in acute services and appropriately skilled staff in specialist mental health services. The guidance highlights the need for specific nursing care plans that address the physical and mental health care required for children and young people with an eating disorder.

The severity of a child or young person's eating disorder and the level of nursing care and supervision they require will influence where they are nursed on a paediatric ward. There are mixed views on the pros and cons of nursing young people with eating disorders in a single room. Although this offers privacy for someone who may struggling with difficult thoughts, it also gives them more opportunity to exercise, dispose of food or purge. As the MARSIPAN guidelines state, nursing in single rooms also runs the risk of overlooking the immediate care needs of young people with anorexia nervosa on a busy children's ward. The guidance therefore recommends that separate nursing should be considered on a case-by-case basis.

The MARSIPAN guidelines recognise that caring for a child or young person with an eating disorder can often be anxiety provoking for nursing staff, particularly in the absence of specialist training and support from CAMHS services. The guidelines describe the more appropriate situation, which is to have nursing staff who have been trained in both children's and mental health nursing. However, such dual training is not common, and nurses with this training are more likely to be working in CAMHS rather than paediatric settings. To overcome this shortfall in the skills base of children's nurses, the MARSIPAN guidance recommends that a core group of nurses should be identified to take care of children and young people with anorexia nervosa during a paediatric hospital admission.

The MARSIPAN guidance also refers to specialist interventions undertaken by nurses working with children and young people with eating disorders. These include insertion of a nasogastric tube and percutaneous endoscopic gastrostomy tube feeding. Before undertaking these interventions, nurses should be trained in safe restraint techniques and be clear about the legal framework for their interventions.

National Collaborating Centre for Mental Health

Recent guidance on community eating disorder services for children and young people makes a number of recommendations that should be taken into consideration by nurses in schools, hospitals, community teams and other practice settings. It specifies that medical and nursing staff need to take responsibility for ensuring that the child or young person's physical state is comprehensively assessed and appropriate medical management plans are put in place. This is alongside the assessment of mental state and psychosocial aspects of the child or young person's presentation and the implementation of appropriate management and support plans. The guidance states that nurses have a key role to play in providing family and group interventions, home treatment and mealtime support. At the end of treatment and at follow-up, nurses play a role in monitoring the full range of domains of functioning. This involves physical and psychological monitoring as well as management of any ongoing risks associated with the young person's eating disorder (NCCMH 2015).

Working with families

Future in Mind (Department of Health 2015) states that eating disorders can have a considerable impact on families and carers, both personally and economically. Eating disorders are costly because, for example, families and carers may be required to make changes to their own employment to care for the child or young person. They can also disrupt family life and activities, and may have a significant effect on siblings. As is pointed out in guidance on commissioning eating disorder services for children and young people, it is usually a worried parent who makes the first contact with their child or young person often reluctant to seek help (NCCMH 2015). Further deterioration can occur in the child or young person if families or carers are unable to support them (Treasure *et al.* 2001). Furthermore, where parents or carers and professionals do not work together, progress can often be lacking (Bryant-Waugh and Lask 2004). It is therefore important that nurses involve families as much as possible and that they understand the potential dynamics and dilemmas involved (Gross and Goldin 2008).

Nurses and other professionals need to be able to respond to the broader needs of families and carers as well as the child or young person with an eating disorder. This may include supporting parents with strategies to help manage their child's eating or providing information about eating disorders or access to specialist services. However, some young people may not want their family to know about their eating disorder, which nurses often find difficult to reconcile in the knowledge that family involvement usually benefits outcomes (NICE 2004; Noller 2005). Here, the challenge for nurses is to get the right balance between the young person's right to privacy and confidentiality and the parent's right to be involved. Whilst it is vital to have a working knowledge of the legal frameworks involved, simply asking the young person and their parents about how they want to manage information sharing can often be helpful and need not involve any breach of confidentiality.

In cases of bulimia nervosa and binge eating disorder, the young person is more likely to be older and to access help alone. The NCCMH (2015) suggests that young people may sometimes not seek help for the eating disorder directly but, instead, present with a range of symptoms secondary to the eating disorder (e.g. menstrual disturbances, gastrointestinal symptoms, fatigue, lethargy, anxiety or depression).

Conclusion

Eating disorders tend to get worse if they are not treated. Without help, young people place both their physical and mental health at risk. In anorexia nervosa, the risks of infertility, damage to internal organs and osteoporosis increase into adult life. In bulimia nervosa, permanent tooth decay and psychological problems in terms of low self-esteem and self-hatred are all long-term risks of untreated eating disorders.

Nursing children and young people with eating disorders can be challenging and emotionally draining. Young people with these conditions invest a lot of their emotional energy and focus on controlling weight and using maladaptive behaviours to avoid eating. The impact of caring for young people also needs to be carefully managed within the wider nursing team. Supporting young people to recover can invoke strong feelings in the nursing team, and splitting is not unusual. Marsden (2001) encourages members of the team to identify and express some of their own feelings, thus making it possible to explore strongly projected feelings and splits in the staff team. Clinical supervision, staff support and training are equally important if nurses are to understand and safely support young people with eating disorders.

References

Ahern, A., Bennett, K. and Hetherington, M. (2008) Internalisation of the ultra-thin ideal: positive implicit associations with underweight fashion models are associated with drive for thinness in young women. *Eating Disorders*, 16(4): 294–307.

Bell, B. T. and Dittmar, H. (2011) Does media type matter? The role of identification in adolescent girls' media consumption and the impact of different thin-ideal media on body image. *Sex Roles*, 65(7–8): 478–90.

Bryant-Waugh, R. and Lask, B. (2004) *Eating Disorders: A Parent's Guide*. Hove: Brunner-Routledge.

Department of Health (2015) *Future in Mind: Promoting, Protecting and Improving Our Children and Young People's Mental Health and Wellbeing*. London: Department of Health.

Fairburn, C. G. (2008) *Cognitive Behaviour Therapy and Eating Disorders*. New York: Guilford Press.

Gallagher, A., Rippon, S., Carthy, J. and Rioga, M. (2015) The effects of contemporary media upon adolescents' body image disturbance. *British Journal of Mental Health Nursing*, 4(5): 214–18.

Gowers, S. G., Wheetman, J., Shore, A., Hossain, F. and Elvins, R. (2000) Impact of hospitalisation on the outcome of adolescent anorexia nervosa. *British Journal of Psychiatry*, 176(2): 138–41.

Gross, V. and Goldin, J. (2008) Dynamics and dilemmas in working with families in inpatient CAMHS services. *Clinical Child Psychology and Psychiatry*, 13(3): 449–61.

Halek, C. (1997) Eating disorders: the role of the nurse. *Nursing Times*, 93(28): 63–6.

Health and Social Care Information Centre (2014) Eating disorders: hospital admissions up by 8% [online] HSCIC, 30 January. Available at: www.hscic.gov.uk/article/3880/Eating-disorders-Hospital-admissions-up-by-8-per-cent-in-a-year (accessed 21 July 2016).

House, J., Schmidt, U., Craig, M., Landau, S., Simic, M., Nicholls, D., Hugo, P., Berelowitz, M. and Eisler, I. (2012) Comparison of specialist and non-specialist care pathways for adolescents with anorexia nervosa and related eating disorders. *International Journal of Eating Disorders*, 45(8): 949–56.

James, A. and Worrall-Davies, A. (2015) Provision of intensive treatment: intensive outreach, day units, and in-patient units. In A. Thapar, D. S. Pine, J. F. Leckman, S. Scott, M. J. Snowling and E. Taylor (eds) *Rutter's Child and Adolescent Psychiatry* (sixth edition). Chichester: John Wiley & Sons, Ltd, pp. 648–60.

Kjelsas, E., Bjornstrom, C. and Gotestam, K. (2004) Prevalence of eating disorders in female and male adolescents (14–15 years). *Eating Behaviours*, 5(1): 13–25.

Lask, B. and Bryant-Waugh, R. (2000) *Anorexia Nervosa and Related Eating Disorders in Childhood and Adolescence* (second edition). Brighton: Psychology Press.

Lewer, L. (2006) Nursing children and young people with eating disorders. In T. McDougall (ed.) *Child and Adolescent Mental Health Nursing*. London: Blackwell, pp. 88–115.

Marsden, P. (2001) Food and violence: childhood violence and emotional abuse as complicating factors in the inpatient treatment of eating disorders. *Psychoanalytic Psychotherapy*, 15(3): 225–42.

Micali, N., Hagberg, K. W., Petersen, I. and Treasure, J. L. (2013) The incidence of eating disorders in the UK in 2000–2009: findings from the General Practice Research Database. *BMJ Open*, 3: e002646.

National Collaborating Centre for Mental Health (NCCMH) (2015) *Access and Waiting Time Standard for Children and Young People with an Eating Disorder: Commissioning Guide*. London: NCCMH.

National Institute for Health and Care Excellence (NICE) (2004) *Eating Disorders in Over 8s: Management* (CG9). Manchester: NICE.

Nicholls, D. and Viner, R. (2005) ABC of adolescence: eating disorders and weight problems. *British Medical Journal*, 330(7497): 950–3.

Noller, P. (2005) Communication with parents and other family members: the implications of family process for young people's wellbeing. In A. Williams and C. Thurslow (eds) *Talking Adolescence: Perspectives on Communication in the Teenage Years* (third edition). New York: Peter Lang, pp. 207–28.

O'Hara, C. (2013) Recognising anorexia nervosa: approaches to treatment. *British Journal of Mental Health Nursing*, 2(1): 22–7.

O'Herlihy, A., Lelliott, P., Bannister, D., Cotgrove, A., Farr, H. and Tulloch, S. (2007) Provision of child and adolescent mental health inpatient services in England between 1999 and 2006. *The Psychiatrist (formerly Psychiatric Bulletin)*, 31(12): 454–6.

Ramjan, L. M. (2004) Nurses and the 'therapeutic relationship': caring for adolescents with anorexia nervosa. *Journal of Advanced Nursing*, 45(5): 495–503.

Royal College of Psychiatrists (2012) *Junior MARSIPAN: Management of Really Sick Patients Under 18 with Anorexia Nervosa (CR 168)*. London: Royal College of Psychiatrists.

Treasure, J., Murphy, T., Szmukler, G., Todd, G., Gavan, K. and Joyce, J. (2001) The experience of caregiving for severe mental illness: a comparison between anorexia nervosa and psychosis. *Social Psychiatry and Psychiatric Epidemiology*, 36(7): 343–7.

Chapter 10

Nursing children and young people with ADHD

Noreen Ryan

Key points:

- The core symptoms of attention deficit hyperactivity disorder (ADHD) are hyperactivity, inattention and impulsivity, which all present in the population as a whole. ADHD as a syndrome is a pervasive, persistent and severe impairment consisting of inattention, motor restlessness and impulsive behaviour that is considered outside of developmental norms.
- ADHD presents with other difficulties. In particular, comorbidity with behavioural difficulties and conduct disorder is very common for those with ADHD, and attention should be paid to this when nurses are assessing children and young people.
- Whilst what causes ADHD is an area of research and controversy, it can be understood within biological, psychological and social paradigms. There is evidence to support genetic, neurological and cognitive mechanisms involved in this disorder.
- Professionals such as nurses, health visitors, teachers, social workers and youth workers working with children and young people are well placed to identify and recognise the symptoms of ADHD with their knowledge and experience of child and adolescent development.
- Interventions for the treatment of ADHD are varied. Nurses and other professionals working with children and young people can offer intervention for the domains that interfere with day-to-day activities. These often involve psycho-education, social skills training, parent training and behaviour management, school-based interventions and psychopharmacology.
- Nurse prescribing has continued to develop, and nurses play a significant role in the pharmacological care of children and young people with ADHD.

Introduction

Attention deficit hyperactivity disorder (ADHD) remains one of the most common presentations in child and adolescent mental health services (CAMHS) and community paediatric clinics. ADHD is a common disorder of childhood, described as a behavioural problem characterised by excessive patterns of hyperactivity, inattention and impulsiveness (National Institute for Health and Care Excellence [NICE] 2008; Barkley 2015a). The core symptoms of ADHD are recognised as having ongoing chronic disabling difficulties for children and young people in achieving day-to-day success in living (NICE 2008; Weyandt and Gudmundstottir 2015).

What is interesting is that these symptoms manifest in typical behaviours seen in all children and adults at any one time and are particularly related to developmental levels. These behaviours and symptoms are not just associated with ADHD but may represent many other mental health problems in children and young people. ADHD places stress on the child or young person within their families and wider social environments, such as school or college, and with friendships and social activities. Research has been ongoing into this complex disorder, and even as our understanding of the validity of the diagnosis evolves, its existence remains in doubt for many (Timimi and Radcliffe 2005).

ADHD is conceptualised as a lifelong condition. It is now recognised that the disorder persists into adulthood with approximately 65 per cent of young people diagnosed as children retaining impairment from ADHD symptoms into adult life (Farone *et al.* 2006). Gournay (2015) identifies ADHD in adults as an under-recognised and under-treated disorder. Thus there is a growing need for adult ADHD services to continue to provide healthcare to those who received a childhood diagnosis and to provide assessments and interventions for adults who were not diagnosed as children but seek an understanding of what contributes to their ongoing adult mental health difficulties.

What is ADHD?

NICE (2008) wrote a clear position statement on the validity of ADHD as a diagnosis, stating that ADHD can be distinguished from coexisting conditions. The disorder is associated with high levels of hyperactivity, inattention and impulsivity that are associated with significant clinical, psychosocial and educational impairments and which are enduring and occur across multiple settings. ADHD is a complex disorder with a strong genetic and developmental basis. There are physical, cognitive, social, emotional, genetic, environmental and spiritual elements that influence the progress of ADHD and the way in which these factors impact on each individual child.

There are different terms used to describe difficulties with poor concentration, hyperactivity and impulsivity; it can be referred to as ADHD or ADD (attention deficit disorder), the latter referring mainly to children with poor concentration without hyperactivity. These behaviours are seen in the whole population all the time, and they can vary from moment to moment, situation to situation and also depending on what we are doing. Therefore, being active, having poor concentration and impulsivity are also 'normal' behaviours. It is normal to be excited around a birthday or holiday. We expect young children to have poor concentration and to be very busy; this is due to them not yet developing the skills or maturity to sit still due to their developmental stage.

Even as adults, we demonstrate impulsive actions – for example, speaking before thinking and buying clothes we never wear! Therefore, we have to consider the behaviour not as something that exists on its own, but understand it with regard to the way that the young person fits into their world. It is sometimes difficult to understand the way children and young people function, which is why assessments can take some time to gather information about the difficulties. It is not unusual for people to mistake behaviour problems for ADHD, but it is really important to be able to separate out the features of hyperactivity, poor concentration and impulsivity.

What causes ADHD?

The causes of ADHD are still not fully understood, but it is now widely agreed that there are various developmental factors that impact on the way in which a child behaves and that children develop at different rates. ADHD is not caused by parents being bad parents or not being good at their 'job'; rather, there is growing evidence that ADHD is a neurobiological problem. Therefore, ongoing research into brain structure suggests that the brains of people with ADHD may be different – grey matter volumes may be smaller and research on neurotransmitters (particularly dopamine and norepinephrine) is providing a new understanding for the presentation of the disorder, moving away from it being thought of a behavioural or environmental issue (Nakao *et al.* 2011). Neurotransmitters help to pass messages around the brain and are thought to help with attention span, organisation and regulation of emotions.

The degree to which young people are affected varies and depends on risk and resilience factors, the existence of other psychosocial difficulties and the support networks available to them. We know that young people inherit their genetic make-up from their parents, so this suggests that, like with other diseases, if a member of your family has a problem then you have a bigger chance of having the same problem. Research continues into whether the symptoms of ADHD could be the result of things that are in the world around us (NICE 2008). The fifth edition of the *Diagnostic and Statistical Manual of Mental Disorders* (DSM) has placed ADHD within the group of neurodevelopmental disorders rather than behavioural disorders, and it highlights that the disorder will change as the young person develops, which means that the disorder needs to be understood in terms of impairment and dysfunction to the individual young person (American Psychiatric Association 2013).

How common is ADHD?

The prevalence rates of ADHD vary from study to study, ranging from as low as 1.5 per cent to 19.8 per cent (NICE 2008). It is currently agreed that approximately 5.0 per cent of children and 2.5 per cent of adults reach criteria for ADHD (Polanczyk *et al.* 2007; American Psychiatric Association 2013). In clinic samples, there are many more boys than girls; but the symptoms presented appear to be similar, as are the deficits (NICE 2008; Owens *et al.* 2015). The course of the ADHD will be particular to each child, but it is thought that the symptom of hyperactivity (and possibly impulsivity) declines more over time than does inattention.

How important is diet?

The role of diet has been implicated in the development of ADHD, possible associations being considered with artificial food additives, food sensitivities, trace element deficiencies, free fatty acid (FFA) deficiencies, Western style of diet and food insecurity. Some families prefer not to have a pharmacological intervention for ADHD, and dietary interventions have been researched using randomised controlled trials, systematic review and meta-analyses (Sonuga-Barke *et al.* 2013):

- Restricted elimination diet – this requires the removal of food stuffs to which the young person is considered to be sensitive by evidence of deteriorating behaviour or increase in ADHD symptoms.
- Exclusion of artificial food colourings (e.g. tartrazine, sunset yellow, brilliant blue, allura red) – this is often referred to as the Feingold diet.
- Supplementing the diet with FFAs – this involves adding FFAs, thought to have a role in brain growth and development, to a diet that is considered to be depleted in them.

The research into dietary interventions remains unclear due to methodological issues with the studies (e.g. low numbers and poor blinding of trials leading to bias). What has been found is that the adverse effects upon behaviour in terms of hyperactivity are seen not only in children with ADHD but in children in general; this means that some additives make normal children hyperactive and hyperactive children even more hyperactive. Supplementing the diets of children with ADHD (e.g. with fish oils and omega-3 fatty acids) has not been found to cause or help the symptoms of ADHD. NICE (2008) suggested that if there is thought to be a direct link between a particular food and a child's symptoms of hyperactivity, this should be discussed and referral to a dietician considered.

Diagnosing ADHD

The task of formulating and diagnosing ADHD is multifaceted and requires a high level of assessment skill and clinical knowledge. We are aware of the core symptoms of ADHD, but what is it that leads us to understand that for some children, these symptoms cause more disruption and impairment to their day-to-day functioning at home with their families and at school and play with their peers? In order to make a diagnosis of ADHD, the core symptoms need to be present in more than one setting (i.e. home and school). There is also a requirement for the symptoms to cause impairment in their psychological, social and educational development and functioning.

ADHD is a disorder that is comorbid and, therefore, is very difficult to assess and diagnose. As yet, there is no test or investigation that will provide a definitive diagnosis. The process of a mental health nursing assessment requires interviewing skills, history taking, an understanding of child development, observations and understanding to help perceive the interaction between biology, environment and family dynamics. This is done using diagnostic frameworks, completing standardised rating scales, taking information from other sources and undertaking comprehensive assessment interviews.

Diagnostic criteria

In the UK, there are two classification systems that are in use – the tenth revision of the International Classification of Diseases (ICD-10; World Health Organization 1992) and DSM-5 (American Psychiatric Association 2013). The American DSM-5 has recently been updated and is now closer to the ICD-10 criteria used here in the UK and Europe. These focus on inattention, hyperactivity and impulsivity. However, many argue that emotion dysregulation should be given more consideration in the assessment of ADHD due to its impact on psychological, physical and social outcomes (Barkley 2015b; Northover et al. 2015).

ICD-10 criteria for diagnosing ADHD

Box 10.1 outlines the diagnostic criteria for ADHD according to the ICD-10.

DSM-5 criteria for diagnosing ADHD

As already noted, there has been a recent update of DSM with the publication of the fifth edition. Although the criteria is not significantly different from DSM-4, the changes now also try to define the symptoms for an adult population. In DSM-5, ADHD is grouped with other neurodevelopmental disorders rather than with behavioural disorders and the presence

Box 10.1 ADHD diagnosis based on ICD-10

In order to make a diagnosis of ADHD, symptoms described below (for inattention, hyperactivity and impulsivity) must have been present in the past six months, these being maladaptive and inconsistent with the developmental level of the child.

There must be evidence of at least six of the nine symptoms of inattention, at least three of the five symptoms of disturbance of motor activity, and at least one of the four symptoms of impulsivity.

Inattention difficulties

- poor attention to detail/careless errors
- often fails to concentrate on tasks or play
- often appears not to listen
- often fails to finish things
- poor task organisation
- often avoids tasks which require sustained mental effort
- often loses things
- often distracted by external stimuli
- often forgetful.

Hyperactivity difficulties

- often fidgets with hands or squirms in seat
- often leaves seat when expected to sit still
- excessive inappropriate climbing or running
- is often unduly noisy in playing or has difficulty in engaging in leisure activities quietly
- persistent overactivity not modulated by request or context.

Impulsivity difficulties

- often blurts out answers before the question is complete
- often fails to wait turn in groups, games or queues
- often intrudes into games or conversations
- often talks excessively without response to social appropriateness.

Source: adapted from World Health Organization (1992).

Box 10.2 ADHD diagnosis for children and young people, based on DSM-5

Conditions A to E must be met for a diagnosis of ADHD.

A   The child or young person must have experienced either six (or more) symptoms of inattention or six (or more) of symptoms of hyperactivity and impulsivity for at least six months; these symptoms must be inconsistent with developmental level and affect social and academic activities.

Symptoms of inattention are:

a)   fails to give close attention to details or makes careless mistakes in schoolwork, at work, or with other activities

b)   has trouble holding attention on tasks or play activities

c)   does not seem to listen when spoken to directly

d)   does not follow through on instructions and fails to finish schoolwork, chores or duties in the workplace (e.g. loses focus, becomes sidetracked)

e)   has trouble organizing tasks and activities

f)   avoids, dislikes, or is reluctant to do tasks that require mental effort over a long period of time (such as schoolwork or homework)

g)   loses things necessary for tasks and activities (e.g. school materials, pencils, books, tools, wallets, keys, paperwork, eyeglasses, mobile telephones)

h)   is easily distracted

i)   is forgetful in daily activities.

Symptoms of hyperactivity and impulsivity are:

a)   fidgets with or taps hands or feet, or squirms in seat

b)   leaves seat in situations when remaining seated is expected

c)   runs about or climbs in situations where it is not appropriate (adolescents may be limited to feeling restless)

d)   unable to play or take part in leisure activities quietly

e)   is 'on the go' acting as if 'driven by a motor'

f)   talks excessively

g)   blurts out an answer before a question has been completed

h)   has trouble waiting his/her turn

i)   interrupts or intrudes on others (e.g. butts into conversations or games).

B   Several inattentive or hyperactive-impulsive symptoms present before age 12.

C   Several symptoms present in two or more settings (e.g. at home, school or work; with friends or relatives; in other activities).

D   Clear evidence that the symptoms interfere with, or reduce the quality of, social, school or work functioning.

E   The symptoms do not happen only during the course of schizophrenia or another psychotic disorder. The symptoms are not better explained by another mental disorder (e.g. mood disorder, anxiety disorder, dissociative disorder or a personality disorder).

Source: adapted from World Health Organisation (1992).

of an autistism spectrum diagnosis can no longer exclude a diagnosis of ADHD, thus reinforcing the perspective that ADHD has a neurobiological base rather than being a behavioural disorder. There is an acknowledgement that severity of symptoms may vary across settings, time of day, activity and level of adult supervision. Importantly, the age of onset has been increased to 12 years of age.

How does ADHD present day-to-day issues for young people?

If we are to consider how to help young people and their families, we need to review the impairments that the condition presents, not just have knowledge of the core symptoms of hyperactivity, inattention and impulsivity (Barkley 2015a). The effects of ADHD on developmental function and cognitive and neurological function include:

1   Developmental function:
    - adaptive skills – difficulties in forming skills for independence, self-help, self-knowledge and social communication;
    - poor motor coordination;
    - speech and language – difficulties with receptive, expressive and pragmatic language skills;
    - learning difficulties;
    - self-perception – children have an inflated self-esteem;
    - emotional dysregulation – inability to inhibit thoughts and actions leading to emotional dysregulation.
2   Cognitive and neuropsychological function:
    - intellectual functioning – children perform lower on IQ tests;
    - executive functioning – issues with impulse control, strategic planning and cognitive flexibility;
    - planning – difficulties with planning, leading to poor task performance and completion;
    - inhibition – difficulties with inhibiting responses to events and stimuli;
    - working memory – difficulties with sense of time and recall of learned information.

Based on these effects on function, it is easy to see the complex nature of the disorder, not just in what is observed but in how the young person tries to make sense of what is happening around them and respond appropriately.

CAMHS nursing assessment

Nurses have a strong role to play in the assessment of ADHD (Ryan and McDougall 2009). The NICE (2008) clinical guideline informs what should be included in a comprehensive assessment. As with any child mental health problem, the process of careful assessment and formulation is key to diagnosis and care planning. The key features of assessment as described by NICE (2008) are:

- a clinical interview;
- a medical examination;
- administration of standardised rating scales to parents and teachers;

- observation in educational settings – cognitive, neuropsychological, developmental and literacy skills assessments may or may not be indicated.

Many of the skills that nurses use are also used by other professionals. Nurses have a duty of care to treat people as individuals, uphold their dignity, listen to their concerns and respect their preferences (Nursing and Midwifery Council [NMC] 2015). The nurse's role with ADHD utilises skills and knowledge in order to undertake the assessment (i.e. create a therapeutic environment, act as a socialising agent and advocate for the child and family). Dogra and Baldwin's (2009) description of the components of a CAMHS nursing assessment (see Box 10.3) is not too dissimilar to that advised by NICE (2008).

Box 10.3 Key components of a CAMHS nursing assessment

- Presenting concerns
- Family history
- Social history
- Developmental history
- Integrating cultural issues
- Mental state examination
- Observation of the young person with their carers
- Risk assessment
- Formulating and agreeing a care plan.

Source: adapted from Dogra and Baldwin (2009: 51).

Nurses have varied roles in the assessment of ADHD from formal interviewing to observation of the child in the structured classroom setting and the unstructured clinic or playground setting. Symptoms of ADHD are often initially detected in primary care by school nurses, teachers or general practitioners, particularly when the child is unable to meet the educational and social demands of the classroom (Schacher and Tannock 2002; Mangle 2011). Mental health, paediatric and school nurses are well placed to identify and recognise the symptoms of ADHD with their knowledge and experience of child development. Teachers often seek the advice of school nurses in relation to disruptive behaviour in the classroom.

The cornerstone of any nursing assessment is to carefully gather a detailed history that includes the presenting concerns of the family/carer, the child's physical, emotional, motor and cognitive development, family history and social development, and school performance. The purpose is to assess the child's difficulties within the context of their normal developmental milestones.

The family interview

The assessment processes for ADHD are complex, requiring the nurse to use extensive communication and observational skills. The aims of the family interview are to build up a picture of the child and their family or carers through a process of inquisitive questioning and to work collaboratively with the young person and family to identify goals and outcomes that they want from contact with services. The choice and partnership approach (CAPA) evidences this (York and Kingsley 2013). The interview not only acts as a medium for gathering information but also allows for a relationship to develop on the basis of a collaborative alliance between the nurse and the child and family. This trusting relationship enables the family and nurse to consider which problems are amenable to change and offers a medium for work with the child and their family to achieve this (Dogra and Baldwin 2009).

The environment for the interview is pivotal to the interaction. The interview room should be quiet, private, free from distractions and well equipped with toys that are appropriate to the developmental age of the child. Observations made during the interview about the child's ability or inability to use the toys appropriately are useful. During the interview, the nurse should take note of the points in Box 10.4.

Box 10.4 The family interview

- The child's activity levels and interactions in a small group and on a one-to-one basis
- The child's ability to concentrate and levels of hyperactivity and impulsivity
- The interactions between family members
- Strategies used by the family members to manage behaviour in the interview.

Information gathered during the interview will allow the parents to bring their concerns forward, and the clinician can rule out any concerns about mood, anxiety, learning and speech and language. There should be opportunity for the nurse to conduct a child-centred interview as well as an opportunity for parents to discuss their concerns with the nurse on a one-to-one basis. During the parental interview, questionnaires that are helpful in assessment of ADHD can be completed. These include the Conners Parent Rating Scale (Conners 1989a) and the Strengths and Difficulties Questionnaire (SDQ; Goodman 1997).

The purpose of taking a detailed family history is to create an understanding of the family's methods of operating and to establish any other family difficulties. The family history may generate important information about parental conflicts, financial problems or difficulties with other family members. It is important to have an understanding of the ways in which the family copes with pressures and their style of communication. It is also useful for the nurse to understand the language, emotions and behaviour exhibited by the family and to explore the social support systems that are in place, using a genogram as a way of enquiring about the extended family. This can help to facilitate a detailed understanding of the family history, the family belief systems and the development of family relationships over a period of time. The family history should be able to identify the information in Box 10.5.

The parent/carer interview

Parents or carers should always be given the opportunity to meet without the young person to describe what their concerns are for their child. As the difficulties can place stress and strain on the family system, relationships can be strained and parents may be negative and critical of their child. This can be difficult to manage in a clinic setting and requires the nurse to manage the emotions and distress of all the participants sensitively. The parental interview should be conducted in order to ascertain the information in Box 10.6.

Box 10.5 The family history

- The people in the family and those who live at home
- Contact with absent parents
- Family relationships and communication style
- The coping style of the family
- Family support systems
- Distressing life events (e.g. family separation, domestic violence, death of relatives, house and school moves).

Box 10.6 The parent/carer interview

- What they require from the assessment, eliciting their main concerns
- Attempts by them to improve the problem
- Impact of the problems on the young person and the family system.

Child interview

Regardless of the child's age or developmental stage, spending time with the young person on an individual basis provides important information about day-to-day functioning. When assessing for ADHD, attention should be given to the presence or absence of the core symptoms of ADHD presented by the child on interview. The child interview should be used to assess the aspects listed in Box 10.7.

Box 10.7 The child interview

- Ability to separate from caregivers
- Physical appearance
- Motor functioning
- Ability to create a rapport and sustain this with concentration skills
- Emotional regulation
- Speech and language comprehension and use of language
- Social interactions with family and interviewer, dependent on the developmental level of the child
- Mood
- Child self-report if appropriate – e.g. Conners Adolescent Self Report (CASR; Conners 1989b) for ages 12 to 18 and Child SDQ (Goodman 1997) for ages 8 to 16.

ADHD Child Evaluation (ACE)

The ADHD Child Evaluation (ACE) is a semi-structured diagnostic interview developed by Young (2015). It is available to download for use in assessing ADHD to provide a structure for the important aspects in the assessment. Clinicians can use it to look for evidence in neurological, biological, cognitive as well as social domains. It provides evidence for the strengths as well as the difficulties for the young person within the context of their day-to-day functioning.

QbTest

The QbTest is a new innovation in the assessment of ADHD. As had been stated, there is no empirical test for ADHD, and reliance on subjective information is often a criticism of the assessments that are carried out. The QbTest addresses this criticism; it is an objective computerised testing system that simultaneously measures attention, impulsivity and motor activity, a core requirement of diagnostic criteria in both DSM-5 and ICD-10.

The test consists of an infrared motion camera combined with a continuous performance test. The test measures the young person's sustained and selective attention and, to a lesser degree, their level of impulsivity. The test consists of rapid presentation of stimuli on a computer screen, among which there is a designated 'target' stimulus; motor activity is recorded by the use of the infrared sensor. The test takes approximately 15 minutes to complete. The individual patient's performance is then compared to an age- and sex-matched control group, and a comprehensive report is produced to use with children and families.

Reports are in a readily understandable format and outline whether a child is more active, impulsive and inattentive than the control group (children without ADHD). The test is FDA cleared as an aid to assessment and treatment follow-up. As with other tools used in the assessment of ADHD, the QbTest does not in itself provide a definitive diagnosis.

The developmental history

As ADHD is now defined as a neurodevelopmental disorder, the need for a comprehensive account of the child's development is of fundamental importance. It may be necessary to seek further information from other professionals such as a health visitor, school nurse, general practitioner or paediatrician if carers are poor historians or, as may be the case for looked-after children, little is known about their developmental history. Das Gupta and Frake (2009) suggest the areas in Box 10.8 are taken into consideration when a developmental history is taken.

Information from other sources

With the consent of the child and family, it is necessary to obtain reports from the child's school or other agencies working with the child (e.g. educational psychologist, youth workers or specialist behaviour workers). A telephone interview will provide the nurse with the necessary information about the child's academic, behavioural, developmental and social functioning in school. Use of standardised rating scales, such as the Conners Teacher Rating Scale (Conners 1989c) and SDQ Teacher report (Goodman 1997), may provide useful information about the child's functioning. If necessary, more detailed information should be sought from speech and language therapists, educational psychologists,

---

Box 10.8 Taking a developmental history

- Maternal health during pregnancy (including information about conception, antenatal history, foetal growth, toxaemia, threatened miscarriage)

- Postnatal history (including birth complications, birth weight, neonatal complications)

- Use of medication (including drugs, alcohol and nicotine)

- Developmental milestones (including motor development, attachment, sleep, language development, growth and temperament)

- Medical history (including other developmental disorders, epilepsy and tics)

- School performance (including learning difficulties, ability to separate from parents at school age and comparison to developmental peer group at school).

Source: adapted from Das Gupta and Frake (2009).

---

paediatricians or voluntary agencies to add important information in relation to the child's overall presentation.

Reaching a conclusion: formulation and diagnosis

The use of clinical skills and judgement and an ability to assimilate complex information to reach a conclusion is crucial, focusing specifically on the symptoms and behaviours listed in the ICD-10 and DSM-5 diagnostic categories. The nurse should consider if there is a another explanation for this presentation of symptoms (i.e. a differential diagnosis). In order to make a diagnosis of ADHD, there needs to be clear evidence of clinically significant impairment in social, academic or occupational functioning (NICE 2008; Barkley 2015a). The use of the term 'impairment' suggests that the symptoms impact pervasively and interfere with the child's day-to-day activities with their family, school and friendships to a greater frequency and severity than would be expected of the child's developmental peer group.

Comorbidity

ADHD rarely exists as a single disorder; there are associations with other mental disorders, specific learning difficulties and a range of psychosocial problems. This generates a need for multidisciplinary assessment and treatment strategies (Pliska *et al.* 1999; Jenson *et al.* 2001; Dalsgaard *et al.* 2002; Green *et al.* 2005). Box 10.9 lists some of the associated difficulties.

How can nurses help children and young people manage their ADHD?

In order to improve the outcomes for children and young people with ADHD, the interventions are varied and a multimodal approach is often required (MTA Cooperative Group 1999). The consequences of the disorder can be wide-reaching and the impact upon the child's life widespread. The needs of each child and family will require different levels of input, and this should be a collaborative task between young person/carer and professional. The mainstay interventions currently used in the management of ADHD are described next.

Box 10.9 ADHD comorbidities

- Oppositional defiant disorder

- Conduct disorder

- Autistic spectrum disorder

- Asperger's syndrome

- Depression and/or anxiety

- Tourette syndrome

- Learning disabilities

- Language impairment

- Dyslexia

- Dyspraxia.

Psycho-educational measures

An important part of the nursing role is to provide education to parents/carers, children and teachers about ADHD and its associated conditions. This will help the child and family to develop an understanding of the nature of the disorder and have more realistic expectations. Teachers may benefit from information about a particular child's needs and difficulties, and they can consult specialists within the education system to enhance the child's learning.

Parent training and behavioural interventions

Parent training programmes have been widely used to help parents and carers of children with ADHD (Taylor *et al.* 2004; NICE 2008). The programmes are based on social learning theories and behaviour modification and are designed to teach parents about the need to reinforce positive behaviour and reduce the number of punitive strategies as well as suggesting techniques to manage inappropriate and defiant behaviour. Parent training programmes have been shown to improve parental management of the child's behaviour, enhance parental self-confidence, reduce family stress and alleviate difficult behaviour (Schacher and Tannock 2002; Zwi *et al.* 2011). However, Zwi *et al.* (2011) found that most of the studies of parent training and behavioural interventions were based on poor methodological processes, which introduces uncertainty about results and means, therefore, that they can not be recommended on the basis of evidenced-based outcomes.

School-based behavioural and psycho-educational interventions

It is important that a child with ADHD is integrated into their peer group as much as possible. Schools may wish to seek advice from their specialist educational colleagues as to how best to help a child with ADHD access their education successfully (NICE 2008). Factors such as classroom structure, providing work based on small tasks that are frequently reviewed by the teacher, having the child placed near the teacher and implementing a range of behavioural strategies to address specific problem behaviours are all helpful. For an outline of classroom management techniques, see the book by O'Regan (2002).

Psychopharmacological interventions

Psychopharmacology is used to relieve the core symptoms of inattention, hyperactivity and impulsivity, and there have been many trials of effectiveness (Heyman and Santosh 2002; Bolea-Alamañac *et al.* 2014; Barkley 2015a). Medications are trialled to assess positive response such as reduction in hyperactivity and impulsivity and improved concentration. The two main groups of medicines used to treat ADHD are stimulants and non-stimulants.

Stimulants are medicines that act on the central nervous system and are designed to increase the levels of dopamine and noradrenaline in synapses in the brain, these being neurotransmitters that are associated with ADHD symptoms. According to NICE (2008), these drugs should be used first-line when considering a psychopharmacological intervention. These are short-acting methylphenidate hydrochloride and long-acting methylphenidate hydrochloride (Concerta XL, Equasym XL, Medikinet XL and Matoride), all available in the UK (British National Formulary 2014).

Non-stimulants include Atomoxetine (Strattera), which is a selective noradrenaline transport blocker indicated for the treatment of ADHD. It is thought to act by increasing the intra-synaptic concentration of noradrenaline (British National Formulary 2014).

Nurses are well placed to offer routine monitoring of medication and to provide other psychosocial interventions. Routine monitoring should focus on general mental health assessment and physical wellbeing (Waldock 2009), particularly focusing on tics, depression, irritability, social withdrawal and lack of spontaneity. The factors given in Box 10.10 should be monitored.

Box 10.10 Monitoring stimulants and non-stimulants

- Blood pressure and pulse, plotted on centile charts
- Height and weight, plotted on centile charts
- Unwanted effects referred to as side effects
- Positive and negative responses to treatment
- Progress at school.

The manufacturers of methylphenidate recommend periodic blood tests to review haematological status, but there is little evidence to support this practice and it can be argued that the benefits of regular blood tests are outweighed by the distress caused to the child (NICE 2008). There is little guidance as to the length of treatment; discontinuation is recommended periodically to assess the child's progress and the need to continue with treatment. Treatment may continue into adult life and further research is required in this area.

Nurse prescribing and ADHD

Non-medical prescribing, referred to as nurse prescribing, is an advancement in the role of nurses working with children and families with a diagnosis of ADHD (National Prescribing Centre, National Institute for Mental Health in England and Department of Health 2005;

Ryan and McDougall 2009; Doran 2013). A high degree of clinical judgement is required to make a diagnosis, and expertise in the field of ADHD is needed in order for both doctors and nurses to make accurate diagnoses of the condition. Changes to legislation has allowed for nurses to prescribe controlled drugs independently (NMC 2012). This has had a major impact on nurses working in ADHD as many of the treatments are controlled drugs; until the legislation change, these were only available through supplementary prescribing, which required an agreement between the child/family, the independent prescriber (a doctor) and a supplementary prescriber (a nurse) in line with the treatment plan. Now, nurses demonstrate the skills and competence and have the training to prescribe controlled drugs independently (Mangle *et al.* 2014).

There are important considerations when prescribing for children and young people. First, they metabolise medicines at different rates to adults; therefore, it is necessary to take into account age, weight, dose calculations and the developmental status of the child (Sutcliffe 1999; Beckwith and Franklin 2007). Second, concordance and compliance with treatment by the child or adolescent and their family or carer is vital and needs to be established by the nurse in order to determine effectiveness of treatment. Third, nurses need to help young people develop self-management skills for their own disorder and medicines. Nurses must assess the ability of the child or adolescent to take care of their own medication and address issues related to supervision and safety of medicines in the home. Finally, depending on the age and wishes of the child or adolescent, they must be involved in the decision-making process about medication along with their family or carers.

Conclusion

ADHD remains a complex disorder to assess and treat. This chapter gives a brief overview and further reading is necessary. This is not helped by the differing classification systems that are currently in use. It is not surprising, therefore, that there continues to be controversy around ADHD despite ongoing research and advances in our understanding of the biological, genetic, psychological and social pathways of the behaviours associated with this disorder. The long-term effects of having a diagnosis of ADHD are widespread. The outcomes for this population can be seen in terms of poor academic performance, family-based difficulties, social exclusion, low self-esteem, increased risk of mental disorder in adult life, occupational failure in adult life and difficulties with long-term relationships (Shaw *et al.* 2012). Further research is required into our understanding of ADHD and what interventions are helpful to children and families.

Nurses have a vital role to play in the assessment, treatment and management of ADHD. They have specific responsibilities in respect of the care of the young person with an ADHD diagnosis. They are required to undertake comprehensive assessments in monitoring medication, which includes physical health monitoring (height, weight, blood pressure and pulse) as well as evaluating the effectiveness of medication and adverse side effects. Nurses are also in key positions to provide psychosocial interventions for the child and family to help ameliorate associated behavioural problems. It is important that nurses continue to update their skills and ensure that their knowledge and practice is evidence-based. Full consideration should always be given to the professional code of conduct (NMC 2015), and nurses should always work within their sphere of competence and acknowledge their limitations of knowledge and skills. This particularly applies to the role of nurse prescribing.

The work that has been undertaken about service users' views (parents/carers and children/young people) is limited; this includes young people's understanding of their disorder and the impact that it has on them.

References

American Psychiatric Association (2013) *Diagnostic and Statistical Manual of Mental Disorders* (fifth edition). Arlington, VA: American Psychiatric Association.

Barkley, R. A. (2015a) *Attention-Deficit Hyperactivity Disorder: A Handbook for Diagnosis and Treatment* (fourth edition). New York: Guildford Press.

Barkley, R. A. (2015b) Emotional dysregulation is a core component of ADHD. In R. Barkley (ed.) *Attention-Deficit Hyperactivity Disorder: A Handbook for Diagnosis and Treatment* (fourth edition). New York: Guildford Press, pp. 81–115.

Beckwith, S. and Franklin, P. (2007) *Oxford Handbook of Nurse Prescribing.* Oxford: Oxford University Press.

Bolea-Alamañac, B., Nutt, D., Adamou, M., Asherson, P., Bazire, S., Coghill, D., Heal, D., Muller, H., Nash, J., Santosh, P., Sayal, K., Sonuga-Barke, E. and Young, S. (2014) Evidence-based guidelines for the pharmacological management of attention deficit hyperactivity disorder: update on recommendations from the British Association for Psychopharmacology. *Journal of Psychopharmacology,* 28(3): 179–203.

British National Formulary (2014) *BNF for Children 2014–2015.* London: BNF Publications.

Conners, C. (1989a) *Conners Parent Rating Scale Manual.* New York: Multi-Health System.

Conners, C. (1989b) *Conners Adolescent Self Report Rating Scale Manual.* New York: Multi-Health System.

Conners, C. (1989c) *Conners Teacher Rating Scale Manual.* New York: Multi-Health System.

Dalsgaard, S., BoMortensen, P., Frydenberg, M. and Thomsen, P. (2002) Conduct problems, gender and adult psychiatric outcome of children with attention-deficit hyperactivity disorder. *British Journal of Psychiatry,* 181(5): 416–21.

Das Gupta, M. and Frake, C. (2009) Child and family development. In N. Dogra and S. Leighton (eds) *Nursing in Child and Adolescent Mental Health.* Maidenhead: Open University Press, pp. 19–32.

Dogra, N. and Baldwin, L. (2009) Nursing assessment in CAMHS. In N. Dogra and S. Leighton (eds) *Nursing in Child and Adolescent Mental Health.* Maidenhead: Open University Press, pp. 55–68.

Doran, C. (2013) *Prescribing Mental Health Medication: A Practitioner's Guide* (second edition). Abingdon: Routledge.

Faraone, S., Biederman, J. and Mick, E. (2006) The age-dependent decline of attention deficit hyperactivity disorder: a meta-analysis of follow-up studies. *Psychological Medicine,* 36(2): 159–65.

Goodman, R. (1997) The Strengths and Difficulties Questionnaire: a research note. *Journal of Child Psychology and Psychiatry,* 38(5): 581–6.

Gournay, K. (2015) Under-recognised and under-treated: ADHD in adults. *British Journal of Mental Health Nursing,* 4(2): 60–3.

Green, H., McGinnity, A., Meltzer, H., Ford, T. and Goodman, R. (2005) *Mental Health of Children and Young People in Great Britain.* London: Office for National Statistics.

Heyman, I. and Santosh, P. (2002) Pharmacological and other physical treatments. In M. Rutter and E. Taylor (eds) *Child and Adolescent Psychiatry* (fourth edition). Oxford: Blackwell, pp. 998–1018.

Jenson, P., Hinshaw, S., Kraemer, H., Lenora, N., Newcorn, J., Abikoff, H., March, J., Arnold, L., Cantwell, D., Conners, K., Elliott, G., Greenhill, L., Hetchman, L., Hoza, B., Pelham, W., Severe, J., Swanson, J., Wells, K., Wigal, T. and Vitiello, B. (2001) ADHD comorbidity findings from the MTA study: comparing comorbid subgroups. *Journal of the American Academy of Child and Adolescent Psychiatry,* 40(2): 147–58.

Mangle, L. (2011) The ADHD integrated care pathway and school nursing. *British Journal of School Nursing*, 6(3): 119–22.

Mangle, L., Phillips, P., Pitts, M. and Laver-Bradbury, C. (2014) Implementation of independent nurse prescribing in UK mental health settings: focus on attention-deficit/hyperactivity disorder (ADHD). *ADHD: Attention Deficit and Hyperactivity Disorders*, 6(4): 269–79.

MTA Cooperative Group (1999) A 14-month randomised clinical trial of treatment strategies for attention-deficit hyperactivity disorder. *Archives of General Psychiatry*, 56(12): 1073–86.

Nakao, T., Radua, J., Rubia, K. and Mataix-Cols, D. (2011) Gray matter volume abnormalities in ADHD: voxel-based meta-analysis exploring the effects of age and stimulant medication. *American Journal of Psychiatry*, 168(11): 1154–63.

National Institute for Health and Care Excellence (NICE) (2008) *Attention Deficit Hyperactivity Disorder: Diagnosis and Management of ADHD in Children, Young People and Adults (GC72)*. London: NICE.

National Prescribing Centre, National Institute for Mental Health in England and Department of Health (2005) *Improving Mental Health Services by Extending the Role of Nurses in Prescribing and Supplying Medication: Good Practice Guide*. London: Department of Health.

Northover, C., Thapar, A., Langley, K. and van Goozen, S. (2015) Emotion regulation in adolescent males with attention-deficit hyperactivity disorder: testing the effects of comorbid conduct disorder. *Brain Sciences*, 5(3): 369–86.

Nursing and Midwifery Council (NMC) (2015) *The Code: Professional Standards of Practice and Behaviour for Nurses and Midwives*. London: NMC.

Nursing and Midwifery Council (NMC) (2012) Amendments to Home Office Misuse of Drugs Regulations 2001, 23 April [online]. Available at: www.nmc.org.uk/news/news-and-updates/amendments-to-home-office-misuse-of-drugs-regulations-2001/ (accessed 27 September 2015).

O'Regan, F. (2002) *How to Teach and Manage Children with ADHD*. Cambridge: LDA.

Owens, E., Cardoos, S. and Hinshaw, P. (2015) Developmental progression and gender differences among individuals with ADHD. In R. A. Barkley (ed.) *Attention-Deficit Hyperactivity Disorder: A Handbook for Diagnosis and Treatment* (fourth edition). New York: Guildford Press, pp. 223–55.

Pliska, S., Carlson, C. and Swanson, J. (1999) *ADHD with Comorbid Disorders: Clinical Assessment and Management*. New York: Guildford Press.

Polanczyk, G., de Lima, M., Hotra, B., Bierderman, J. and Rohde, L. (2007) The worldwide prevalance of ADHD: a systematic review and meta-regression analysis. *American Journal of Psychiatry*, 164(6): 942–8.

Ryan, N. and McDougall, T. (2009) *Nursing Children and Young People with ADHD*. Abingdon: Routledge.

Schacher, R. and Tannock, R. (2002) Syndromes of hyperactivity and attention deficit. In M. Rutter and E. Taylor (eds) *Child and Adolescent Psychiatry* (fourth edition). Oxford: Blackwell, pp. .399–418.

Shaw, M., Hodgkins, P., Young, S., Kahle, J., Woods, A. and Arnold, L. (2012) A systematic review and analysis of long-term outcomes in attention deficit hyperactivity disorder: effects of treatment and non-treatment. *BMC Medicine*, 10: 99.

Sonuga-Barke, E., Brandeis, D., Cortese, S., Daley, D., Ferrin, M., Stevenson, J., Danckaerts, M., van der Oord, S., Dopfner, M., Dittmann, R. W., Simonoff, E., Zuddas, A., Banaschewski, T., Buitelaar, J., Coghill, D., Hollis, C., Konofal, E., Lecendreux, M., Wong, I. and Sergeant, J. (2013) Non-pharmacological interventions for ADHD: systematic review and meta-analyses of randomized controlled trials of dietary and psychological treatments. *American Journal of Psychiatry*, 170(3): 275–89.

Sutcliffe, A. J. (1999) Prescribing medicines for children. *BMJ*, 319(7202): 70–1.

Taylor, E., Doepfner, M., Sergeant, J., Asherson, P., Banaschewski, T., Buitelaar, J., Coghill, D., Danckaerts, M., Rothenberger, A., Sonuga-Barke, E., Steinhausen, H. and Zuddas, A. (2004) European clinical guidelines for hyperkinetic disorder – first upgrade. *Journal of European Child and Adolescent Psychiatry*, 13(1): 1–30.

Timimi, S. and Radcliffe, N. (2005) The rise and rise of ADHD. In C. Newnes and N. Radcliffe (eds) *Making and Breaking Children's Lives*. Ross-on-Wye: PCCS Books, pp. 63–70.

Waldcock, H. (2009) The essence of physical health care. In P. Callaghan, J. Playle and L. Cooper (eds) *Mental Health Nursing Skills*. Oxford: Oxford University Press, pp. 96–110.

Weyandt, L. and Gudmundsdottir, B. (2015) Developmental and neuropsychological deficits in children with ADHD. In R. A. Barkley (ed.) *Attention-Deficit Hyperactivity Disorder: A Handbook for Diagnosis and Treatment* (fourth edition). New York: Guildford Press, pp. 116–39.

World Health Organization (1992) *The ICD-10 Classification of Mental and Behavioural Disorders: Clinical Descriptions and Diagnostic Guidelines*. Geneva: World Health Organization.

York, A. and Kingsley, S. (2013) *Choice and Partnership Approach: Service Transformation Model*. London: CAMHS Network.

Young, S. (2015) ADHD child evaluation: a diagnostic interview of ADHD in children [online]. Available from: www.psychology-services.uk.com/resources.htm (accessed 28 September 2015).

Zwi, M., Jones, H., Thorgaard, C., York, A. and Dennis, J. (2011) Parent training interventions for attention deficit hyperactivity disorder (ADHD) in children aged 5 to 18 years. *Cochrane Database of Systematic Reviews*, 12: CD003018.

Chapter 11

Nursing children and young people with psychosis and schizophrenia

Tim McDougall and Sally Sanderson

Key points:

- The phrase 'early intervention' is used in two ways when referring to children and young people with psychosis or schizophrenia. Generally, it refers to intervention at the earliest stage in order to minimise cognitive, psychological and social impairments and to optimise outcomes. Specifically, it is used to describe 'early intervention services', which aim to reduce both the duration and severity of psychosis or schizophrenia and to improve a young person's interpersonal and social functioning.
- Nurses are in key positions to provide psychological interventions to young people, their families and carers across a range of practice settings. Nurses who have been trained to use cognitive behaviour therapy for psychosis can apply this approach to assess individual symptoms such as auditory hallucinations, delusions and paranoia.
- A thorough multidisciplinary assessment is the foundation on which an accurate diagnosis of psychosis or schizophrenia can be made, and it is essential before planning care, treatment and management. Assessing children and young people as soon as possible, and preferably within 24 hours, may have a positive impact on the developmental trajectory and prognosis of their condition.
- Treatment for psychosis and schizophrenia involves the use of pharmacology, individual psychological support and a range of psychosocial and family-based interventions. Most appropriately, it comprises a combination of evidence-based interventions from all these treatment modalities.
- The parents of carers of children and young people with psychosis or schizophrenia usually have a key role to play, and they should be involved according to the age and wishes of their child or young person.

Introduction

This chapter explores what we mean by psychosis and schizophrenia. Individual and family-based assessment and treatment approaches are covered as well as a description of how services are organised and provided for children, young people and their families. The importance of a careful and thorough nursing assessment, collaborative care planning and engagement to support the process of recovery are also discussed.

Perhaps more than in any other child and adolescent mental health services (CAMHS), the language that is used to describe children and young people with serious mental illness, their experiences and the services to help and support them contains a lot of jargon. A number of terms are explained in this chapter.

Background

Schizophrenia has been identified as the ninth leading cause of disability among all known diseases, and it is the most persistent and disabling of all the major mental disorders (Murray and Lopez 1996). Longitudinal studies suggest that on average, people with schizophrenia die 16–25 years sooner than the general population due to higher rates of cardiovascular, respiratory and infectious diseases (Brown *et al.* 2010). This is of course unacceptable. *No Health Without Mental Health* (Department of Health 2011) aims to ensure that emotional health and wellbeing and physical health are viewed as equally important in the commissioning and provision of modern health services.

It is a decade since the Chief Nursing Officer's report on mental health nursing (Department of Health 2006) announced that more had to be done to increase knowledge among nursing staff of the physical health implications for people with a mental health condition such as schizophrenia. Nurses are well placed to help reduce physical and mental comorbidity through mental and public health interventions, and there have been significant improvements in the provision of holistic care in the last ten years. However, there is still much to do to ensure that care for young people with mental health problems is on an equal footing with care for physical problems.

Childhood or preadolescent onset schizophrenia is very rare with an estimated incidence of between 0.14 and 1.0 per 10,000 (Hafner *et al.* 1998; Hollis 2000). However, the rate of onset for all psychotic disorders rises steeply during adolescence, particularly during the teenage years (Hafner *et al.* 1998). Within this younger age range, schizophrenia is more common amongst males than females by a ratio of approximately 2:1, although this difference becomes less marked with a later age of onset (Russell *et al.* 1989). It is now known that half of all mental disorders begin before the age of 14 (Maughan and Kim-Cohen 2005), and this has been a compelling driver in making 'invest to save' policy statements (Department of Health 2011).

As psychotic symptoms often emerge during the crucial developmental period of adolescence, young people can experience considerable disruption to their academic, vocational and social development. Adolescence is a crucial life stage that involves the consolidation of identity, the quest for independence, mastery of educational and vocational endeavours and the development of important peer relationships (McGorry and Edwards 1997). It also represents a time of development and change when young people begin to realise their potential. Thus when the development of psychosis and schizophrenia occurs during adolescence or young adulthood, the effects can be profound, far-reaching and often life changing (Yung and McGorry 1996; McGorry and Edwards 1997).

Until relatively recently, most community CAMHS teams stopped working with children when they reached the age of 16, which is just at the time when the incidence of psychotic disorders increases and services are required most (Kirkbride *et al.* 2006). Indeed, the vast majority of mental illness starts in the teenage years (Kim-Cohen *et al.* 2003), precisely when most child and adolescent services stop and adult services start.

What do we mean by psychosis and schizophrenia?

Schizophrenia and psychosis in children and young people refers to a major psychiatric disorder or cluster of disorders characterised by so-called 'positive' psychotic symptoms such as hallucinations, delusions and thought disorders and 'negative' symptoms such as loss of motivation and social withdrawal. Some of these terms can be confusing and require clarification.

Positive symptoms are those that most individuals do not normally experience but are present in people with schizophrenia. They can include delusions, disordered thoughts and speech, and hallucinations. Negative symptoms refer to deficits of normal emotional responses or of other thought processes. They commonly include flat or blunted emotional expressions, difficulty experiencing pleasure, lack of desire to form relationships and a general lack of motivation. Perhaps more than positive symptoms, negative symptoms can contribute to poor quality of life and functional disability.

Hallucinations are experiences of seeing, hearing or feeling things that have no basis in reality. They can be tactile, auditory, visual, olfactory or gustatory and can often be anxiety provoking and troubling for people, particularly when they interfere with everyday functioning. Delusions are fixed or falsely held beliefs that are unusual, not shared by the majority of society and generally regarded as not being based in reality. (Strategies to support children and young people with psychotic symptoms are discussed later in this chapter.)

In the years following Kraepelin's and Bleuler's initial work on *dementia praecox* at the turn of the twentieth century (see Bleuler 1911), there was a great deal of pessimism associated with schizophrenia. The diagnosis was often regarded as a 'life sentence' with little hope for improvement, let alone recovery (Albiston *et al.* 1998). This view of hopelessness was reflected in successive government policies that were weak and lacking in hope and ambition. The deteriorating developmental course of schizophrenia that was initially proposed by Kraepelin started to come into question in the 1970s and 1980s. Ciompi (1980) noted a high degree of variability in the course of this disorder with only one-third of individuals displaying the chronic course described by Kraepelin as a defining feature.

The 1990s witnessed a growing optimism regarding improved outcomes for individuals experiencing a psychotic episode together with a drive to reform access to and quality of the available treatments and services. Whilst this was in some way due to the development of novel antipsychotic medicine, which reported improved efficacy whilst inducing fewer side effects, there was also a renewed interest in the psychological and psychosocial management of psychotic symptoms. In their book on early onset psychosis, Birchwood and colleagues (1998) note that a plateau of psychopathology and disability is reached early in the illness, a finding which has since been replicated in numerous studies. Deterioration, although variable, occurs early in the course of schizophrenia, often stabilising within two to five years from onset (Birchwood *et al.* 1998).

Although attitudes to people with psychosis and schizophrenia have modernised since the seminal work of Kraepelin and Bleuler, present-day stigma remains rife and there is much to do to develop care and treatment services further. The ability to foster hope and optimism are now seen as important qualities of the professional nursing role (Dusseldorp *et al.* 2011). Bowers and colleagues (2009) describe the moral foundation on which nursing practice is formed and refer to a number of qualities and values including encouragement, empathy, honesty and respect.

What causes these conditions?

No common cause of psychosis and schizophrenia has been established for all children and young people. However, there is broad agreement that these conditions result from a combination of genetic factors and life events. The stress-vulnerability model, as first coined by Zubin and Spring (1977), is used to view and understand how symptoms of psychosis and schizophrenia develop in the context of life events. Some propose that the timing of onset leads this to be understood as a disorder of adolescence and the consequence of severe disruption in this normally difficult psychological maturational process in vulnerable individuals (Harrop and Trower 2001).

We have heard that the discourse of psychosis and schizophrenia uses a vast range of terms and phrases that may at first seem bewildering to the nurse or other professional. Whilst we do not qualify all those in use, the following terms are explained in everyday language.

Prodrome

Yung and McGorry (1996) describe the prodromal phase of schizophrenia as a period of change from premorbid functioning that generally precedes active symptoms, which can last weeks, months and even years. During this period, day-to-day functioning may become progressively impaired and the young person is at risk of developing psychosis or schizophrenia.

At risk mental state

Cannon *et al.* (2008) identify a group of young people who have a complex array of psychological, emotional and social problems that they refer to as an 'at risk mental state' (ARMS). The link between ARMS and transition to psychosis or schizophrenia is perhaps the most widely researched area within the field (Demjaha *et al.* 2012).

Duration of untreated psychosis

The duration of untreated psychosis refers to the period of time following prodromal onset or the development of psychotic symptoms until treatment is started. This is another area which has received extensive research attention, the outcomes of which have influenced policy and treatment guidance (see Marshall *et al.* 2005; National Institute for Health and Care and Excellence [NICE] 2013).

Attenuated psychotic symptoms

Attenuated psychotic symptoms can be defined as unusual perceptual experiences or beliefs that are similar to psychotic symptoms such as hearing voices, seeing visions or being convinced that strangers intend to cause harm. They happen less often and are less intense than psychotic symptoms, and there is sometimes uncertainty in the person's mind about whether these experiences are happening or not.

NICE (2013) points out that most children and young people with transient or attenuated psychotic symptoms do not go on to develop psychosis or schizophrenia. However, those with such symptoms are at higher risk of developing psychosis and schizophrenia up to ten years after onset of attenuated symptoms. It is therefore important that a child or young person who is experiencing transient or attenuated psychotic symptoms associated with distress or impairment is assessed by CAMHS or an early intervention in psychosis (EIP) service without delay.

Recovery

The principles of the recovery approach, which emphasises the equal importance of good relationships, education, employment and purpose alongside reduction in clinical symptoms, apply equally to children and young people (Department of Health 2011). During the later stages of treatment, specific symptoms including positive psychotic symptoms, underlying depression and social anxiety together with strategies aimed at substance use are often key components of treatment. Sanderson (2006) argues that one of the most important parts of supporting recovery from psychosis or schizophrenia is enabling the young person to make sense of their experiences, which can also assist with relapse prevention. This is because early recovery is an important indicator of outcome. Young people who remain psychotic after six months of onset have only a 15 per cent chance of achieving full remission, whilst half of those who make a full recovery have psychotic symptoms for less than three months (Hollis and Rapoport 2011).

Relapse prevention

Another priority in supporting children and young people who have experienced a first episode of psychosis is concentration on the prevention of subsequent episodes. The identification of idiosyncratic relapse signatures through the recognition of early warning signs enables individuals to access support at the earliest sign of symptoms re-emerging (Birchwood *et al.* 2000). This helps manage problems early, and a relapse of psychotic symptoms or transition to schizophrenia may sometimes be averted. Involving young people and parents or carers in relapse prevention also helps tackle the feelings of powerlessness that psychotic disorders can often generate in young people and families. Dusseldorp and colleagues (2011) describe how mental health nurses can help decrease the risk of relapse through the preparation of a relapse prevention plan and the provision of psycho-education for the young person and their family.

The importance of early intervention

The phrase 'early intervention' is used in two ways when discussing children and young people with psychosis or schizophrenia. First, it refers to the principle of intervention at the earliest stage in order to optimise outcomes. Since children and young people with this condition have greater cognitive, psychological and social impairments, early detection and intervention is crucial. Early intervention aims to reduce both the duration and severity of acute psychosis and to improve a young person's social functioning and assist them in staying in or returning to school, college or university. Second, it is used to describe 'early intervention services', which are discussed throughout this chapter.

The importance of early intervention in the life course of psychosis and schizophrenia has been recognised for over 70 years (Cameron 1938; McGorry 1998). Generally speaking, the earlier treatment can be started, the quicker and better the process of recovery. A growing body of research evidence has continued to demonstrate the efficacy of early detection and intervention in helping to enable positive outcomes and recovery for people living with this condition (McGorry *et al.* 2002; McGorry 1998). In contrast, late intervention can be associated with severe impairments for young people and their families (Royal College of Psychiatrists 2010).

Coining the phrase 'the critical period', Birchwood *et al.* (1998) proposed that focused interventions within the early years following onset had a disproportionate impact relative to interventions later in the course of the disorder. This was found to result in a substantial reduction in morbidity together with a better quality of life for individuals and their families.

What is the policy context?

Early intervention in psychosis (EIP) services originated in *The NHS Plan* (Department of Health 2000). They were intended to provide community interventions for people aged between 14 and 35 who were in prodromal and early phase psychosis or schizophrenia (Department of Health 2001). The model of care that has since evolved is now part of healthcare systems across the UK, Europe and North America. Engagement with families is an important element, particularly for children and young people who are living with one or both parents or carers. EIP teams offer specialised psychosocial and pharmacological interventions and generally use a recovery-based model to help optimise social, education and vocational outcomes. Some key requirements of EIP are summarised in Box 11.1.

Box 11.1 Key requirements of early intervention in psychosis services

- Reduce the length of time that young people remain undiagnosed and untreated.

- Provide a seamless service available for people aged 14 to 35 that effectively integrates child, adolescent and adult mental health services and works in partnership with primary care, education, social services, youth and other services.

- Develop meaningful engagement, provide evidence-based interventions and promote recovery during the early phase of illness.

- Increase stability in the lives of service users, facilitate development and provide opportunities for personal fulfilment.

- Ensure that the care is transferred thoughtfully and effectively at the end of the treatment period.

- Reduce stigma associated with psychosis and improve professional and lay awareness of the symptoms of psychosis and the need for early intervention.

Source: adapted from Department of Health (2001).

NICE (2013) states that regardless of the age of onset of psychosis or schizophrenia, children and young people with psychosis or schizophrenia who are being treated in an EIP service should have access to that service for up to three years or until their eighteenth birthday, whatever period is longer. Unfortunately, this is not always the case and this standard has been diluted in recent years.

Despite policy and associated guidance, the roles and responsibilities of CAMHS and EIP teams for local children and young people with psychosis and schizophrenia tend to be inconsistent, and access to these vary across the UK (Rethink 2011). EIP teams generally form part of adult mental health services with just a minority located in CAMHS. In 2004, a group of international experts put forward recommendations for the essential elements of EIP services and their relationship with CAMHS. There was consensus that the two services should be better integrated and that EIP teams should have dedicated input from a child and adolescent psychiatrist and other professionals with training to support young people (Marshall *et al.* 2004). In practice, however, only a minority of EIP teams include input from CAMHS, and despite the national policy directives (Department of Health 2001) and NICE (2013) guidance, some do not see young people under 16 at all (Pinfold *et al.* 2007).

How effective are EIP services?

There is evidence that EIP services are clinically effective and cost-effective and that they play a vital part in shifting the focus of services towards prevention and early identification and intervention (Department of Health 2011; NICE 2013). They have also been shown to be effective in preventing full psychosis and reducing relapse (Knapp *et al.* 2014). This is why NICE (2013, 2015) recommends that if a child or young person experiences transient psychotic symptoms or other experiences suggestive of possible psychosis, they should be referred to a specialist mental health service for assessment without delay.

The national mental health strategy, *No Health Without Mental Health* (Department of Health 2011), states that EIP services for young people aged 14 to 35 with the first onset of psychosis have been shown to reduce relapse, improve employment and educational outcomes and reduce risk of suicide and homicide. The NHS Confederation (2011) suggests that EIP services offer mental health providers opportunities to support the delivery of key objectives within the mental health strategy. The Confederation adds that through their innovative practice, EIP teams have evidenced substantial clinical improvements, met productivity targets, reduced costs and, most importantly, have been positively received by the clients, families and the referral agencies that have experienced them.

Despite the evidence base, EIP services have been cut in recent years (Rethink Mental Illness 2014). This has had a major impact on the ability of teams to provide NICE-concordant interventions, and timely access by young people with a first episode of psychosis or schizophrenia has been significantly compromised. *Achieving Better Access to Mental Health Services by 2020* (Department of Health 2014) outlines waiting time standards for mental health. This includes a standard which will ensure that by 2016, at least 50 per cent of children, young people and adults referred for Early Intervention in Psychosis services will start treatment within two weeks.

Assessment

A thorough multidisciplinary assessment is the foundation for accurate diagnosis of psychosis or schizophrenia and is essential before planning care, treatment and management. Assessing all young people with first-episode psychosis as soon as possible, and preferably within 24 hours, may have a positive impact on the course and prognosis of their illness. Whether a child or young person is being assessed in CAMHS or EIP services, some general principles apply. The assessment should be multidisciplinary, comprehensive and holistic, and undertaken by those with skills and competencies in working with children and young people with psychosis and schizophrenia.

The assessment should be paced according to the child or young person's level of understanding, emotional maturity and cognitive abilities. A detailed developmental and neurodevelopmental history, including birth history and speech and language development as well as information about attachment, behaviour and any sexual, physical, or emotional abuse, should be undertaken. The areas of need in Box 11.2 should be covered during the assessment.

A thorough multidisciplinary assessment should include a comprehensive mental state examination, a medical review to exclude physical causes for psychotic symptoms, and further neuropsychological and neurological evaluation as appropriate. It is important to evaluate risk during the assessment process. This is particularly important for children and young people who are at risk of suicide, exploitation or severe self-neglect and those who present a risk to others.

Box 11.2 Key areas for assessment

- Developmental history

- Mental health and disorder including comorbidity

- Psychological and psychosocial functioning

- Functioning in education, training or employment

- Physical health and history

- Risk and needs

- Family needs.

Care planning

The NICE guidance on service user experience of adult mental health has been adapted to the needs of children and young people. This states that children and young people with psychosis or schizophrenia should be routinely able to access care from a single multidisciplinary team and not be passed from one team to another and have to go through multiple assessments (NICE 2013). In order to help ensure continuity of access and to avoid disruptive transitions, care and treatment should be carefully planned and organised with all involved parties. For example, children and young people who are taking antipsychotic medication are at heightened risk of adverse events (Kumra *et al.* 2008), and responsibility for physical care, baseline assessments and monitoring needs to be clear to all those involved in the care plan.

The care plan for a child or young person with psychosis or schizophrenia should always include a crisis element. This should be developed in conjunction with the young person, their parents or carers and all the professionals involved in the care package. This is so that intervention in crisis is timely and hospital admission is avoided wherever possible. The crisis plan should include a focus on 'relapse signatures' (i.e. signs that a young person may be becoming unwell), and the details of the support network and the roles, responsibilities and contact details of all professionals who are involved should be clearly stated.

Depending on the age of the child or young person and where they live, services may be available to avoid hospital admission. For young people over 16, crisis resolution and home treatment (CRHT) teams are usually available where support can be provided in the community or at home. For children under 16, the options are much more limited. CRHT teams in CAMHS are virtually non-existent, and children in psychiatric crisis are usually admitted to hospital only where the option of emergency admission exists, which is not in all areas of the UK. This means that children and young people in mental health crisis may sometimes be admitted to inappropriate settings such as paediatric wards, adult mental health wards or police custody (McDougall and Bodley-Scott 2008; McDougall 2014).

Treatment

Treatment for psychosis and schizophrenia involves the use of antipsychotic medication, individual psychological support and a range of psychosocial and family interventions. Most appropriately, it comprises a combination of all these modalities. It is not possible to describe the full range of interventions that are provided as well as a discussion of their relative evidence or lack of evidence within the scope of this chapter. Therefore, some general principles as well as information in relation to where the evidence is most robust are summarised.

Most antipsychotic medication does not have a UK marketing authorisation specifically for children and young people. NICE (2013, 2015) recommends offering oral antipsychotic medication in conjunction with psychological interventions for children and young people with first-episode psychosis. The choice of medication should be made by the parents or carers of younger children or jointly with the young person and their parents or carers and healthcare professionals. There should be a full discussion about the risks and potential benefits of medication including side effects. Children, young people and parents should be aware that there is a risk of weight gain and diabetes with many drugs and that extrapyramidal side effects including akathisia, dyskinesia and dystonia may be possible. Additionally, cardiovascular and hormonal risks should be discussed.

Whilst drug treatment is often the mainstay of treatment for psychosis and schizophrenia, NICE (2013) states that antipsychotic medication should not be offered where psychotic symptoms or mental state changes are insufficient for a psychosis or schizophrenia diagnosis. It should also not be offered with the aim of decreasing the risk of psychosis.

Like all treatment goals, those to support children and young people with psychosis or schizophrenia should be SMART (i.e. specific, measurable, achievable, realistic and timely) and ideally framed in the child or young person's own words. Such aims or goals should also be flexible so that they can change if necessary during the treatment programme.

Psychological interventions

Psychological interventions are often set in the context of the stress-vulnerability model, although this is not the only paradigm to explain and treat people with psychosis and schizophrenia. Psycho-educational interventions based on the stress-vulnerability model have been described for use with children and families in primary care settings (Asarnow et al. 2001). This intervention is designed to enhance understanding of symptoms through a working model that links stress to effects on feelings, thoughts and behaviour which, if left unchallenged, can lead to deterioration in mental health.

Research findings indicate that psychotic symptoms can be conceptualised with reference to normal psychological processes, and this then makes the content of symptoms understandable and suitable for cognitive behaviour therapy (CBT; Chadwick et al. 1996). CBT with children and young people with psychosis or schizophrenia involves a combination of techniques for distraction from persistent voices or auditory hallucinations and techniques where the primary aim of intervention is anxiety reduction (Bentall et al. 1994). Nurses are in key positions to provide psychological interventions to young people, their families and carers across a range of practice settings. Those who have been trained to use CBT for psychosis can apply this approach to assess individual symptoms such as auditory hallucinations, delusions and paranoia. A number of validated psychometric tools can assist nurses in this process and Table 11.1 lists a few.

In order to use CBT with young people with psychosis, it is necessary to first perform a thorough assessment. Box 11.3 includes a summary of the areas that should be explored.

The primary aim of CBT for psychosis is to enable the young person to cope with their psychotic symptoms, reappraise their meaning and make them less distressing. Positive psychotic symptoms such as command auditory hallucinations can be assessed and managed

Table 11.1 Validated psychometric tools for psychosis and schizophrenia

Tool	Focus	Reference
Cognitive Assessment Schedule	Used to assess the nature of auditory hallucinations, the evidence young people attribute to their beliefs, and emotional and behavioural responses to delusions, voices and paranoia	Chadwick *et al.* (1996)
Beliefs About Voices Questionnaire	Measure of key beliefs about auditory hallucinations that enables the nurse or other mental health professional to evaluate the malevolence, benevolence or relative benignity of voices as well as the dimensions of coping such as resistance and engagement	Birchwood and Chadwick (1997)
Topography of Voices Rating Scale	Used to measure the frequency, audibility and intrusiveness of voices reported by young people	Hustig and Hafner (1990)
Positive and Negative Syndrome Scale	A brief scale to measure positive symptoms, such as delusions, hallucinations and grandiosity, and negative symptoms, such as blunted affect, social withdrawal and apathy	Kay *et al.* (1987)
Comprehensive Assessment of At Risk Mental States	Measures positive and negative symptoms and cognitive and behavioural changes as well as general psychopathology	Yung *et al.* (2005)

Box 11.3 *Cognitive behaviour therapy with young people with psychosis: areas for assessment*

- Activating events prior to psychotic symptoms
- Levels of conviction, control and distress associated with psychotic symptoms
- Meaning that the young person attributes to their psychotic symptoms
- Functional assumptions and beliefs about others
- Adaptive and maladaptive coping strategies
- Risk of violence to self or others arising from psychotic symptoms
- History of trauma.

---

within a CBT framework. Close attention is paid to the voices themselves, the meaning a young person attaches to their voices, and how they subsequently feel and behave as a consequence. Coping strategy enhancement is formulated from the work of Yusupoff and Tarrier (1996) and involves ways of empowering young people to cope with symptoms that may be distressing or upsetting. Alternative ways of thinking and behaving are explored.

Children and young people with psychosis or schizophrenia have often had experiences of trauma (Kilcommons and Morrison 2005; Read *et al.* 2005; Morrison 2009). It is therefore important that the treatment programme includes psychotherapeutic interventions where these are indicated. Separate provision of this can be problematic and may lead to fragmented care. It is not just individual therapies that can be helpful. In 2015, NICE reviewed the evidence that had become available since the guideline for children and young people with psychosis or schizophrenia had been published. The review team found that structured psycho-educational group intervention for young people with psychosis and their parents or carers, comprising problem-solving activities and provision of written materials, appeared to reduce visits to the emergency department (NICE 2015).

Family-based interventions

The early stages of psychosis or schizophrenia can be a frightening and bewildering time for children or young people and their families or carers. There is a relatively good evidence base for family interventions with parents, carers and siblings often fulfilling invaluable roles in the assessment, treatment and recovery process. Like any serious disorder in the family, the development of psychosis or schizophrenia during childhood or adolescence usually results in extention of the caregiver role, which is a process that needs to be fully supported. The stress-vulnerability model (Zubin and Spring 1977) reinforces the maintenance role of social, familial and environmental stressors upon the course of serious mental illnesses. Psychosocial family interventions based on the stress-vulnerability model have been shown to be clinically effective and of value to the family (Brooker *et al.* 1994).

One commonly occurring but often overlooked area of need is in relation to the ongoing parenting of children and young people with psychosis or schizophrenia. This is even more important to review if they have spent a period of time in hospital. It is not unusual for parents and carers to struggle with identifying what is part of their child's illness and what is part of the normal course of adolescence or early adulthood. One commonly cited reason for this situation is the wish to avoid a potentially distressing or stress-provoking confrontation. Sanderson (2006) suggests that this may arise from an incomplete explanation of the stress-vulnerability model with emphasis placed upon the avoidance of stress-provoking situations rather than encouraging stress management strategies.

The use of a framework such as the stress-vulnerability model to explain the development of psychotic experiences has been beneficial in terms of aiding greater understanding of the disorder. However, if the model is not properly understood or misapplied then it can reinforce unhealthy family dynamics, which in turn may compound social isolation, exclusion and the maintenance of psychotic symptoms. Therefore, supporting parents and carers with stress management and goal setting strategies is crucially important and can assist with confidence building.

Hospital admission

Children and young people with psychosis use primary, secondary and tertiary health services and receive care and treatment in hospital and community settings. Most will not require hospital admission and can instead be safely and effectively supported by community CAMHS or EIP teams. Until the early 1990s, most adolescents with psychosis and schizophrenia were admitted to inpatient CAMHS units. This was partly because EIP teams were not in existence and also because there were very few alternatives to hospital admission for young people with serious mental health problems (Lamb 2009). There are no efficacy studies but Gowers *et al.* (2001) suggest that young people with psychosis may be effectively managed as day patients, with key determinants being level of risk to self or others, degree of psychosocial complexity and the likely compliance and engagement with investigation and treatment.

Children and young people with psychosis or schizophrenia should usually only be admitted to hospital if the risks associated with their care and treatment mean that care and treatment in the community is likely to be unsafe or if they require intensive 24-hour nursing care. This is because hospital admission can have a negative impact on family life, education and social relationships. It can compromise the mastery of developmental tasks of adolescence such as separating from parents, increasing autonomy and forming a supportive peer network. Admission to hospital in crisis should be to an appropriate hospital environment which is usually an adolescent unit. There may be occasions when an adult ward is more appropriate than a CAMHS unit. This might be where the young person is experiencing a first episode of psychosis and their care in hospital is likely to go beyond their eighteenth birthday. However, a young person's care on an adult ward should take account of their developmental needs. In some areas of the UK, access to adolescent hospital beds is very limited or completely lacking; this means that children and young people have to travel many miles from family and friends, which is unacceptable.

The NICE (2013) guidance on psychosis and schizophrenia confirms that hospital admission can be disruptive and inpatient admission should be seen as one part of a care pathway rather than an end in itself. This is particularly important if it means the child or young person will be admitted a long way from home, which is becoming increasingly common (McDougall 2014). To minimise the risks of hospital admission, there should be close liaison and collaboration with community CAMHS and EIP services; and the Care Programme Approach (CPA) should be used to help optimise the length of hospital stay and support a carefully planned discharge.

Discharge from hospital must be in conjunction with community services. The transition from hospital to CAMHS or EIP services should be supported as evidence shows that this is a time of vulnerability for relapse. Furthermore, the treatment gains made through hospital admission can be diminished or lost as a result of inadequate or failed transition to community EIP, CAMHS or adult services.

Summary

When it comes to care and treatment planning, psychological treatments are just as important as pharmacological therapies. Like all mental health treatments for children and young people, psychological interventions should be planned and delivered collaboratively. Nurses and other professionals should provide verbal and written information which is developmentally appropriate. This is to help gain informed consent, where appropriate, and in order to support the care and treatment goals, help ensure treatment adherence and support recovery. In practice, this involves adapting adult models to suit the needs of children and young people. However, not all children and young people can work with a CBT model so other therapies may need to be explored.

The NICE (2013) guidance suggests that CBT may be helpful in conjunction with antipsychotic medication to both reduce symptoms and prevent relapse. CBT works by enabling the child or young person to recognise the interconnection between their thoughts, feelings and behaviours and to appraise and monitor these in the context of their current or past experiences. This may assist them to reappraise perceptions and challenge unhelpful beliefs. In turn, this may lead to a reduction in distress or anxiety. However, it is important to note that the evidence base for CBT comes predominantly from adult studies and as such it is not generally transferable.

The parents of carers of children and young people with psychosis or schizophrenia usually have a key role to play and should be involved according to the age and wishes of their child or young person. However, it has been suggested that nurses working in CAMHS require further training in working with families (Shannon and Cusack 2015).

Strong links with schools, colleges and higher education institutions are vital to promote and maintain recovery, social inclusion and reduce the stigma associated with psychosis and schizophrenia. Nurses in hospital, community settings and schools are well placed to form effective networks to help optimise outcomes for children and young people with these conditions.

References

Albiston, D., Francey, S. and Harrigan, S. (1998) Group programmes for recovery from early psychosis. *British Journal of Psychiatry*, 172(33): 117–21.

Asarnow, J., Jaycox, L. and Thompson, M. (2001) Depression in youth: psychosocial interventions. *Journal of Clinical Child Psychology*, 30(1): 33–47.

Bentall, R., Haddock, G. and Slade, P. (1994) Psychological treatment for auditory hallucinations: from theory to therapy. *Behaviour Therapy*, (25): 51–66.

Birchwood, M. and Chadwick, P. (1997) The omnipotence of voices: testing the validity of a cognitive model. *Psychological Medicine*, 27(6): 1345–53.

Birchwood, M., Spencer, E. and McGovern, D. (2000) Schizophrenia: early warning signs. *Advances in Psychiatric Treatment*, 6(2): 93–101.

Birchwood, M., Todd, P. and Jackson, C. (1998) Early intervention in psychosis: the critical period hypothesis. *British Journal of Psychiatry*, 172(33): 53–9.

Bleuler, E. (1911) *Dementia praecox oder Gruppe der Schizophrenien*. Leipzig: Franz Deuticke.

Bowers, L., Brennan, G., Winship, G. and Theodoridou, C. (2009) *Talking with Acutely Psychotic People: Communication Skills for Nurses and Others Spending Time with People who are Very Mentally Ill*. London: City University London.

Brooker, C., Falloon, I., Butterworth, T., Goldberg, D., Graham-Hole, V. and Hillier, V. (1994) The outcome of training CPNs to deliver psychosocial interventions. *British Journal of Psychiatry*, 165(2): 122–30.

Brown, S., Kim, M., Mitchell, C. and Inskip, H. (2010) Twenty-five year mortality of a community cohort with schizophrenia. *British Journal of Psychiatry*, 196(2): 116–21.

Cameron, D. (1938) Early schizophrenia. *American Journal of Psychiatry*, 95(3): 567–78.

Cannon, T. D., Cadenhead, K., Cornblatt, B., Woods, S. W., Addington, J., Walker, E., Seidman, L. J., Perkins, D., Tsuang, M., McGlashan, T. and Heinssen, R. (2008) Prediction of psychosis in youth at high clinical risk: a multisite longitudinal study in North America. *Archives of General Psychiatry*, 65(1): 28–37.

Chadwick, P., Birchwood, M. and Trower, P. (1996) *Cognitive Therapy of Delusions, Voices and Paranoia*. Chichester: John Wiley & Sons.

Ciompi, L. (1980) Catamnestic long-term study of the course of life and aging of schizophrenics. *Schizophrenia Bulletin*, 6(4): 606–18.

Demjaha, A., Valmaggia, L., Stahl, D., Byrne, M. and McGuire, P. (2012) Disorganization/cognitive and negative symptom dimensions in the at-risk mental state predict subsequent transition to psychosis. *Schizophrenia Bulletin*, 38(2): 351–9.

Department of Health (2014) *Achieving Better Access to Mental Health Services by 2020*. London: Department of Health.

Department of Health (2011) *No Health without Mental Health: A Cross-Government Mental Health Outcomes Strategy for People of All Ages*. London: Department of Health.

Department of Health (2006) *From Values to Action: The Chief Nursing Officer's Review of Mental Health Nursing*. London: Department of Health.

Department of Health (2001) *Policy Implementation Guidance for Early Intervention Services*. London: Department of Health.

Department of Health (2000) *The NHS Plan: A Plan for Investment, a Plan for Reform*. Cm 4818-I. London: The Stationery Office.

Dusseldorp, L., Goossens, P. and van Achterberg, T. (2011) Mental health nursing and first episode psychosis. *Issues in Mental Health Nursing*, 32(1): 2–19.

Gowers, S., Clarke, J., Alldis, M., Wormald, P. and Wood, N. (2001) In-patient admission of adolescents with mental disorder. *Clinical Child Psychology and Psychiatry*, 6(4): 537–44.

Hafner, H., Hambrecht, M., Loffler, W., Munk-Jorgensen, P. and Riecher-Rossler, A. (1998) Is schizophrenia a disorder of all ages? A comparison of first episodes and early course across the life-cycle. *Psychological Medicine*, 28(2): 351–6.

Harrop, C. and Trower, P. (2001) Why does schizophrenia develop at late adolescence? *Clinical Pyschology Review*, 21(2): 241–65.

Hollis, C. (2000) Adolescent schizophrenia. *Advances in Psychiatric Treatment*, 6(2): 83–92.

Hollis, C. and Rapoport, J. (2011) Child and adolescent schizophrenia. In D. Weinberger and P. Harrison (eds) *Schizophrenia* (third edition). Wiley: London, pp. 24–46.

Hustig, H. and Hafner, R. (1990) Persistent auditory hallucinations and their relationship to delusions of mood. *Journal of Nervous and Mental Disease*, 178(4): 264–7.

Kay, S., Fiszbein, A. and Opler, L. (1987) The positive and negative syndrome scale (PANSS) for schizophrenia. *Schizophrenia Bulletin*, 13(2): 261–76.

Kilcommons, A. and Morrison, A. P. (2005) Relationships between trauma and psychosis: an exploration of cognitive and dissociative factors. *Acta Psychiatrica Scandinavica*, 112(5): 351–9.

Kim-Cohen, J., Caspi, A. and Moffitt, T. (2003) Prior juvenile diagnoses in adults with mental disorder: developmental follow-back of a prospective longitudinal cohort. *Archives of General Psychiatry*, 60(7): 709–17.

Kirkbride, J. B., Fearon, P., Morgan, C., Dazzan, P., Morgan, K., Tarrant, J., Lloyd, T., Holloway, J., Hutchinson, G., Leff, J. P., Mallett, R. M., Harrison, G. L., Murray, R. M. and Jones, P. B. (2006) Heterogeneity in incidence rates of schizophrenia and other psychotic syndromes: findings from the 3-center AeSOP study. *Archives of General Psychiatry*, 63(3): 250–8.

Knapp, M., Andrew, A., McDaid, D., Iemmi, V., McCrone, P., Park, A., Parsonage, M., Boardman, J. and Shepherd, G. (2014) *Investing in Recovery: Making the Business Case for Effective Interventions for People with Schizophrenia and Psychosis*. London: Rethink Mental Illness.

Kumra, S., Oberstar, J. V., Sikich, L., Findling, R. L., McClellan, J. M., Vinogradov, S. and Charles Schulz, S. (2008) Efficacy and tolerability of second-generation antipsychotics in children and adolescents with schizophrenia. *Schizophrenia Bulletin*, 34(1): 60–71.

Lamb, C. (2009) Alternatives to admission for children and adolescents: providing intensive mental healthcare services at home and in communities: what works? *Current Opinion in Psychiatry*, 22(4): 345–50.

McDougall, T. (2014) Improving quality and safety in inpatient CAMHS. *British Journal of Mental Health Nursing*, 3(4): 148–50.

McDougall, T. and Bodley-Scott, S. (2008) Too much too young: under 18s on adult mental health wards. *Mental Health Practice*, 11(6): 12–15.

McGorry, P. (1998) Preventative strategies in early psychosis: verging on reality. *British Journal of Psychiatry*, 172(33): 1–2.

McGorry, P. and Edwards, J. (1997) *Social Treatments: The Early Psychosis Training Pack*. Macclesfield: Gardiner-Caldwell Communications.

McGorry, P. D., Yung, A. R., Phillips, L. J., Yuen, H. P., Francey, S., Cosgrave, E. M., Germano, D., Bravin, J., McDonald, T., Blair, A., Adlard, S. and Jackson, H. (2002) Randomized controlled trial of interventions designed to reduce the risk of progression to first-episode psychosis in a clinical sample with sub-threshold symptoms. *Archives of General Psychiatry* 59(10): 921–8.

Marshall, M., Lewis, S., Lockwood, A., Drake, R., Jones, P. and Croudace, T. (2005) Association between duration of untreated psychosis and outcome in cohorts of first-episode patients: a systematic review. *Archives of General Psychiatry*, 62(9): 975–83.

Marshall, M., Lockwood, A. and Lewis, S. (2004) Essential elements of an early intervention service for psychosis: the opinions of expert clinicians. *BMC Psychiatry*, 4: 17.

Maughan, B. and Kim-Cohen, J. (2005) Continuities between childhood and adult life. *British Journal of Psychiatry*, 187(4): 301–3.

Morrison, P. (2009) A cognitive behavioural perspective on the relationship between childhood trauma and psychosis. *Epidemiologia e Psichiatria Sociale*, 18(4): 294–8.

Murray, C. and Lopez, A. (1996) *The Global Burden of Disease: A Comprehensive Assessment of Mortality and Disability from Diseases, Injuries and Risk Factors in 1990 and Projected to 2020*. Cambridge, MA: Harvard University Press.

National Institute for Health and Care Excellence (NICE) (2015) *Psychosis and Schizophrenia in Children and Young People: Evidence Update*. London: NICE.

National Institute for Health and Care Excellence (NICE) (2013) *Psychosis and Schizophrenia in Children and Young People: Recognition and Management*. London: NICE.

NHS Confederation (2011) *Early Intervention in Psychosis Services: Briefing*. London: NHS Confederation.

Pinfold, V., Smith, J. and Shiers, D. (2007) Audit of early intervention in psychosis service development in England. *Psychiatric Bulletin*, 31(1): 7–10.

Read, J., van Os, J., Morrison, A. P. and Ross, C. (2005) Childhood trauma, psychosis and schizophrenia: a literature review with theoretical and clinical implications. *Acta Psychiatrica Scandinavica*, 112(5): 330–50.

Rethink (2011) *Joint Working at the Interface: Early Intervention in Psychosis and Child and Adolescent Mental Health Services*. London: Rethink.

Rethink Mental Illness (2014) *Lost Generation: Why Young People with Psychosis are Being Left Behind, and What Needs to Change*. London: Rethink Mental Illness.

Royal College of Psychiatrists (2010) *Psychiatric Services for Children and Adolescents with Learning Disabilities (CR163)*. London: Royal College of Psychiatrists.

Russell, A., Bott, L. and Sammons, C. (1989) The phenomenology of schizophrenia occurring in childhood. *Journal of the American Academy of Child and Adolescent Psychiatry*, 28(3): 399–407.

Sanderson, S. (2006) Young people and early onset psychosis: a nursing perspective. In T. McDougall (ed.) *Child and Adolescent Mental Health Nursing*. London: Blackwell, pp. 116–30.

Shannon, M. and Cusack, E. (2015) An *Education and Training Review of Nurses Working in Child and Adolescent Mental Health Services in the Republic of Ireland*. Dublin: Office of the Nursing and Midwifery Services Director.

Yung, A. and McGorry, P. (1996) The prodromal phase of first-episode psychosis: past and present conceptualisations. *Schizophrenia Bulletin*, 22(2): 353–70.

Yung, A., Yuen, H., McGorry, P., Phillips, L., Kelly, D., Dell'Olio, M., Francey, S., Cosgrave, E., Killackey, E., Stanford, C., Godfrey, K. and Buckby, J. (2005) Mapping the onset of psychosis: the Comprehensive Assessment of At-risk Mental States. *Australian and New Zealand Journal of Psychiatry*, 39(11–12): 964–71.

Yusupoff, I. and Tarrier, N. (1996) Coping strategy enhancement for persistent hallucinations and delusions. In G. Haddock and P. Slade (eds) *Cognitive Behavioural Interventions with Psychotic Disorders*. Hove: Routledge, pp. 86–102.

Zubin, J. and Spring, B. (1977) Vulnerability: a new view of schizophrenia. *Journal of Abnormal Psychology*, 86(2):103–26.

Part 3

Service provision

Nursing and school-based mental health services

Tim McDougall

Key points:

- School nurses are in key positions to work in partnership with teachers to deliver activities related to emotional health and wellbeing with a focus on self-awareness, emotional intelligence, mindfulness and resilience.
- School nurses have been identified as crucial in terms of helping children and young people choose healthy lifestyles. This can be in relation to diet and exercise, personal health and hygiene, healthy sexual behaviour and the harmful effects of drugs and alcohol, through life skills teaching.
- Several factors are associated with the success of school-based mental health services. These include consistent programme implementation, the use of multiple modalities, involvement of parents, teachers and peers, the integration of programme content into the general curriculum and approaches that are developmentally appropriate.
- School nurses in particular encounter children and young people who are being exploited or bullied. Here their role is to help develop whole school approaches to prevent and tackle bullying as well as to support individual children and young people who are involved in bullying.
- School nurses require support and time to discuss any concerns they may have about the mental health of pupils and students as well as resources to develop their knowledge, skills and confidence in relation to supporting the mental health of children in school. Primary mental health workers have an important bridging role in supporting their colleagues in schools and ensuring pathways to specialist child and adolescent mental health services are clear and easily accessible.

Introduction

There is now compelling evidence that investment in promoting the mental health and wellbeing of children in the preschool and early years can avoid health and social problems in adolescence and adulthood (McCrone *et al.* 2010; Allen 2011; Khan *et al.* 2015). Leighton (2006) suggests that schools are the ideal place to begin to address the crisis in child and adolescent mental health. Layard (2015) goes further, stating that the whole expansion in mental health therapy should be on school premises, which provide a much more acceptable location for early intervention than traditional CAMHS settings (British Youth Council 2011). As The Children's Society (2015) points out, school-based counselling services could go a long way in tackling the poor satisfaction children in England have with their school and overall life experience. This is in relation to helping to address high rates of bullying and general unhappiness in school. Unlike school-based counselling in Wales and Northern

Ireland where this is a legal requirement, schools in England are not required to provide this service. This chapter describes the role of schools in supporting the mental health of children and discusses the specific contribution that school nurses can make, including practical strategies that can be employed at an individual, group and whole school level.

Why are schools important?

Good schools recognise that the wellbeing of children is linked to positive outcomes across all life domains. The central role that schools play and the potential for them to enable and optimise positive health outcomes has been recognised for many years (Rutter 1999). This is as well as the recognised connection between good mental health and academic attainment and achievement (Jamal *et al.* 2013). Schools play a vital role by supporting children to develop autonomy, relationships and emotionally enriching routines. They set high expectations for children to aspire towards and provide opportunities for children to achieve and enjoy success (McDougall 2010). Concepts such as 'emotional literacy', 'self-talk' and 'circle time' have resilience at their core and have been introduced into the national curriculum in recent years (Weare 2004).

According to Newman (2002), the resilient child or young person can resist adversity, cope with uncertainty and recover more successfully from traumatic life events. McDougall (2010) describes a number of practical ways in which school nurses and other professionals can support children and young people to develop resilience (Box 12.1).

Box 12.1 Ten things to do and say that support children and young people to develop emotional resilience

1 Think positively and remain optimistic – people have little or no control over negative events, but they can influence how they feel about them.

2 Take a different perspective – there are many different ways to consider things.

3 Embrace challenges – things which at first may seem difficult may be easy to overcome.

4 Do something to help someone else – prosocial behaviour such as community involvement helps build resilience.

5 Encourage play and creativity – this enables children and young people to learn about themselves, their relationship with others and the world around them.

6 Identify and nurture strengths – by recognising positive qualities and reinforcing them, children will grow in self-esteem, pride and confidence.

7 Promote self-esteem and self-efficacy – these are the fundamental building blocks of resilience and can be enhanced by participating in valued activities.

8 Make connections – good relationships create a climate of support.

9 Explore opportunities for self-discovery – children who have experienced trauma or loss often grow and develop as a result of their experiences.

10 Look after yourself – eat healthily, sleep properly and exercise regularly; looking after oneself helps individuals to keep their mind and body resilient.

Source: adapted from McDougall (2010).

Successive governments have launched a plethora of policies, strategies and projects designed to improve mental health outcomes as well as educational achievement. Some have been discontinued in their entirety while for others, elements remain or have been adapted. Others have their roots in behaviour improvement programmes that have been refined to address the causes rather than effects of behaviour problems. A good example of this was the government's Behaviour and Education Support Teams programme (see Department for Education and Skills 2005) with the focus on promoting emotional wellbeing and preventing difficulties. The main programmes and initiatives that have had an influence on the mental health in schools agenda are shown in Box 12.2.

Box 12.2 *National policies and initiatives to improve educational attainment as well as emotional health and wellbeing*

- National Healthy Schools Programme – this aimed to improve health, raise academic attainment, increase social inclusion and encourage better joint working between health and education agencies.

- Social and Emotional Aspects of Learning (SEAL) – this referred to resources for primary and secondary schools to deliver a whole school approach to promoting social, emotional and behavioural skills. SEAL was operating in 80 per cent of primary schools and 30 per cent of secondary schools across England in 2008 (Institute of Education 2010). Elements of SEAL continue to be used in schools, and the resources have been widely evaluated (Evans et al. 2003; Durlak et al. 2011).

- Targeted Mental Health in Schools (TaMHS) – this was a three-year government-funded programme that ran between 2008 and 2011. It aimed to help schools deliver timely support to pupils with mental health problems and those considered at increased risk of developing them.

- Connexions – this was an information, advice and guidance service for young people aged 13–25.

- Extended Schools Programme – this focused on extracurricular services and activities for children, young people and the wider community.

- Young People's Development Programme – this involved working with schools to identify and provide targeted support to 'at risk' young people aged 13–15.

- Full-service extended schools – these provided a comprehensive range of health services, adult learning and community activities, study support and wrap-around childcare.

- AcSEED Award – this quality assurance scheme was founded by young people with direct experience of mental health problems and provides accreditation for schools that have made a substantial effort to provide emotional health and wellbeing support for pupils.

Children who are unhappy or struggling with problems do not do well either academically or socially. Greenhalgh (1994) suggests that some emotions (such as sadness and anger) can block learning whereas others (such as a sense of wellbeing, feeling safe and feeling valued) promote learning. It therefore follows that learning to manage emotions can assist learning in itself. Cemalcilar (2010) agrees, observing that positive relationships both between school staff and pupils and among pupils themselves are crucial in promoting emotional wellbeing and in helping to foster a sense of belonging to and liking of school or college.

The Good Childhood Report (The Children's Society 2015) is an international study of childhood wellbeing. It suggests that children in England are unhappier with their school life than children in almost all of the other 14 countries taking part in the international study. England ranked in the bottom third of countries for liking going to school as well as satisfaction with their school experience in general, and there was a sharp decline between Year 6 (10- to 11-year-olds) and Year 8 (12- to 13-year-olds) in satisfaction with most aspects of school. Children in England also reported relatively low satisfaction with their relationships with classmates, ranking twelfth (The Children's Society 2015).

Public Health England (2015) suggests that in an average secondary school classroom of 30 pupils, 3 are likely to have mental disorder, 10 are likely to have experienced their parents separate and 1 may have experienced the death of a parent. Additionally, 7 are likely to have been bullied and 6 may be self-harming. The report of the Children and Young People's Mental Health and Wellbeing Taskforce, *Future in Mind*, (Department of Health 2015) identified a national commitment to encouraging schools to develop whole school approaches to promoting mental health and wellbeing. Public Health England (2015) uses the diagram in Figure 12.1 to represent eight principles that help them achieve this.

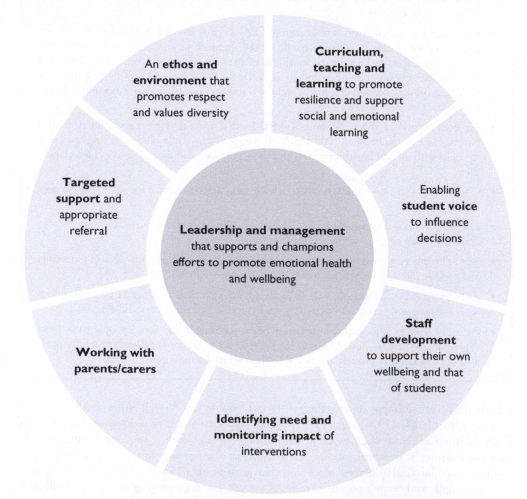

Figure 12.1 Eight principles to support emotional health and wellbeing in schools
Source: Public Health England (2015: 6).

Why are school nurses important?

Like nurses in CAMHS more generally, school nurses are the 'single biggest workforce specifically trained and skilled to deliver public health for school-aged children' (Department of Health and Public Health England 2014a: 6). They are recorded on Part 3 of the Nursing and Midwifery Council Register under the title of specialist community public health nurse. School nurses work with pupils and students aged 5–19 in schools and colleges. They are often the first point of professional contact for children and young people with mental health problems, and they are particularly well placed to identify mental health problems and difficulties and to provide effective support for pupils or students (Department of Health and Public Health England 2014a). Unlike many other professionals, they work across education, health and social care boundaries, which puts them in key positions of leadership and influence with multi-agency colleagues.

School nurses require good networks and working relationships with other health and social care professionals. They often liaise with health visitors, speech and language therapists, paediatricians and specialist nurses for children with complex health needs as well as GPs, practice nurses, psychologists and mental health workers. To network effectively, they need good working knowledge of other statutory agencies and voluntary organisations such as early years' provision, youth services, youth offending teams, drug and alcohol teams, social services and the police (Skills for Health 2010).

It has been suggested that during term time, school-based professionals spend more time with children than even their parents (Wolk 2008). This of course enables them to form positive and meaningful relationships with pupils and students as well as helping to reduce health inequalities. School nurses have also been identified as crucial in terms of helping children and young people choose healthy lifestyles. In addition to emotional health and wellbeing, this can focus on issues such as diet and exercise, personal health and hygiene, healthy sexual behaviour or the harmful effects of drugs and alcohol through life skills teaching (Moore 2000).

School nursing services are universal, and there are reports that young people see them as less stigmatising than specialist CAMHS (British Youth Council 2011; Department of Health 2015). Despite the key positions school nurses occupy, the Royal College of Nursing ([RCN] 2012) has been concerned that their value has not been recognised in many areas of the UK, which limits the potential public health contribution they can make. Additionally, school nurses recognise that supporting pupils in relation to emotional health and wellbeing is an important aspect of their work, but often lack relevant additional training and support to take on this role (Haddad *et al.* 2010).

What resources are available for school nurses?

School nursing practice is influenced by several National Institute for Health and Care Excellence (NICE) guidelines focusing on physical and mental health, including overarching standards such as those related to children in care (2015a) and guidance on social and emotional wellbeing in the early years (2012), primary (2008a) and secondary (2009a) education.

The NICE guidance on social and emotional wellbeing in primary education (2008a) encourages head teachers, governors and teachers to demonstrate leadership and commitment to children's mental health. This is by ensuring that social and emotional wellbeing is a key part of school improvement plans, policies and curriculum activities. The guidance for primary schools recommends the development of a curriculum that integrates the development of social and emotional skills within all subject areas with a focus on problem-solving, conflict resolution and managing feelings.

A systematic review of approaches designed to promote mental wellbeing in schools (Wells *et al.* 2003) concluded that studies which focused mainly on pupil behaviour were less likely to be effective than those that took a whole school approach. Therefore, NICE recommends a whole school approach to children's social and emotional wellbeing to provide an emotionally secure and safe environment that prevents any form of bullying or violence, support all pupils and, where appropriate, their parents or carers. Additionally, the guidance sets standards for helping pupils who are most at risk or already showing signs of social, emotional and behavioural problems.

The guidance for secondary schools builds on the primary school advice but is more extensive. In this, NICE (2009a) recommends that the curriculum should promote positive behaviours and successful relationships and help to reduce disruptive behaviour and bullying. Skills that should be developed in addition to those in the guidance for primary schools include motivation, self-awareness, collaborative working and how to manage relationships with parents, carers and peers. In addition, secondary schools are encouraged to tailor social and emotional skills education to the developmental needs of young people.

As well as guidelines on social and emotional wellbeing and mental health, school nurses can refer to a wide range of quality standards that keep them up to date with evidence-based practice. These include NICE publications on prevention and lifestyle weight management programmes for obesity (2015b) and guidance on a range of public health issues such as school-based interventions for alcohol (2007); smoking prevention in schools (2010); and physical activity for children and young people (2009b).

A number of disorder-specific NICE guidelines also have relevance for the day-to-day practice of school nurses: the identification and management of attention deficit hyperactivity disorder (ADHD; 2008b), depression (2005) and antisocial behaviour and conduct disorder (2013). In addition to NICE guidance, school nurses and other professionals can consult resources on mental health and behaviour in schools (Department for Education 2014a) and advice on counselling in schools (Department for Education 2015).

More broadly, the Department for Education (2014b) provides advice and guidance for head teachers, staff and governing bodies in relation to preventing and tackling bullying, including cyberbullying, in schools. This includes a focus on whole school approaches as well as strategies to support and safeguard individual pupils and is directly applicable to nurses and other school-based professionals. O'Brien and Moules (2010) studied the impact of cyberbullying on young people's mental health and made a number of recommendations relevant to nursing practice (see Box 12.3).

The Department of Health and Public Health England (2014b) produced joint guidance on promoting emotional wellbeing and positive mental health of children and young people. This includes using a whole school approach and encouraging health-promoting schools. The guidance (Box 12.4) identifies a number of important factors to consider.

It should be noted, however, that the ability of school nurses to act on the various sources of guidance is limited because of their role and the authority they have, and there is a responsibility on public health commissioners and school governing bodies. To fulfil their mental health roles effectively, Bartlett (2015) suggests that school nurses require further postgraduate training and regular supervision from a mental health specialist.

Box 12.3 Recommendations for practice and policy in relation to cyberbullying

- Develop educational programmes around awareness for young people, parents/carers and schools.

- Deliver education that brings together young people and their families to enhance communication in relation to online media.

- Educate young people about what constitutes acceptable behaviour online.

- Support young people to report incidents of cyber-bullying through other young people who could help change attitudes and provide a source of support to young people.

- Develop policies that take a holistic approach and which stress the importance of developing values of care and kindness amongst young people.

Source: O'Brien and Moules (2010: 52).

Box 12.4 Guidance for schools on promoting emotional wellbeing and positive mental health of children and young people

- Ensuring early identification of risk factors based on the demographics of the school population

- Providing advice and guidance to address health and wellbeing concerns

- Providing multi-agency drop-in services within schools

- Providing support and information for parents whose children are starting primary school

- Providing signposting for parents and carers to local services, support groups and interest groups

- Ensuring early identification of emotional health and wellbeing needs

- Providing health checks to indicate developmental concerns and delays

- Ensuring support for health promotion and change management around issues such as obesity, smoking, drugs and alcohol, sexual health and relationship issues

- Providing support where behavioural difficulties are present

- Using evidence-based interventions or specific packages of care for identified health needs

- Using local assessment teams to inform and assist judgement and to work across partnerships

- Ensuring early intervention with partner agencies and working with voluntary agencies

- Providing referral to support services such as CAMHS

- Providing primary school drop-ins to support parents

- Providing on-site counselling services with links to CAMHS

- Using evidence-based targeted programmes promoting health in the school and community settings

- Providing continued intervention and support to prevent deterioration

- Informing other professionals about the health needs of the child and family.

Source: adapted from Department of Health and Public Health England (2014b).

What kind of activities can be helpful?

School nurses are in key positions to work in partnership with teachers to deliver activities related to emotional health and wellbeing with a focus on self-awareness, emotional intelligence, mindfulness and resilience. These often come under the overall umbrella of the Personal, Social, Health and Economic (PSHE) education curriculum and include wider public health priorities such as Sex and Relationships Education and Social, Moral, Spiritual and Cultural education. Various interventions can be helpful, including awareness raising, assertiveness training, peer support and mentoring (Ryan 2006). Rones and Hoagwood (2000) cite several factors associated with the success of school-based mental health services. These include consistent programme implementation, the use of multiple modalities, involvement of parents, teachers and peers, the integration of programme content into the general curriculum and approaches that are developmentally appropriate.

Numerous school-based interventions have been shown to prevent and reduce mental health problems in children. Some of these are summarised in Box 12.5, but this list is far from exhaustive.

Box 12.5 School-based interventions

- The Good Behaviour Game has been shown to improve behaviour problems by focusing on social and emotional learning and reinforcing positive or prosocial behaviour (Embry 2002). This is suitable for children aged 6 to 8. By reducing aggressive behaviour, it helps prevent problem behaviours in adolescence and adulthood (Washington State Institute for Public Policy 2014).

- The Circle of Friends initiative originated in the US as one of a range of strategies to promote the inclusion into mainstream school of students with disabilities and difficulties. This has been used in many UK settings and has been found to be helpful with children and young people with and without mental health problems, developmental disorders and learning disabilities (Newton et al. 1996; Whittaker et al. 1998). The use of Nurture Groups for pupils who are showing signs of behavioural, social or emotional difficulties can be helpful, particularly for children who are experiencing disruption or distress outside of school. Nurture groups work with individual children or small groups and provide targeted support.

- Circle Time has been used in many British primary schools. Discussions facilitated by the teacher encourage cooperation and the sharing of feelings between pupils. Exponents of Circle Time see it as a powerful method that has a key place in emotional and social competence and in building empathy, respect and a sense of mutual support in the whole school community (Weare and Gray 2003).

- The FRIENDS programme has also been positively reported (Public Health England 2015). This is an evidence-based cognitive behaviour therapy (CBT) programme delivered by school nurses. Children and young people with anxiety or with low self-esteem or confidence are offered intervention and support; sessions are co-facilitated between school nurses and teaching staff, helping to build the capacity of the school to offer early intervention at a whole school level.

- Improving the quality of mental health in schools (QUEST) was a project led by the Institute of Psychiatry and King's College London (The Health Foundation 2012). The project leads recognised that school nurses played a pivotal role in identifying children and young people with mental health problems but were concerned that they did not always have access to CAMHS training. The QUEST project trained school nurses to undertake mental health screening assessments, manage low-level difficulties and make referrals to specialist CAMHS for more serious mental health problems. A range of training materials and resources were developed including video-based learning for intervention with depressed adolescents and a facilitated network for school nurses to enable peer support. The results demonstrated that the QUEST project had a positive effect on the knowledge, skills and attitude of school nurses, and their confidence working with pupils who had mental health difficulties was shown to greatly improve (The Health Foundation 2012).

- The Penn Resilience Programme (Challen *et al.* 2011) was a licenced project in three UK local authorities that focused on the development of emotional intelligence, self-efficacy and assertive communication amongst Year 7 and Year 8 pupils. To deliver the programme, teachers accessed a five-day training course called How to Thrive. This equipped them with the knowledge, skills and confidence to deliver the programme. It included a focus on their own resilience and emotional wellbeing – a key part of the whole school ethos and approach to emotional health and wellbeing, which is recommended in current policy. Outcomes of the project demonstrated a reduction in symptoms of low mood and depression and better school attendance.

- The Leicester Child Behaviour Intervention Initiative commenced in 1999, providing services to children up to the age of 13 by working with schools, groups of pupils and individual children and their families. Primary mental health workers (PMHWs) and school nurses were involved.

- The Total Learning Challenge in Tyneside focused on both mainstream and so-called disaffected pupils using whole school approaches. Teaching skills were combined with group therapy and input from child psychologists.

- Promoting Alternative Thinking Strategies is a CBT-based approach that uses acronyms, visual images and mnemonics. It has been shown to be effective in helping adolescent boys with anxiety (Hains 1992).

- Total Learning Challenge is a brief, targeted group work approach for up to eight children aged 11–16. It combines teaching skills with group and individual therapy, the development of emotional literacy through creative expression and reflection on real-life situations, and the use of drama.

- Me First is funded by Health Education England and produced by Common Room Consulting. It is an education and training resource designed to help healthcare professionals and front-line staff develop their knowledge, skills and confidence in communicating with children and young people. It does this by encouraging a child-centric mentality in staff and by providing tools and advice to support this. The Me First website contains a resource hub for the sharing of tools and ideas from throughout the UK as well as practical advice from children, young people and healthcare professionals.

Public Health England (2015) reference a number of useful resources in their guidance on promoting children and young people's emotional health and wellbeing through whole school and college approaches (see Box 12.6).

Box 12.6 *Resources to promote children's emotional health and wellbeing*

Feeling Good activity sheets – for primary pupils aged 4–7

How to Get Up and Go When You Are Feeling Low – booklets for Year 4 children when they are feeling upset or stressed

Stop, Breathe and Be – intervention for secondary school students that uses mindfulness as part of the Mindfulness in Schools project

Stop Stigma – used in classrooms to help address mental health stigma and raise awareness about emotional health and wellbeing

What's on Your Mind? – produced as part of the Scottish anti-stigma campaign (See Me), this is a resource pack that includes a video and downloadable lesson plans to help teachers introduce the subject of emotional wellbeing and mental health to students

I Gotta Feelin – a booklet that offers Year 7 students top tips on how to feel good.

Source: adapted from Public Health England (2015).

Bullying

School nurses in particular encounter children and young people who are being exploited or bullied in a range of settings. Here, their role is to help develop whole school approaches to prevent and tackle bullying as well as to support individual children and young people who are involved in bullying (Offler 2000). Children who have been bullied are more likely to have mental health problems than other children. *The Good Childhood Report* (The Children's Society 2015) suggests that children in England experienced the highest levels of emotional bullying out of all of the 15 countries surveyed, with half of children reporting being left out by their classmates and over a third of children having been hit by other children in the last month.

Bullying is a common risk factor for poor emotional wellbeing, but it can be targeted through whole school interventions. Despite this, there is surprisingly little guidance for UK school nurses with much of the good practice advice coming from the US. Research has shown that whole school approaches with multiple components are more effective than teaching or learning-based activities (Knapp *et al.* 2011). One high-quality study of a whole school intervention found a 21–22 per cent reduction in the proportion of children victimised (Evers *et al.* 2007). Outcomes included improvements in emotional, physical and social health as well as better school attendance and attainment in students who had been bullied.

How can school nurses be supported by specialist CAMHS?

It is important that nurses and other school-based professionals recognise and understand their roles and responsibilities in relation to pupil and student emotional health and wellbeing. They have traditionally been described as Tier 1 professionals, which means that they are not expected to possess specialist skills in child and adolescent mental health but should be able to recognise when a child or young person may be struggling to cope. *Future in Mind* (Department of Health 2015) proposed that local CAMHS develop links to schools through named contacts with the aims of making mental health support more visible and easily accessible and improving communication. It also makes clear that staff working with children and young people in universal settings such as schools should receive training in children and young people's development and behaviours and know how to support those who have less serious difficulties, but they should not be expected to replace specialist CAMHS.

The Common Assessment Framework (CAF) and a range of NICE guidelines state that children who are showing early signs of anxiety, emotional distress or behavioural problems should have access to stepped care pathways that include referral and access to top specialist CAMHS. These are known as 'early help assessments'. There is national guidance for school nurses and other professionals in universal settings on how they can seek advice from or make a referral to specialist CAMHS (Department for Education 2014a). This may result in a formal consultation and referral of the young person for a specialist CAMHS assessment.

School nurses require support, time to discuss any concerns they may have about the mental health of pupils and students, and resources to develop their knowledge, skills and confidence in relation to supporting the mental health of children in school. However, Pryjmachuk *et al.* (2012) surveyed school nurses and found there was often frustration about referrals being rejected from CAMHS without explanation, long waiting times, scant feedback on the progress of children accepted by CAMHS and a general lack of communication.

Primary mental health workers

PMHWs are often nurses (Baldwin 2005) who are in key positions to support their colleagues in schools to address the mental health needs of children. PMHWs also act as the link between schools and specialist CAMHS, and their positive impact has been evaluated and reported widely (Gale and Vostanis 2003; Clarke *et al.* 2003; MacDonald *et al.* 2004). Despite the evidence for these important and effective roles, PMHWs have been steadily reduced in recent years. A review of the PMHW role by the National Foundation for Educational Research (Atkinson *et al.* 2010) identified several important key roles (see Box 12.7).

Box 12.7 The primary mental health worker role

- Liaison – network, instigate effective multi-agency working and collaboration and increase access to and signpost other services that support children and young people's mental health needs.
- Consultation – identify a child's mental health needs and discuss appropriate ways of meeting their needs in partnership with other professionals.
- Training – provide training programmes for school based professionals to increase and build on their understanding of mental health issues.
- Supervision – improve the ability of school based professionals to manage child mental health needs by increasing their skills and knowledge, and facilitating reflection on their work.
- Intervention – work with school based professionals and directly intervene when a child has not responded to the measures undertaken by the school based staff. Ensure access to specialist CAMHS for more serious, complex or persistent mental problems
- Strategic planning – proactively inform and influence children and young people's mental health strategies, develop protocols, engage in joint planning and facilitate collaborative working relationships
- Service development – identify service needs and any gaps across different agencies, obtain service users' views and involve them in the design, delivery and evaluation of CAMHS services.

Source: adapted from Atkinson *et al.* (2010: 6).

School nurses often have important roles to play in the assessment and treatment of suspected or actual mental health or developmental disorders. For instance, when a child is being assessed for ADHD, school nurses are able to make observations and assessments of functioning in the school environment and help evaluate the child's development in comparison with their peer group. This helps give an indication of the severity of the key symptoms of ADHD (hyperactivity, inattention and impulsivity) and the impact these may be having on the child's academic and social progress (Ryan 2006).

Many specialist CAMHS have developed resources, support and close working relationships with schools, though the quality of some of these working relationships has been challenged during the recession and with cuts to local authority and health budgets. One good example is in Birmingham through the Solihull Approach Training, which has been evaluated (Milford et al. 2006) and recommended by Public Health England (2015) as a framework for supporting schools to respond to the emotional health and wellbeing of students.

Summary

There is much that school nurses and other school-based professionals can do to improve mental health outcomes for pupils and students. They play a crucial leadership, coordination and delivery role as part of the wider Healthy Child Programme (see Department of Health 2014b). However, there is widespread concern that school nurses are overstretched. Safeguarding and child protection activities and tackling wider public health priorities, such as reducing drug and alcohol use and obesity, often overshadows their mental health work.

The immunisation and vaccinations programme has also grown in recent years. The National Child Measurement Programme and the Human Papilloma Virus immunisation programme have each had a major impact on the capacity of school nurses to fulfil their wider health promotion roles in schools (Thomas Coram Institute 2010). Additionally, school nurses are often the lead professional for CAF meetings, which can be very time-consuming and intensive. Furthermore, school nurses are now expected to play a greater role in supporting children and young people who are not in education, employment or training. However, Wilson et al. (2008) report that their public health role should not be at the expense of their important contribution to mental health and wellbeing.

Thus there is a risk that school nurses are pulled in all directions and that expectations are too great. Indeed, despite the key positions school nurses occupy, the RCN (2012) has been concerned about the breadth of their role and argues that their value has not been recognised in many areas of the UK, which limits the potential public health contribution they can make. Given the breadth of their role, it is perhaps unsurprising that there is wide variation in the emphasis placed on mental health and emotional wellbeing. It is unfortunate that the important and effective PMHW role has not been expanded to help meet the mental health problems facing pupils and students in schools and colleges. This role is key to promoting good emotional health, preventing mental health problems and identifying mental health problems early. In other words, it holds the key to early intervention, which is at the heart of all government policy affecting children and young people today.

References

Allen, G. (2011) Early Intervention: The Next Steps. London: The Cabinet Office.
Atkinson, M., Lamont, M. and Wright, B. (2010) NFER Review: The Role of Primary Mental Health Workers in Education. Slough: National Foundation for Educational Research.

Baldwin, L. (2005) Multidisciplinary post-registration education in child and adolescent mental health services. *Nurse Education Today*, 25(1): 17–22.

Bartlett, H. (2015) Can school nurses identify mental health needs early and provide effective advice and support? *British Journal of School Nursing*, 10(3): 126–34.

British Youth Council (2011) *Our School Nurse: Young People's Views on the Role of the School Nurse*. London: British Youth Council.

Cemalcilar, Z. (2010) Schools as socialisation contexts: understanding the impact of school climate factors on students' sense of school belonging. *Applied Psychology*, 59(2): 243–72.

Challen, A., Noden, P., West, A. and Machin, S. (2011) *UK Resilience Programme Evaluation: Final Report*. London: Department for Education.

Children's Society, The (2015) *The Good Childhood Report*. London: The Children's Society.

Clarke, M., Coombs, C. and Walton, L. (2003) School based identification and intervention service for adolescents: a psychology and school nurse partnership model. *Child and Adolescent Mental Health*, 8(1): 34–9.

Department for Education (2015) *Counselling in Schools: A Blueprint for the Future: Departmental Advice for School Staff and Counsellors*. London: Department for Education.

Department for Education (2014a) *Mental Health and Behaviour in Schools: Departmental Advice for School Staff*. London: Department for Education.

Department for Education (2014b) *Preventing and Tackling Bullying: Advice for Headteachers, Staff and Governing Bodies*. London: Department for Education.

Department for Education and Skills (2005) *Evaluation of Behaviour and Education Support Teams*. London: Department for Education and Skills.

Department of Health (2015) *Future in Mind – Promoting, Protecting and Improving Our Children and Young People's Mental Health and Wellbeing*. London: Department of Health.

Department of Health and Public Health England (2014a) *Maximising the School Nursing Team Contribution to the Public Health of School-Aged Children: Guidance to Support the Commissioning of Public Health Provision for School Aged Children 5–19*. London: Department of Health and Public Health England.

Department of Health and Public Health England (2014b) *Health Visiting and School Nurse Programme: Supporting Implementation of the New Service Offer: Promoting Emotional Wellbeing and Positive Mental Health of Children and Young People*. London: Department of Health and Public Health England.

Durlak, J., Weissberg, R., Dymnicki, A., Taylor, R. and Schellinger, K. (2011) The impact of enhancing students' social and emotional learning: a meta-analysis of school-based universal interventions. *Child Development*, 82(1): 405–32.

Embry, D. (2002) The good behavior game: a best practice candidate as a universal behavioral vaccine. *Clinical Child and Family Psychology Review*, 5(4): 273–97.

Evans, J., Harden, A., Thomas, J. and Benefield, P. (2003) *Support for Pupils with Emotional and Behavioural Difficulties (EBD) in the Mainstream Primary Classrooms: A Systematic Review of the Effective Interventions*. London: EPPI-Centre, University of London.

Evers, K. E., Prochaska, J. O., Van Marter, D. F., Johnson, J. L. and Prochaska, J. M. (2007) Transtheoretical-based bullying prevention effectiveness trials in middle schools and high schools. *Educational Research*, 49(4): 397–414.

Gale, F. and Vostanis, P. (2003) The primary mental health worker within child and adolescent mental health services. *Clinical Child Psychology and Psychiatry*, 8(2): 185–99.

Greenhalgh, P. (1994) *Emotional Growth and Learning*. London: Routledge.

Haddad, M., Butler, G. and Tylee, A. (2010) School nurses' involvement, attitudes and training needs for mental health work: a UK-wide cross-sectional study. *Journal of Advanced Nursing*, 66(11): 2471–80.

Hains, A. (1992) Comparison of cognitive behavioral stress management techniques with adolescent boys. *Journal of Counseling and Development*, 70(5): 600–5.

Health Foundation, The (2012) *Involving Primary Care Clinicians in Quality Improvement: An Independent Evaluation of the Engaging with Quality in Primary Care Programme*. London: The Health Foundation.

Institute of Education (2010) *Childhood Wellbeing: A Brief Overview*. London: Institute of Education.

Jamal, F., Fletcher, A., Harden, A., Wells, H., Thomas, J. and Bonell, C. (2013) The school environment and student health: a systematic review and meta-ethnography of qualitative research. *BMC Public Health*, 13(798): 1–11.

Khan, L., Parsonage, M. and Stubbs, J. (2015) *Investing in Children's Mental Health: A Review of Evidence on the Costs and Benefits of Increased Service Provision*. London: Centre for Mental Health.

Knapp, M., McDaid, D. and Parsonage, M. (eds) (2011) *Mental Health Promotion and Mental Illness Prevention: The Economic Case*. London: Department of Health.

Layard, L. (2015) *A New Priority for Mental Health*. London: Centre for Economic Performance, London School of Economics and Political Science.

Leighton, S. (2006) Nursing and school-based mental health services. In T. McDougall (ed.) *Child and Adolescent Mental Health Nursing*. London: Blackwell, pp. 207–21.

McCrone, P., Park, A-L. and Knapp, M. (2010) *Economic Evaluation of Early Intervention (EI) Services: Phase IV Report. PSSRU Discussion Paper 2745*. Canterbury: Personal Social Services Research Unit.

MacDonald, W., Bradley, S., Bower, P., Kramer, T., Sibbald, B., Garralder, E. and Harrington, R. (2004) Primary mental health workers in child and adolescent mental health services. *Journal of Advanced Nursing*, 46(1): 78–87.

McDougall, T. (2010) Continuing professional development: fostering resilience in children and young people. *British Journal of Wellbeing*, 1(4): 35–43.

Milford, R., Kleve, L., Lea, J. and Greenwood, R. (2006) A pilot evaluation of the Solihull Approach. *Community Practitioner*, 79(11): 358–62.

Moore, D. (2000) Pathways to better health. *Learning Disability Practice*, 3(4): 11–16.

National Institute for Health and Care Excellence (NICE) (2015a) *Looked-after Children and Young People (PH28)*. London: NICE.

National Institute for Health and Care Excellence (NICE) (2015b) *Obesity in Children and Young People: Prevention and Lifestyle Weight Management Programmes (QS94)*. London: NICE.

National Institute for Health and Care Excellence (NICE) (2013) *Antisocial Behaviour and Conduct Disorders in Children and Young People: Recognition and Management (CG158)*. London: NICE.

National Institute for Health and Care Excellence (NICE) (2012) *Social and Emotional Wellbeing: Early Years (PH40)*. London: NICE.

National Institute for Health and Care Excellence (NICE) (2010) *Smoking Prevention in Schools (PH23)*. London: NICE.

National Institute for Care Excellence (NICE) (2009a) *Social and Emotional Wellbeing in Secondary Education (PH20)*. London: NICE.

National Institute for Health and Care Excellence (NICE) (2009b) *Physical Activity for Children and Young People (PH17)*. London: NICE.

National Institute for Health and Care Excellence (NICE) (2008a) *Social and Emotional Wellbeing in Primary Education (PH12)*. London: NICE.

National Institute for Health and Care Excellence (NICE) (2008b) *Attention Deficit Hyperactivity Disorder: Diagnosis and Management (CG72)*. London: NICE.

National Institute for Health and Care Excellence (NICE) (2007) *Alcohol: School-based Interventions (PH7)*. London: NICE.

National Institute for Health and Care Excellence (NICE) (2005) *Depression in Children and Young People: Identification and Management (CG28)*. London: NICE.

Newman, T. (2002) *Promoting Resilience: A Review of Effective Strategies for Child Care Services*. Exeter: Centre for Evidence Based Social Services, University of Exeter.

Newton, C., Taylor, G. and Wilson, D. (1996) Circles of friends: an inclusive approach to meeting emotional and behavioural difficulties. *Educational Psychology in Practice*, 11(4): 41–8.

O'Brien, N. and Moules, T. (2010) *The Impact of Cyber-bullying on Young People's Mental Health: Final Report*. Chelmsford: Anglia Ruskin University.

Offler, E. (2000) Bullying: everybody's problem. *Paediatric Nursing*, 12(9): 22–6.

Pryjmachuk, S., Graham, T., Haddad, M. and Tylee, A. (2012) School nurses' perspectives on managing mental health problems in children and young people. *Journal Of Clinical Nursing*, 21(5–6): 850–9.

Public Health England (2015) *Promoting Children and Young People's Emotional Health and Wellbeing: A Whole School and College Approach*. London: Public Health England.

Rones, M. and Hoagwood, K. (2000) School-based mental health services: a research review. *Clinical Child and Family Psychology Review*, 3(4): 223–41.

Royal College of Nursing (RCN) (2012) *The RCN's Position on School Nursing*. London: RCN.

Rutter, M. (1999) Resilience concepts and findings: implications for family therapy. *Journal of Family Therapy*, 21(2): 119–44.

Ryan, N. (2006) Nursing children and young people with attention deficit hyperactivity disorder. In T. McDougall (ed.) *Child and Adolescent Mental Health Nursing*. London: Blackwell, pp. 29–49.

Skills for Health (2010) *CAMHS in Context: Helping You to Achieve Better Outcomes for Children, Young People and Families*. London: Skills for Health.

Thomas Coram Institute (2010) *Promoting the Health of Children and Young People through Schools: The Role of the Nurse. Final Research Report*. London: Thomas Coram Institute.

Washington State Institute for Public Policy (2014) Benefit-cost results [online]. Available at www.wsipp.wa.gov/BenefitCost (accessed 25 May 2016).

Weare, K. (2004) *Developing the Emotionally Literate School*. London: Paul Chapman Publishing.

Weare, K. and Gray, G. (2003) *What Works in Developing Children's Emotional and Social Competence and Wellbeing? Research Report No 456*. London: Department for Education and Skills.

Wells, J., Barlow, J. and Stewart-Brown, S. (2003) A systematic review of universal approaches to mental health promotion in schools. *Health Education*, 103(4): 197–220.

Whitaker, P., Barratt, P., Joy, H., Potter, M. and Thomas, G. (1998) Children with autism and peer group support: using circles of friends. *British Journal of Special Education*, 25(2): 60–4.

Wilson, P., Furnivall, J., Barbour, R., Connelly, G., Bryce, G., Phin, l. and Stallard, A. (2008) The work of health visitors and school nurses with children with psychological and behavioural problems. *Journal of Advanced Nursing*, 61(4): 445–55.

Wolk, S. (2008) Joy in school. *The Positive Classroom*, 66(1): 8–15.

Chapter 13

Managing behaviours that challenge nurses in CAMHS inpatient settings

Tim McDougall and Terri-Anne Nolan

Key points:

- There has been much political, organisational and professional focus on inpatient units for children and young people in recent years. The staffing, skill mix and quality of care for children and young people requiring inpatient care has also been under public scrutiny. As nurses make up the biggest professional group in inpatient child and adolescent mental health services (CAMHS) settings, they have key roles to play in addressing these challenges.
- There are a number of key topics that nurses in inpatient settings need to understand and apply in their day-to-day practice. These include the importance of therapeutic engagement; the need for comprehensive assessment and clear care planning; and the principle of least restrictive practice.
- The practice of inpatient CAMHS nurses and the care environments within which they work should be influenced by national quality standards and professional practice guidelines. The Quality Network for Inpatient CAMHS sets a number of minimum quality and best practice standards that apply directly to registered nurses and the practice of healthcare assistants or support workers, who currently provide the majority of direct care in CAMHS inpatient units.
- Inpatient CAMHS environments can be challenging to work in. Supporting children and young people who may use aggression and violence or self-harm to communicate distress, solve problems or compete for adult attention is no easy task. Nurses working in inpatient settings need to seek to understand why children or young people behave in particular ways and achieve a careful balance of authority, responsibility and risk-taking in helping them to recover.

Introduction

There has been major public and political interest in access to inpatient beds for children and young people over the last few years. Scandal stories about children in police cells and parents travelling many miles from home to visit their children in hospital have prompted debate and concern about access to help for young people in crisis. However, it is not just a lack of beds that has been in the spotlight. The staffing, skill mix and quality of inpatient care for children and young people has also been called into question. As nurses make up the biggest professional group in inpatient CAMHS, they have key roles to play in addressing these concerns.

This chapter discusses a number of the key practice issues associated with managing behaviours that challenge the nursing team in CAMHS inpatient settings. These include the importance of therapeutic engagement; the need for thorough assessment and focused care planning; risk assessment and management; and the principle of 'least restrictive practice' which is becoming more important and topical within CAMHS inpatient settings.

Self-harm is another aspect that nurses often find challenging to manage within the hospital environment. This is covered in Chapter 8 with the present chapter primarily discussing the management of violence and aggression. Of course, these are not the entirety of issues that are important for inpatient CAMHS nurses to understand. Some of these are discussed elsewhere in this book, and for a fuller discussion of inpatient care in general, readers are directed to McDougall and Cotgrove (2014).

What are child and adolescent inpatient units?

The vast majority of children and young people with severe, complex or persistent mental health problems never require hospital admission. Instead, they can be safely and successfully treated in primary services or by community-based specialist teams. However, inpatient admission is an essential part of the care pathway, and evidence of effectiveness has been demonstrated for some groups (McDougall 2014).

There are currently 7 child and adolescent inpatient units for children and 80 adolescent inpatient units in England. This is in addition to a number of Psychiatric Intensive Care Units and several medium secure units. Inpatient units are generally commissioned to provide mental health assessment and treatment for children and young people with complex, persistent or severe mental disorders. Factors that lead to hospital admission are not only the acuity or chronicity of the child or young person's mental health difficulties but also the lack of response to community treatment, breakdown in therapeutic relationships, and level of risk to self or others (O'Herlihy et al. 2009).

Children and young people who are admitted to child and adolescent mental health services (CAMHS) inpatient units often have backgrounds characterised by high levels of psychosocial adversity. Commonly, they have suffered from substantial trauma, abuse and loss which has contributed to their mental health difficulties and risk-taking behaviours. This group of young people includes:

- those with poor attachments and complex needs, whose severe and persistent behaviour problems are difficult to manage in community services;
- those who engage in serious self-harming or suicidal behaviour;
- those whose aggressive or violent behaviour places other people at risk.

Whilst hospital admission is often ineffective for children and young people with psychosocial difficulties or conduct disorder, these problems can often coexist with mental disorder. Additionally, regardless of the basis of a child or young person's difficulties, there is often the need for a brief admission, particularly if they are acutely suicidal.

How are CAMHS inpatient units staffed?

Numerous national reports, reviews and public inquiries have demonstrated that the numbers and skill mix of nurses makes a difference to the quality of care, patient experience and clinical outcomes in hospital settings. The Francis (2013) inquiry highlighted the risks of low staffing levels and too few nurses to provide safe care. Poor skill mix contributed to the failings at Mid Staffordshire NHS Foundation Trust, and the inquiry team recommended a more systematic and responsive approach to determining nurse staffing levels.

The *Five Year Forward View for Mental Health* (Mental Health Taskforce 2016) reports that staff shortages have contributed to deaths on inpatient wards, and they have also been linked to the rise in Mental Health Act detentions. There are not only staff shortages in inpatient services. According to The King's Fund (2015) report *Mental Health Under Pressure*, almost half of community mental health services had staffing levels judged to be less than adequate in 2014, and many more were unable to provide a full multidisciplinary team.

Published in response to the Francis report, *The Cavendish Review* (Department of Health 2013) called for formal training for healthcare assistants and support workers. This group makes up the majority of the nursing workforce in inpatient and secure CAMHS settings. Published around the same time, the Keough (2013) review found high use of temporary staff, low levels of night staff and high registered nurse vacancies. This picture is mirrored in many CAMHS inpatient settings today. The Berwick (2013) review made recommendations to improve patient safety in the NHS, partly through adequate staffing levels, the introduction of nurse to patient ratios and the use of evidence-based acuity tools to help calculate safe and effective staffing levels.

Following concern about access to inpatient mental health care for children and young people, NHS England commissioned a national review in 2013. The report of the review highlighted nursing workforce development as a key strategic priority for attention, and identified nurse recruitment, retention and training as a significant area of challenge for stakeholders (NHS England 2014). Senior healthcare managers are acutely aware that recruitment and retention is an ongoing problem affecting inpatient CAMHS units. As Sergeant (2009) points out, there are increased opportunities for promotion and greater flexibility in community CAMHS. There have also been concerns about access to appropriate training and induction. The Alice Reeves Independent Research (2011) team observed that it appears to be common for nurses and support workers who are working directly with young people to have received little or no CAMHS-specific training. This was in relation to skills to assess and manage suicidal risk, skills in therapeutic intervention and more general skills such as active listening.

In recent years, there has been a gradual drift of staff members away from inpatient services. This has contributed to a situation where the care of young people with the most complex, serious or challenging needs are being cared for and managed by the most inexperienced staff. This concern has been shared by the Quality Network for Inpatient CAMHS (2007), which noted a negative impact on both staff morale and effectiveness. In their report, both young people and their carers expressed concern about the over-reliance of agency staff and the impact on safety and quality of care.

A programme of work looking at safe staffing in inpatient mental health settings led by the National Institute for Health and Care Excellence (NICE) commenced in 2014, including CAMHS in its scope. However, the NICE safe staffing programme was abandoned early in 2015 when a decision was taken by the then Health Secretary to refer the issue of safe staffing and professional skill mix to the Mental Health Taskforce, expected to report in 2016/17.

National quality standards

The practice of inpatient CAMHS nurses and the care environments within which they work should be influenced by best practice quality standards. The Quality Network for Inpatient CAMHS (QNIC) is a European peer review and accreditation network focused on quality improvement in inpatient CAMHS. The network sets a number of minimum standards that apply directly to registered nurses and the practice of healthcare assistants. QNIC also recommends core training for those working in CAMHS inpatient units, including management of imminent and actual violence, breakaway techniques and restraint measures. The Care Quality Commission (CQC) focuses on safe staffing levels as part of their current inspection regime, and QNIC standards are recognised as an official information source. The CQC standards (2012) state that there must be sufficient numbers of suitably qualified, skilled and experienced staff to safeguard people's health, safety and welfare.

National public and political debate about the lack of access to inpatient beds for children and young people as well as an increase in those being admitted to adult wards culminated in the publication of national quality standards in relation to safe and appropriate care on adult mental health wards (O'Herlihy *et al.* 2009). These cover environment and facilities; staffing and training; assessment, admission and discharge; care and treatment; education and further learning; consent, confidentiality and advocacy; and other safeguards.

What do we mean by challenging behaviours?

Research on anger, aggression and violence in children and young people is extensive and varied. Factors such as trauma, abuse and loss (Boswell 1997), early exposure to violence (Calouste Gulbenkian Foundation 1995), harsh and inconsistent discipline (Withecomb 1997) and drug and alcohol use (Christian *et al.* 2001) have each been strongly correlated to violent behaviour by young people.

The relationship between anger, aggression and violence is complex. Whilst anger is a normal, healthy emotion with expressive qualities, it is neither necessary nor sufficient for aggression to occur. Aggression may be either hostile and angry or instrumental and lack anger. For example, a child may use aggression instrumentally and without anger to achieve a particular goal such as robbery. By comparison, hostile aggression may erupt in response to provocation whilst a child is angry. Violence refers to behaviour that may cause physical or psychological harm.

The goal of individual work with children is to help them make sense of their angry, aggressive or violent behaviour. This means that by understanding how thoughts, feelings and actions relate to each other, children can be helped to replace violence with non-violent choices. However, this is rarely a straightforward process.

The importance of therapeutic engagement

Care and treatment is only effective if it is delivered with knowledge, empathy and compassion and in a way that the child or young person can engage with. Too little has been published on the impact of nursing care for young people who exhibit behaviours that challenge nurses. Where treatment strategies have been evaluated, reporting tends to focus on interventions such as behavioural management or multimodal treatment strategies (Fonagy *et al.* 2002) rather than the therapeutic relationship between the nurse and the young person per se. Much of what is known to be helpful in inpatient CAMHS settings is anecdotal or what might more accurately be called practice-based evidence. Green (2006) describes the importance of the therapeutic alliance, which he calls a 'significant but neglected variable in child mental health treatment studies'.

Assessment and care planning

Before attempting to embark on management strategies to address challenging behaviours, it is important for the nurse to undertake a thorough assessment of what are invariably complex or entrenched difficulties. This process often takes time and cannot be addressed in a short or superficial assessment. It requires the collation of information from a number of sources in multiple settings using a variety of methods (Mitchell 2014). The purpose of undertaking a thorough assessment is to understand the scope, frequency, duration and severity of the behaviour in question. For some young people, aggression or violence may have become a way of managing difficult emotions or controlling their environment and the people around them. Introducing a particular management approach without assessment, detailed planning and preparation may simply lead to a repetition or escalation of the oppositional and challenging behaviour it is intended to reduce (Higgins and Burke 1998). The assessment process will involve not only the child or young person but also the parents or carers and other professionals who know them.

Risk assessment and management

Like all assessment tools, risk assessment tools have utility in informing clinical decision-making and are not an end in themselves. They should be structured, draw on multiple information sources and be dynamic rather than static. Just as capacity for moral reasoning, empathy and understanding consequences all increase as a child gets older, so too do risk behaviours. Additionally, since young people are prone to sudden mood changes and tend to be sensitive to environmental changes, the factors that combine to produce risk can also change rapidly (Mitchell 2006). It is therefore important that nurses working with children and young people in inpatient settings reassess risk on a regular basis.

There is no point doing any risk assessment unless this is to inform a risk management plan. For children and young people in hospital, this will involve a care plan which should form part of a wider multi-agency strategy. Similarly, it is difficult to evaluate the effectiveness of a risk management plan unless this has been based on an individualised assessment of risk. In general, risk assessment tools explore how specific factors affect the likelihood of future adverse events occurring within a defined population. Numerous risk assessment tools have been developed for use in a wide variety of adult mental health settings. However, these are not generally transferable for use with children and young people; indeed, nurses only have access to a limited number of risk assessment tools specifically designed for children or adolescents. One of these is the Structured Assessment of Violence Risk in Youth (SAVRY; Borum *et al.* 2002), which assesses the risk of aggression based on a combination of historical and current factors. Additionally, the Early Assessment Risk List (Augimeri *et al.* 2001) has been devised for violence risk assessment in boys (EARL-20B) and girls (EARL-20G).

Principle of least restrictive practice

Inpatient CAMHS environments can be challenging for nurses to work in. Supporting children and young people who may use aggression and violence to communicate distress, solve problems or compete for adult attention is no easy task. Nurses working in inpatient settings need to achieve a careful balance of authority, responsibility and risk-taking. If the inpatient team operates an ethos that is overly controlling and oppressive, Sergeant (2009) warns that it is likely that young people may adopt an oppositional stance. They may 'act out' by withdrawing or become overly hostile.

The concept of least restrictive practice derives from the Mental Health Act code of practice (Department of Health 2008). However, the philosophy of least restriction has been documented in the mental health literature over many years (Carr *et al.* 1999; Huckshorn 2004; Smith *et al.* 2005). The government's Positive and Safe programme outlines key requirements for organisations in relation to promoting the development of therapeutic environments and minimising all forms of restrictive practices (Department of Health 2014). The Positive and Safe programme aims to radically transform culture, leadership and professional practice. This is to deliver care and support that keeps people safe and promotes recovery. The approach encompasses models such as Safewards (Bowers 2014).

Figure 13.1 illustrates 'how restrictive practices and restrictive interventions can be seen within a human rights-based model of positive and proactive support' (Department of Health, Skills for Health and Skills for Care: 12).

Strategies for the management of aggression and violence must always be underpinned by a thorough assessment with the young person, their family or carers. This is to understand the scope, frequency, duration, severity and function of the aggressive or violent behaviour. Positive support plans or behaviour support plans (Allen *et al.* 2012) are increasingly used within mental health settings including CAMHS wards. These involve a skilled assessment in order to understand the reasons why a young person might be acting the way they are, what predicts the occurrence of behaviours and which factors maintain and sustain them. The behaviour support plan, which should be located within the care plan, should include primary, secondary and tertiary preventative strategies that aim to prevent the need for restrictive practice and support the therapeutic environment.

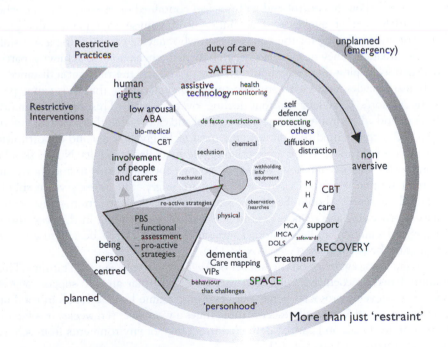

Figure 13.1 Positive and proactive care
Source: Department of Health, Skills for Health and Skills for Care (2014: 12).

Verbal de-escalation

All too often, management of violence and aggression (MVA) programmes focus more on reactive physical interventions than proactive psychological interventions. In an attempt to address this, some organisations describe PMVA programmes that include prevention. Whilst most programmes usually comprise both physical intervention skills and verbal de-escalation techniques, the former is usually disproportionate to the latter. This is a missed opportunity since the most effective skills to successfully manage anger, aggression and violence in the context of behaviour problems are likely to be psychological rather than physical (McDougall 1997).

Indeed, various nurses have asserted that the most valuable tool for working with children and young people who have mental health problems is the self (Leighton *et al.* 2001; Holyoake and Fitzgibbon 2002), and this is pertinent when working with children and young people who may be angry, aggressive or violent. Verbal de-escalation is a proactive approach that aims to manage anger or aggression before the young person becomes physically aggressive or violent. It is an interactional process, and whilst the young person's anger is the focus, attention is also paid to the use of self through posture, intention movements, touch and the use of space. Nurses should be aware of their non-verbal communication at all times and particularly when a young person is angry or aroused. They should avoid sudden movements and allow a wide personal space. This is because sudden movements can be perceived as an attack and because young people who are highly aroused, angry or aggressive command an enlarged sense of personal space.

Understanding of the theoretical principle of containment and its application to nursing care is essential. As Higgins and MacDougall (2006) point out, the ability of the nurse to remain calm in a challenging situation is crucially important. Young people who are angry or aggressive may feel out of control and will not feel contained or reassured by staff who are frustrated, frightened or avoidant. The ability of the nurse to remain calm provides containment and modelling for the young person who may be experiencing a stressful and bewildering situation. They may expect their challenging behaviour to achieve a particular purpose, such as helping them get their own way or keeping the nurse at a distance. This approach also provides nurses with an opportunity to demonstrate that they can cope with the young person's behaviour without feeling overwhelmed. This provides emotional containment and an environment that is thoughtful and calm rather than reactive and tense.

Drury (2005) commented that adolescents need to be given space and opportunities to discuss their views in a way that is appropriately role-modelled by adults. Nurses should pay attention to what they say and how they say it. Young people are likely to find short, simple, non-abstract sentences easier to process if they are angry. The nurse's voice should be lowered and sentences should be short, simple and lack abstraction. This simplifies information processing and reduces cognitive workload. Responding in this way also lacks high expressed emotion and heightened arousal and is likely to be appraised as non-threatening to the young person (see Box 13.1).

There is emerging evidence on the impact of Aggression Replacement Training. This is a programme based on cognitive behaviour therapy (CBT) that aims to support aggressive adolescents to develop prosocial behaviour. The programme lasts 30 hours in total and is delivered to groups of 8 to 12 adolescents three times a week over ten weeks. It is facilitated by trained professionals and can be delivered in a range of environments from schools to youth justice settings (Khan *et al.* 2015).

Box 13.1 *Verbal de-escalation strategies*

- Remain calm – young people who are angry or aggressive will not feel contained and reassured by staff who appear anxious or frightened.

- Keep your posture relaxed and open – sudden movements can sometimes be interpreted by young people as aggressive or attacking.

- Maintain eye contact and avoid looking downwards to the young person – this reduces the sense of powerlessness the young person may feel.

- Lower the pitch and tone of your voice – reduced levels of expressed emotion are potentially less threatening to the young person.

- Communicate clearly – short, simple, non-abstract statements are easier to process when you are angry. In contrast, long, convoluted instructions are difficult to process and may therefore be misunderstood.

- Repeat important information – young people in a heightened state of arousal will have difficulty thinking and processing information. It is important that one rather than several people speak to them during the de-escalation process.

- Don't argue – by presenting one side of the argument, you invite the young person to take up the other. The more a young person defends their position, the more they become committed to it. The potential for positive change is subsequently reduced.

- Make positive 'do' statements rather than saying 'do not'.

- Monitor your arousal – if you are angry with the young person, this will be communicated non-verbally and the young person may respond defensively and aggressively. Angry staff are more likely to be assaulted.

- Maintain space – young people who are angry, aggressive or paranoid may be sensitive to interpersonal distance and have an enlarged sense of personal space. Invading their personal space may be seen as provocative.

- Provide 'face-saving' alternatives – young people who are highly aroused, angry or threatening may need to be given a way of backing down without losing face.

- Reduce the audience factor – pride, status within the group and the possibility of humiliation mean that young people are unlikely to back down in the face of their peers, staff or visitors. Wherever possible, encourage young people who may be present to engage in other activities.

- Set fair and consistent rules and boundaries – like any residential setting for young people, the CAMHS inpatient unit requires consistent boundaries, clear expectations and the application of consequences to function effectively. When expectations are clearly stated and consequences are known in advance, the organisational structure is perceived as safe, supportive and containing.

- Apply appropriate and effective limit setting – fair and consistent rules and boundaries are important external controls that enable young people to develop internal controls and learn alternative coping strategies.

- Help young people to structure their time – boredom, frustration and restriction of liberty are all antecedents to aggression and violence in inpatient settings. Staff should provide young people with a balance of therapeutic activity, leisure and quiet time alone.

- Enable effective distraction, diversion and relaxation strategies – these should be identified in conjunction with the young person and in advance of the de-escalation process. Helpful strategies should be in the young person's care plan.

- Do not encourage young people to take out their anger or aggression on inanimate objects – the use of 'cathartic' methods, such as 'punch-bags', helps maintain levels of physiological and psychological arousal and may actually increase aggression and violence. It also gives young people a message that problems can be solved aggressively.

- Do not encourage angry or aggressive young people to spend too much time alone – allowing young people time to ruminate and become preoccupied can increase anger reactions.

- Reflect positive progress – young people with chronically low self-esteem may have little regard for damaging consequences and may seek punishment.

- Positively role model – some young people may have had limited exposure to prosocial behaviour, but learn how to resolve conflict using interpersonal skills.

Self-awareness and clinical supervision

The strategies outlined in this chapter require the nurse to have insight into their own strengths, vulnerabilities and weaknesses as well as an awareness of how these may affect their management of children and young people in their care. This is dependent on the nurse having sufficient support and access to regular and skilled clinical supervision. Utilised with skill and compassion, supervision can enable nurses to explore issues of parenting, limit setting, authority, discipline and how they may respond to particular behaviours.

The ability to self-reflect is central to the successful management of behaviours that challenge nurses. For example, if the nurse is aware that they have strong views about physical abuse due to their own personal experiences, they can be supported to accommodate this into how they approach and respond to a young person who may be physically abusing others. Developing and sharing self-awareness is part of healthy and effective team functioning and can directly impact on how a young person's behaviour problems are managed. If a nurse is able to share with colleagues those situations they find challenging, support and understanding can be given.

Self-awareness and enabling insights of this nature also help to challenge the unhelpful notion that all nurses should be able to cope equally well with all young people in all situations. It is important that nurses are able to acknowledge that they find some young people more challenging and harder to work with than others. As Higgins and MacDougall (2006) remind us, this is neither uncaring nor unprofessional if it is acknowledged with insight and understanding and explored and reflected on within supervision.

Johns (2004) writes of the importance of nurses being reflective practitioners. Nurses and managers in CAMHS inpatient settings need to develop supervision and reflective practice as core components of the unit philosophy and service development strategy. It is the responsibility of nurse managers and leaders to establish a culture of sharing practice and concerns. Nurses need to feel confident that they can question each other's practice in an open and supportive way. Most important, however, is the establishment of a culture where discussion, dialogue and open debate are valued as key components of safe and effective care.

Physical restraint

It would be remiss to write a chapter about the management of behaviour that challenges nurses without acknowledging that in some situations verbal de-escalation may be insufficient or ineffective in reducing the potential for harm. Physical restraint may be appropriate and required when:

- the young person has actually been violent and there are immediate concerns that the violence may continue;
- the young person makes a specific threat of violence and violence appears to be imminent;
- the young person is at risk of coming to immediate harm.

Where physical restraint is used, nurses should be trained in the use of approved methods. Following any episode of physical restraint, it is necessary to focus on several key areas. The order in which these issues are addressed will depend on the circumstances, but all need to be addressed in a timely way (see Box 13.2).

Box 13.2 *Important issues to consider following physical restraint*

- Physical harm to child or young person – if there have been any injuries sustained during the restraint, the priority is to seek appropriate medical attention.

- Debrief with the young person – this gives young people an opportunity to say how they feel about being restrained and receive appropriate support. It also provides an opportunity to reflect on the behaviour of the young person that led to restraint and to discuss alternative coping strategies and interventions.

- Undertake a risk assessment to help prevent further aggression or violence – this should be discussed with the young person, their parents or carer and the multidisciplinary team.

- Inform person with parental responsibility – this is to communicate any ongoing concerns about their child, seek their views about ongoing management and generally keep them involved in all aspects of care, treatment and management.

- Review care plans – this should take account of the young person's behaviour that led to restraint in order to identify triggers.

- Report details of restraint – this should contain clear information about antecedents, the behaviour that led to restraint and the steps taken afterwards. This is to assist the clinical and management teams to decide whether additional action is required. Where injuries have been sustained during restraint, reporting should be specific about the nature of injuries.

- Debrief staff – restraining a young person can evoke strong feelings in staff, including upset, anger or fear. Left unaddressed, these feelings can interfere with care delivery and can be potentially harmful for staff themselves. The nurse in charge should seek to support all staff members who have been involved in restraint, either alone or in a group.

- Raise any immediate concerns about the welfare of the young person according to local safeguarding protocols – this is about being open and transparent and helps ensure that appropriate steps are taken to safeguard and promote the welfare of the young person concerned. Whilst the restraint of young people is not usually a safeguarding matter, there are sometimes circumstances that require involvement of the organisations safeguarding team. These include physical injury to a young person arising from physical restraint; violence between service users; prolonged restraint; and repeated restraint of individual young people.

Physical interventions should only be used as part of a wider strategy to prevent and manage behaviours that challenge nurses in inpatient settings. Whilst the option for physical management of aggression and violence is an important part of the overall approach, equally crucial are the values and culture of the organisation and the therapeutic milieu.

Interestingly, the term 'milieu' is derived from the French word for environment. The term 'therapeutic milieu' implies that the environment is an important part of treatment; this is, of course, an important factor in inpatient care. Sergeant (2009) observes that milieu therapy has been used with children since the late 1800s when so-called moral treatment and therapeutic communities were the key approaches in the treatment of choice for psychiatric problems and disorders.

Summary

Nurses and other professionals must be aware of the challenging behaviours with which young people may present in the context of their specific developmental needs. It can be a complex and challenging task for a busy inpatient nurse to maintain a therapeutic alliance with a young person who may exhibit challenging behaviours, and the inpatient team has to be skilled in using negotiation and compromise whist being effective in maintaining limits and boundaries. This chapter summarises the range of skills required by nurses working with children whose behaviour may be challenging within the inpatient setting.

Nurses must develop skills, knowledge, self-awareness and attitudes that enable them to remain positive, nurturing and accepting of the young person as an individual whilst setting and maintaining fair boundaries and expectations. The range of skills required to manage challenging behaviour and at the same time meet the needs of a diverse group of other young people cannot be underestimated. The ultimate tool, however, is the individual nurse's use of their self. How they interact, how they model their behaviour and the degree to which they understand their responses to the young people in their charge will ultimately make the greatest difference – not completing a training course that favours physical interventions alone.

References

Alice Reeves Independent Research (2011) *An Analysis of the Training Needs of Frontline Staff in Inpatient CAMHS.* London: Foundation for Professionals in Services to Adolescents.

Allen, D., Kaye, N., Horwood, S., Gray, D. and Mines, S. (2012) The impact of a whole-organisation approach to positive behavioural support on the use of physical interventions. *International Journal of Positive Behavioural Support,* 2(1): 26–30.

Augimeri, L., Webster, C., Koegl, C. and Levene, K. (2001) *Early Assessment Risk List for Boys: EARL-20B, Version 2.* Toronto: Earlscourt Child and Family Centre.

Berwick, D. (Chair) (2013) *A Promise to Learn – A Commitment to Act: Improving the Safety of Patients in England* (Berwick review into patient safety). London: Department of Health.

Borum, R., Bartel, P. and Forth, A. (2002) *Manual for the Structured Assessment of Violence Risk in Youth (SAVRY).* Tampa, FL: Florida Mental Health Institute.

Boswell, G. (1997) The backgrounds of violent young offenders. In V. Varma (ed.) *Violence in Children and Adolescents.* London: Jessica Kingsley Publishers, pp. 22–36.

Bowers, L. (2014) *Safewards: A New Model of Conflict and Containment on Psychiatric Wards.* London: Institute of Psychiatry.

Calouste Gulbenkian Foundation (1995) *Children and Violence: Report of the Commission on Children and Violence Convened by the Gulbenkian Foundation.* London: Calouste Gulbenkian Foundation.

Care Quality Commission (2012) *The Essential Standards*. London: Care Quality Commission.

Carr, E. G., Horner, R. H., Turnball, A. P., McLaughlin, D. M., McAtee, M. L., Smith, C. E., Ryan, K., Ruef, M., Doolabh, A. and Braddoch, D. (1999) *Positive Behaviour Support for People with Developmental Disabilities: A Research Synthesis*. Washington, DC: American Association of Mental Retardation.

Christian, J., Crome, I., Gilvarry, E., Johnson, P., McArdle, P. and McCarthy, S. (2001) *The Substance of Young Needs: Review 2001*. London: Health Advisory Service.

Department of Health (2014) *Positive and Proactive Care: Reducing the Need for Physical Intervention*. London: Department of Health.

Department of Health (2013) *The Cavendish Review: Review of Health Care Assistants and Support Workers in NHS and Social Care*. London: Department of Health.

Department of Health (2008) *Code of Practice: Mental Health Act 1983*. London: The Stationery Office.

Department of Health, Skills for Health and Skills for Care (2014) *A Positive and Proactive Workforce: A Guide to Workforce Development for Commissioners and Employers Seeking to Minimise the Use of Restrictive Practices in Social Care and Health*. Leeds: Skills for Care; Bristol: Skills for Health.

Drury, J. (2005) Young people's communication with adults in the institutional order. In A. Williams and C. Thurlow (eds) *Talking Adolescence: Perspectives on Communication in the Teenage Years* (third edition). New York: Peter Lang, pp. 229–44.

Fonagy, P., Target, M., Cottrell, D., Phillips, J. and Kurtz, Z. (2002) *What Works for Whom? A Critical Review of Treatments for Children and Adolescents*. New York: Guilford Press.

Francis, R., QC (Chair) (2013) *Report of the Mid Staffordshire NHS Foundation Trust Public Inquiry*. London: The Stationery Office.

Green, J. (2006) The therapeutic alliance: a significant but neglected variable in child mental health treatment studies. *Journal of Child Psychology and Psychiatry*, 47(5): 425–35.

Higgins, I. and McDougall, T. (2006) Nursing children and adolescents who are aggressive or violent: a psychological approach. In T. McDougall (ed.) *Child and Adolescent Mental Health Nursing*. London: Blackwell, pp. 131–49.

Higgins, I. and Burke, M. (1998) Managing oppositional and aggressive behaviour. In J. Green and B. Jacobs (eds) *In-patient Child Psychiatry: Modern Practice, Research and the Future*. Hove: Routledge, pp. 189–200.

Holyoake, D. and Fitzgibbon, S. (2002) *Discussing Child and Adolescent Mental Health Nursing*. Salisbury: APS.

Huckshorn, K. (2004) *Reducing the Use of Seclusion and Restraint: A National Initiative for Culture Change and Transformation*. Lincoln, NE: Roman Hruska Law Centre.

Johns, C. (2004) *Becoming a Reflective Practitioner: A Reflective and Holistic Approach to Clinical Nursing, Practice Development and Clinical Supervision* (second edition). London: Blackwell Science.

Keough, B. (2013) *Review into the Quality of Care and Treatment provided by 14 Hospital Trusts in England*. London: NHS England.

Khan, L., Parsonage, M. and Stubbs, J. (2015) *Investing in Children's Mental Health: A Review of Evidence on the Costs and Benefits of Increased Service Provision*. London: Centre for Mental Health.

King's Fund, The (2015) *Mental Health Under Pressure*. London: The King's Fund.

Leighton, S., Smith, C., Minns, K. and Crawford, P. (2001) Specialist child and adolescent mental health nurses: a force to be reckoned with? *Mental Health Practice*, 5(2): 8–13.

McDougall, T. (2014) Improving quality and safety in inpatient CAMHS. *British Journal of Mental Health Nursing*, 3(4): 148–50.

McDougall, T. (1997) Coercive interventions: the notion of the 'last resort'. *Journal of Psychiatric Care*, 4(1): 19–21.

McDougall, T. and Cotgrove, A. (2014) *Specialist Mental Healthcare for Children and Adolescents: Hospital, Intensive Community and Home Based Services*. Abingdon: Routledge.

Mental Health Taskforce (2016) *Five Year Forward View for Mental Health*. London: Mental Health Taskforce.

Mitchell, P. (2014) Forensic interventions. In T. McDougall and A. Cotgrove (eds) *Specialist Mental Healthcare for Children and Adolescents: Hospital, Intensive Community and Home Based Services.* Abingdon: Routledge, pp. 123–39.

Mitchell, P. (2006) Child and adolescent forensic mental health nursing. In T. McDougall (ed.) *Child and Adolescent Mental Health Nursing.* London: Blackwell, pp. 172–87.

NHS England (2014) *Child and Adolescent Mental Health Services (CAMHS) Tier 4 Report.* London: NHS England.

O'Herlihy, A., Pugh, K., McDougall, T. and Parker, C. (eds) (2009) *AIMS – SC4Y: Safe and Appropriate Care for Young People on Adult Mental Health Wards.* London: Royal College of Psychiatrists.

Quality Network for Inpatient CAMHS (2007) *QNIC Annual Report – Quality Network for Inpatient CAMHS.* London: Royal College of Psychiatrists' Research Unit.

Sergeant, A. (2009). *Working within Child and Adolescent Inpatient Services: A Practitioner's Handbook.* Wigan: National CAMHS Support Service.

Smith, G., Davis, R., Bixler, O., Lin, H., Altenor, A., Altenor, R., Hardenstine, B. and Kopchick, G. (2005) Pennsylvania State Hospital system's seclusion and restraint reduction program. *Psychiatric Services,* 56(9): 1115–22.

Withecomb, J. L. (1997) Causes of violence in children. *Journal of Mental Health,* 6(5): 433–42.

Chapter 14

Nursing children and young people in secure and forensic settings

Paul Mitchell

Key points

- The number of young people placed in the secure estate has reduced by over 60 per cent during the last 12 years. The full reasons for this are not clear, but effective early intervention and diversion, better case management and interventions for those young people who do enter the system are all likely to be major factors.
- It can be argued therefore that, providing risk management is addressed, young people within the youth justice system should access the same interventions and services as their peers in other settings. By addressing issues of risk assessment and management, mental health nurses can play a key role in ensuring this happens.
- Nurses and other professionals working with young people in the justice system should be mindful of their likely trajectories and need for services into adulthood. It is therefore important to establish links with adult mental health and forensic services to ensure that transitional arrangements are in place before young people become adults.
- Young people from black and minority ethnic (BME) groups continue to be over-represented within the justice system. Nurses should, therefore, be aware that there may be a higher than anticipated prevalence of unmet mental health needs among young people of BME origin and that the recognition of these needs may be hampered by cultural bias or misattributions.
- Any intervention or case management by nurses with young people in the justice system should be informed by a robust and comprehensive needs and risk assessment process. It is important that nurses are able to justify the decisions they make, which is why the assessment process should be structured, systematic and evidence-based.

Introduction

Over the last ten years, there have been significant changes in our understanding of the needs of young people in the justice system, both from a mental health and social policy perspective. Increasing attention has been paid to their mental health needs; this has been driven by the realisation that these needs often go unrecognised and unmet (Chitsabesan *et al.* 2006; Vreugdenhil *et al.* 2004) and also because of the long-term psychosocial implications which arise from failure to recognise and address these needs (Maughan and Kim-Cohen 2005; Coid *et al.* 2006).

The two biggest changes in our understanding have been in relation to neuro-disability and attachment. There has been increasing awareness of often unrecognised neurodevelopmental needs such as learning difficulties and difficulties with communication (Hughes *et al.* 2012). We know that young people in the justice system have experienced high levels of trauma (Abram *et al.* 2004) and multiple placements (Chitsabesan *et al.* 2006) and that these often impact on their capacity for self-regulation and ability to form and maintain relationships. It has been argued that these can best be understood using attachment theory (Casswell *et al.* 2012), and there is evidence that this model can be the basis of successful intervention (Ryan and Mitchell 2011).

Internationally there are differences in the legislative framework and the way in which services for young people are configured. In England and Wales, the *National Service Framework for Children, Young People and Maternity Services* (Department of Health 2004) emphasises the need for equality of access to services, particularly for groups such as young offenders who often have complex health needs and find it difficult to access services. More recently in England and Wales, there have been changes in the commissioning and delivery arrangements for mental health services for young people in the justice system in order to better align them with other services for young people. However, there are still concerns regarding the availability and quality of mental health services for young people within the justice system (Department of Health 2009a, 2009b).

This chapter does not address the highly specialised needs of the relatively small population of young people with serious and enduring mental disorders who are cared for in conditions of medium security. Nor does it look at the needs of the very small group of preadolescent children who come into contact with youth justice agencies. Rather, it concentrates on the interface between child and adolescent mental health services (CAMHS) and the youth justice system. Mental health nurses are in key positions to play a prominent role in the development and delivery of these services. This is due both to their specialist knowledge of mental health problems affecting young people and their broad-based understanding of the holistic needs of children and young people.

When looking at the mental health needs of young people in contact with the youth justice system, we can see that their needs are often the same as those of their peers. It can be argued therefore that, providing risk management is addressed, young people within the youth justice system should access the same interventions and services as their peers in other settings. By addressing issues of risk assessment and management, mental health nurses can play a key role in ensuring this happens.

The youth justice system

The youth justice system in England and Wales is overseen by the Youth Justice Board (YJB). The YJB is responsible for custodial provision for young people under 18 years of age. The majority of secure places for under-18s are in young offender institutions (YOIs), but younger offenders or those considered to be particularly vulnerable are placed in local authority secure children's homes (LASCHs), which are smaller than YOIs and staffed by residential care workers. Secure training centres are intermediate in size between YOIs and LASCHs. The YJB also oversees the work of local youth offending teams (YOTs), which are responsible for working with young offenders in the community. YOTs have staff from multiple agencies (probation, social services, education, police and health) and are expected to form part of a 'joined-up' service to meet the wider needs of young offenders as well as supervising their noncustodial sentences. The number of young people placed in the secure estate has reduced by over 60 per cent during the last 12 years. The full reasons for this are not clear, but effective early intervention and diversion (i.e. reducing the number of first-time entrants) and better case management (including multi-agency working) and interventions (i.e. alternatives to custody) for those young people who do enter the system are major factors.

Young people within the youth justice system

The information in this and the following two sections is based partly on a study of young people referred to an adolescent forensic service in the north-west of England and partly on broader studies of the health needs of young people within the justice system.

It is often assumed that young people within the youth justice system have highly specialised mental health needs that are profoundly different to those of their peers. For a small number of young people, this is undoubtedly true; for example, young people who have committed serious acts of violence in response to command auditory hallucinations or paranoid delusions require highly specialised interventions. Particular differences relate to the legal process and include the young person's fitness to stand trial and status as a remanded or sentenced offender. However, for most young people in contact with the youth justice system, their mental health needs should be regarded as one element of their wider range of needs.

For some of these young people, particular concerns may exist in relation to risk. This often justifies referral to a specialised service for assessment and intervention. However, for many young people, there may not be a complex interrelationship between their high-risk or offending behaviour and their mental health needs (although risk will have to be assessed and managed). Here, mental health nurses can play a pivotal role; their skills in determining how specific mental health needs and problems relate to a wider range of personal and social needs is invaluable in devising an appropriate assessment and intervention strategy.

Over half of young people referred for mental health assessment within the justice system are likely to be in current contact with CAMHS services or will have had previous CAMHS contact. Referral is often prompted by a general increase in severity of need, unanticipated change in behaviour or increase in risk. There is often an interaction between a young person's offending behaviour and their current needs, and this interaction can be in either direction. Their unmet needs may have precipitated offending behaviour; conversely, the consequences of offending behaviour can result in new or more severe unmet needs. It is also worth noting that a number of young people will have their mental health needs identified for the first time when they come into contact with the justice system. Sometimes these needs have recently arisen (e.g. first-episode psychosis), but more frequently, they are long-standing needs that have been unrecognised. This is either because the young person has been 'under the radar' and not visible to services or because their manifestation of unmet needs is perceived as a behavioural difficulty. Under such circumstances, the initial concerns are likely to be raised by non-health professionals such as teachers, social workers or youth justice practitioners.

The average age of young people within the justice system is higher than those referred to mainstream CAMHS. Typically, three-quarters of them will be aged 15 or over. Nurses working in the justice system need to be mindful that this will influence both the nature of their problems and how these problems will present. In some areas, there is still effectively a 'service gap' for 16- to 18-year-olds despite the requirement for services to be provided up to the age of 18 (Department of Health 2004). Nurses working with young people in the justice system should be mindful of their likely trajectories and need for services into adulthood; it is important to establish links with adult mental health services (including forensic services) in order to ensure that transitional arrangements are in place before young people reach adulthood.

Boys constitute about 80 per cent of all young people in contact with the justice system and 95 per cent of all those in secure settings (Youth Justice Board 2014). There are undoubtedly some differences in the type of mental health problems that girls present with compared to boys. However, it is important to avoid stereotypes based on gender; there is increasing recognition of conduct disorder in girls (Storvoll and Wichstrom 2002; Delligatti *et al.* 2003), and at the same time, there are indications that the prevalence of self-harming behaviour amongst boys may be increasing (Hawton *et al.* 2003). Historically, the principle task of the criminal justice system has been to manage adult male offenders. Young people, particularly young women and girls, constitute a minority group within the system. As such, nurses need to remain aware of how their specific needs can remain unmet.

Young people belonging to black and minority ethnic (BME) groups continue to be over-represented within the justice system. The prevalence of mental health problems among young people appears to vary with ethnicity (Meltzer *et al.* 2000) although it has been argued that cultural bias and other social factors influence the recognition and reporting of mental health problems within different ethnic groups (Ramchandani 2004). There is also evidence that uptake of services by young people varies with ethnicity (Kodjo and Auinger 2004). Nurses should, therefore, be aware that there may be a higher than anticipated prevalence of unmet mental health needs among young people of BME origin and that the recognition of these needs may be hampered by cultural bias or misattributions.

What kind of mental health problems do they have?

Mental health problems can be categorised either diagnostically or using a needs-based approach. Both have their merits although a needs-based approach is generally more helpful for nurses as it enables a more holistic approach to assessing and meeting needs. Diagnostic frameworks such as ICD-10 – the World Health Organization's (1996) multiaxial classification of child and adolescent psychiatric disorders – can be helpful when young people need to be categorised in order to access specific or specialised services (for instance, when they have psychosis or a learning disability) or if they have rarer disorders. Regardless of how they are assessed, it is generally acknowledged that young people within the justice system have higher levels of mental health problems than their peers – see, for instance, Chitsabesan *et al.* (2006). The same study identified higher levels of unmet need for young people in the community compared with those in secure care. Immediate needs such as accommodation and managing substance misuse issues may be more effectively managed in secure settings, but it should be borne in mind that it is young people with the most unmet needs who are likely to be in custody in the first place and also that secure environments are highly stressful and can generate further needs for young people who are admitted.

Although there is some disagreement between studies regarding the prevalence of specific types of mental health problem, it is generally acknowledged that overall prevalence is at least two-thirds in custodial samples, with mood disorders, anxiety and post-traumatic stress disorder (PTSD) being the most common. Some studies have reported high levels of personality disorder although these figures also include over-18s and are usually based on the use of adult personality measures. Caution should be exercised before using such diagnoses with young people under 18, although some of them will be on a trajectory that will justify that diagnosis in adulthood. A very high proportion of young people in contact with the justice system meet the criteria for a diagnosis of conduct disorder.

It has already been noted that there are high levels of unmet (and generally unrecognised) neurodevelopmental needs among young people in the justice system. These include learning disabilities, communication difficulties, attention deficit hyperactivity disorder (ADHD), autistic spectrum disorders and traumatic brain injury. It is difficult to be clear about specific levels of unmet need in these domains, but the available information suggests prevalence levels between three and ten times higher than those of other populations of young people (Hughes *et al.* 2012).

Prevalence levels for these and other problems depend on how high the bar is set; diagnostic frameworks will typically not identify many young people who score highly on a needs assessment (Mitchell and Shaw 2011). This is often because they do not present with a 'full set' of symptoms for any given diagnosis (although they often have symptoms crossing many diagnostic boundaries) or because some of the symptoms are 'sub-threshold' for diagnosis. Finally, diagnostic frameworks are less effective at identifying levels of impairment or distress, which are often clinically significant and indicate that an intervention is needed. Thus from a nursing perspective, a robust and comprehensive needs assessment is more useful in identifying young people who are in need of support or intervention.

How can we best understand the wider social, personal and health needs of young people in contact with the youth justice system?

Over 10 per cent of young people referred to services in the north-west of England were found to have unmet physical health needs, and over half were identified as having unmet needs in relation to sexual functioning; this includes some young people with potentially serious sexually harmful behaviour but also many young people who put themselves at risk or had unmet needs regarding psychosexual education. A systematic review (Chitsabesan *et al.* 2006) identified high levels of unmet needs in many domains, including drugs (20 per cent) and alcohol (11 per cent), relationships with family (29 per cent) and peers (35 per cent), education or work (36 per cent) and accommodation (11 per cent). We know from other sources (Callen and Walton 2004) that young people in secure settings are highly likely to have a previous history of school exclusion (80 per cent) or of having been a looked-after child (40 per cent).

Thus there are multiple unmet needs across many domains, and it is recognised that these unmet needs are associated with reoffending (National Association for the Care and Resettlement of Offenders 2007). In fact, there are now interventions available for young offenders that adopt a more holistic approach to their needs and risks and explicitly address these to reduce reoffending (see, for instance, Henggeler *et al.* 2006). This model is also consistent with a recovery-based approach to mental health, which seeks to identify the factors that contribute to wellbeing rather than focusing on symptom reduction. Overall, these are significant developments from a nursing perspective as they support the principle of addressing a young person's total needs rather than just addressing their identified problems.

The other model that is particularly helpful in this respect is based on attachment theory. We know that many young people in the justice system have had multiple placements (both inside and outside the care system) and, therefore, have had multiple attachment figures. We also know they have often experienced high levels of trauma, often from an early age. Together, these result in young people who have had difficulty learning to regulate their emotions (and therefore present with unstable moods and behaviour) and have difficulty in engaging with other people (and therefore have relationship difficulties, including difficulty engaging with professionals). The model's value is as an integrated approach with an underlying theoretical framework that uses primary carers such as residential workers or nurses as the key agents of intervention. It is not possible to do attachment theory justice in this chapter, but it has been helpful for meeting the needs of young people within the care system (Golding 2008) and there is emerging evidence regarding its utility for meeting the needs of young people in the justice system (Ryan and Mitchell 2011).

Screening young people in the youth justice system

Bearing in mind the high levels of unmet need that young people in the justice system have plus the additional stresses and loss of family support for those placed in custody, it has been increasingly acknowledged that it is good practice to undertake screening for health and other needs. Internationally, the most widely used screening tool for young people in secure placements is the Massachusetts Youth Screening Instrument-2 (MAYSI-2; Kerig *et al.* 2011). This has generally proven effective in identifying mental health needs, but it only addresses mental health needs and is a self-report tool rather than an interview tool. Other tools have a wider scope and are designed for use by professionals at interview with the young person. For example, the BasisRaadsOnderzoek (BARO) is a more general assessment of mental health and emotional needs that was designed to be administered by a youth justice worker (Doreleijers *et al.* 2011).

In England and Wales, the Comprehensive Health Assessment Tool (CHAT) has recently been rolled out in both secure and community settings (Offender Health Research Network 2014). CHAT consists of five sections: immediate needs, physical health, mental health, substance misuse and neurodevelopmental needs. Each segment of the tool is designed to be administered by suitably trained and experienced practitioners, usually nurses, and collectively provides an integrated overview of a young person's healthcare needs. The tool is designed to be administered within a few days of initial contact except for the immediate needs section, which should be completed as soon as possible, particularly for young people received in to the secure estate. This section is time-critical as it assesses for unmet needs such as suicidal intent, physical dependence on drugs or alcohol, and medical conditions such as diabetes that require continuous treatment. CHAT is derived from the two-stage mental health assessment tool Screening Questionnaire Interview for Adolescents (SQUIFA) and Screening Interview for Adolescents (SIFA), which has been used in the youth justice system for a number of years (Kroll *et al.* 2003) and was originally based on the Salford Needs Assessment for Adolescents (S-NASA; Kroll *et al.* 1999). It should be noted that CHAT is a screening tool designed to assist practitioners in identifying those young people with unmet needs who require support; it is not a comprehensive clinical assessment – that is the next stage in the process.

Clinical assessment of needs and risk: general principles

Any intervention or case management by nurses with young people in the justice system should be informed by a robust and comprehensive needs and risk assessment process. It is important that nurses are able to justify the decisions they make, which is why the assessment process should be structured, systematic and evidence-based. The structured approach of screening tools is useful in that they are evidence-based and assess needs in a systematic way. As such, they are a helpful part of the framework for a more comprehensive assessment. However, it is important to view such tools as an aid to clinical judgement, not a replacement for it. A structured approach used in conjunction with clinical judgement and experience incorporates the best elements of both approaches.

To be robust, assessments should be based on multiple and independent sources of information. Although young people within the justice system have often been subjected to multiple assessments during their journey, these assessments may have had a narrow focus or be of unknown quality. Because of the number of transitions some of them have experienced, there is a risk that there are significant gaps in the narrative. It is also sometimes the case that assessments draw on earlier assessments without establishing the accuracy of the information, which leads to inaccuracies being perpetuated and accepted as fact. Using multiple sources enables the nurse to create a more complete narrative and check different information sources for contradictions or inaccuracies. As a minimum, a robust assessment should include interview with the young person, interview with the parent/carer, and review of documentary evidence provided by, for example, ASSET and medical and social care records/reports. The young person themself is a crucial source of information. They may not always be able to provide a coherent life narrative and may also be prone to minimising, exaggerating or discounting as irrelevant some aspects of their life history. Nevertheless, the young person's understanding of their own life and needs is central to any care planning or intervention. Active involvement of the young person from the outset is the first step in effectively engaging them in their own care and building a therapeutic alliance. It is not uncommon for young people in the justice system to feel like passive recipients of other people's decisions rather than active agents in their own care.

Finally, the information arising from any assessment process has a relatively short shelf life as young people's needs and risks change rapidly over time. Therefore, nurses should regularly review the findings of their assessments and be willing to re-evaluate needs/risks and goals in the light of any changes.

Needs assessment

Needs assessment should be based on multiple information sources, be comprehensive and use a structured format (such as S-NASA). However, young people's lives and narratives do not easily conform to a categorical format, which is why the clinical experience of the nurse is important to the overall quality of the assessment. Some young people will present with potentially unmet needs in particular domains, such as low mood, psychosis or ADHD. In such cases, the structured assessments that would be used in other settings should be used here. Examples of tools that have been used effectively with this population include the Trauma Symptom Checklist (Briere 1996) for trauma, the KGV (Krawiecka, Goldberg and Vaughan, 1977) for psychosis and Conners for ADHD (Conners et al. 1998).

Bearing in mind the multiple unmet needs of this population, it is important to use specialised tools following a comprehensive assessment to ensure accurate identification. It should also be borne in mind that young people in the justice system are generally older than the typical CAMHS population, and this may affect the choice of assessment tool. It may also be necessary to consider how the immediate environment may influence the presentation of problems and to be flexible in how tools are used to complete the assessment. For instance, assessment of ADHD within a secure environment should take into account the generally high level of stimulus in these environments, and it is advisable to get reports from current carers as well as the young person's regular parents/carers.

Assessing and managing risk

As with needs assessment, risk assessment should be viewed as a comprehensive and ongoing process, not a one-off. It should also be undertaken with the purpose of subsequently implementing a risk management strategy; without taking action in response to identified risks, it is pointless assessing risk in the first place. A risk management strategy should seek to identify precipitators and mitigators of risk, indicators or warning signs of increasing risk, and strategies to reduce and manage risk.

It is important that nurses recognise that risk assessment is a dynamic process; risk changes over time and even factors that appear to be consistent do not necessarily occur on either a regular or a purely random basis. For instance, a young person may have a two-year history of persistent aggression in their care placement. Although the frequency of aggressive incidents may have been generally uniform during that period, closer scrutiny of the incidents is likely to reveal patterns within the young person's behaviour. The time of day, the gender and personalities of staff on duty and the presence of peers are just a few of the idiosyncratic factors that could influence the likelihood of acts of aggression occurring.

Generally speaking, the more information that can be gathered about risk, the better the assessment is likely to be. It is important to record specific details about specific aggressive incidents, particularly those which lead either to criminal charges or a change to the way the young person is perceived by those who know them. Bold statements such as 'he tried to stab him' should not be accepted at face value as an assessment of risk and reveal little about the act itself. It is critically important to contextualise the event. Did the young person use a carving knife or butter knife? Whereabouts on the body and how many times did the young person attempt to strike? Was there evidence of provocation or premeditation? What was the intention of the young person making the attack? Did they understand the potential consequences of their actions? These are just a few of the questions a nurse might ask before making any statements regarding the likelihood of future risk. As well as exploring specific risk events in detail, it is important to consider these in the context of the young person's behaviour and social functioning. The wider context may highlight factors that appear to increase risk. Conversely, factors that may reduce the likelihood of future risk behaviour may be identified.

There are a number of tools for assessing specific areas of risk that may be relevant to nursing practice. For assessing the risk of violence, the Structured Assessment of Violence Risk in Youth (SAVRY) is in widespread use and assesses risk on the basis of both historical and current factors (Borum *et al.* 2002). It also incorporates preservative or resilience factors. It is not intended to provide a numerical rating of risk in clinical practice but, rather, to identify areas where intervention is needed in order to manage risk – in other words, to be a structured aid to clinical judgement. It has demonstrated good levels of predictive ability in practice (Dolan and Rennie 2008). The Early Assessment Risk List for Boys (EARL-20B) has been developed for assessing the risk of violence in younger boys, and there is also a version for girls (EARL-20G) (Augimeri *et al.* 2001).

There are a number of tools that have been developed for the assessment of sexually harmful behaviour. These should only be used by nurses with the appropriate training and in the context of a specialised team or service. One such tool is AIM (Print *et al.* 2007; Griffin *et al.* 2008), a structured assessment developed through the Assessment, Intervention and Moving-on Project and used by a number of specialised services in the UK. Internationally, other tools have been developed, such as the Estimate of Risk of Adolescent Sexual Offence Recidivism (ERASOR; Worling 2004) and the Juvenile Sex Offender

Assessment Protocol-II (J-SOAP-II; Prentky and Righthand 2003). These tools have been shown to have some predictive validity but should be used in the context of a comprehensive approach to risk management (Hempel *et al.* 2013).

The assessment of personality problems and, in particular, personality disorder among young people under the age of 18 is a contentious issue partly because of the stigmatising effect of such a label (Edens 2006) and also because the validity of using such constructs with this age group has been challenged (Seagrave and Grisso 2002). If the use of such tools is being contemplated then thought should be given as to how the findings may affect the young person's future trajectory and access to services. The Millon Adolescent Clinical Inventory (Millon 1993) was developed specifically for use with adolescents, and the Psychopathy Checklist: Youth Version (Forth *et al.* 2003) is an adaptation of a widely used adult tool.

There are a number of caveats and other factors that should be considered in relation to the use of risk assessment tools. First, although they may have some predictive validity in analysis of populations, there is also evidence that clinicians' risk judgements may have better predictors in clinical practice (de Vogel *et al.* 2004; Douglas *et al.* 2003). Second, adolescence is a time of major developmental change and judgements about risk should take this into consideration, particularly in relation to the use of personality measures (Dolan and Rennie 2008). Third, specialised tools for assessing particular areas of risk, such as sexual offending and fire-setting, should only be used by trained practitioners working in specialised teams. Finally, robust risk assessment should also take resilience and preservative factors into consideration as there is emerging evidence regarding their importance (Rennie and Dolan 2010).

Interventions and case management

Bearing in mind that the needs of young people in the justice system are similar in many respects to those of other young people, they should have access to the same interventions (i.e. they should have equity of access – or not be denied access because they are in the justice system). Interventions such as cognitive behaviour therapy (CBT), systemic or family interventions, non-verbal therapies such as art therapy, and counselling should be offered if clinically indicated and if effective case management is in place. There is evidence from research and from general clinical practice that such interventions can be used effectively with this population. Some of these interventions require highly specialised training, but increasing numbers of mental health nurses are acquiring skills in modalities such as CBT. However, there are challenges with interventions such as CBT; verbal and non-verbal communication skills may be underdeveloped, as may the capacity for introspection. Motivation may also be low (often based on their overall experience of contact with professionals), and their lifestyle may be unstable.

Despite these challenges, there is evidence that young people within the justice system can be effectively engaged in interventions such as CBT if the model of delivery is adapted to their needs (Mitchell *et al.* 2011). The changes required are variable (depending on circumstances and individual need), but consideration should be given to the frequency, duration and location of sessions, the length of therapy and the development of 'core skills' such as emotional literacy before undertaking any work on higher-order cognitive skills. Therapeutic materials should be tailored to the capacities and preferences of each young person. It is important that goal setting is highly collaborative as the young person's therapeutic goals (i.e. defining the 'problem') may be very different to those of the adults caring for them.

There is also growing interest in models of therapeutic engagement and intervention that are more flexible and adaptive to the needs of individual young people or the needs of specific groups who may not have accessed more 'traditional' services and interventions. These include dialectical behaviour therapy (DBT), originally developed for working with suicidal adults but which has shown some effectiveness with adolescent girls within the justice system (Trupin et al. 2002). Adolescent Mentalisation-Based Integrative Therapy has recently been developed as a more flexible resource to support professionals working with 'hard to reach' young people and their immediate care system (Bevington et al. 2013).

Case management should be based on several key principles. Some of these, including effective engagement with the young person and carers and a comprehensive needs and risk assessment, have been discussed above. Other key elements include robust processes for sharing information and a regularly reviewed inter-agency care plan. These are important as there is often multi-agency involvement and risks and needs can change rapidly. The complexity involved in the care plan and the care planning process will depend on the complexity of each case but should include identified goals and interventions to meet needs, identification of factors that may increase or reduce risk, warning signs of the risk increasing and a safety plan in the event of a rapid change in needs/risk. The care plan should also specify individual and organisational responsibilities clearly.

In the UK, there are two key policy documents relevant for the planning and coordination of care for this population. The Common Assessment Framework (Children's Workforce Development Council 2007) was developed explicitly to guide and coordinate inter-agency working for young people who are disadvantaged, who are potentially at risk or who have complex needs. The guidance does not replace local safeguarding processes but should sit alongside them to support young people who could 'fall through the gaps' or be missed by services. From a mental health perspective, the Care Programme Approach (CPA) was developed to ensure mental health care is coordinated and effectively involves service users and their families. It is not possible here to cover in detail all aspects of CPA implementation. National policy documents are available (Department of Health 2008) and local guidance should also be sought. The CPA Handbook is also a valuable source of information and guidance for nurses (The Care Programme Approach Association 2001).

Case example: Jason

Jason is 15 years old and has just come into contact with the justice system for the first time after being sentenced to a Referral Order in Youth Court for motor vehicle offences. The offence occurred while Jason was in the company of two peers with whom he has spent time since he stopped attending school. He lives at home with his older brother and his mother, a single parent. Jason has not been in education for over 12 months and is currently under the care of CAMHS, who have diagnosed him with ADHD and commenced him on stimulant medication. Jason and his mother lead a disorganised lifestyle, meaning they often miss appointments with the CAMHS team and any other professionals, and Jason often forgets to take his medication.

At his first Youth Offending Service (YOS) meeting, in advance of his Referral Order Panel, Jason only engaged superficially with his YOS worker Desmond, and he did not appear very remorseful for his behaviour. Jason also had a health screen using CHAT. This included a screening by Karen, the mental health nurse attached to the YOS, who is also aware of his ADHD diagnosis. Karen has not identified any other mental health problems, such as low mood or self-harm, but has noted that he scored positively for substance misuse (cannabis and alcohol) and also for possible learning difficulties. There is little education information on ASSET due to the time he has been out of school, but his last school have confirmed that Jason had scored poorly on psychometric testing although he did not meet the criteria for a statement of special educational needs. Karen noted from ASSET that Jason's maternal grandmother died 18 months ago, and he became distressed when this was raised at interview.

Desmond was unsure how to proceed, this being Jason's first contact with the justice system combined with Desmond being aware of his health needs from talking to Karen. However, his offence was potentially serious and Jason did not appear very concerned.

Karen was able to establish a rapport with Jason during the screening, and he agreed to a further interview jointly with his mother and Desmond. Because of the difficulties engaging the family, Karen and Desmond saw Jason and his mother at the family home. The interview went well with both Jason and his mother engaging with Desmond better than at the YOS office. Jason's mother was clearly concerned regarding his behaviour, and she was supportive of Desmond. Karen noted that Jason's mother was also having difficulty coming to terms with the death of her mother.

As a result of the meeting, Desmond felt confident in proposing a number of actions to the Referral Order Panel. The plan included the following:

- Jason and his mother to attend CAMHS appointments to ensure treatment for his ADHD was at an effective level and that he was complying with treatment. (Karen to liaise with CAMHS and support family in attending.)
- Jason to undertake some work regarding bereavement and expressing feelings of loss. (Karen to facilitate.)
- Jason to attend local education support team regarding getting back into education. (Desmond to liaise and support attendance.)
- Jason to undertake work (with Desmond) regarding the following areas:
  - consequential thinking, managing peer pressure and cannabis and alcohol awareness.
- This work to be informed by advice from Karen regarding length and frequency of sessions and the type of materials to use.

The plan also included warning signs that Jason's behaviour may be escalating. These included:

- not taking his stimulant medication;
- associating with the boys he had offended with;
- evidence of cannabis and alcohol use.

If any of these happened then Jason's mother was to contact Desmond and Karen. In addition, Desmond referred Jason's mother, at her request, to the YOS Parenting Team for some support for herself in relation to her parenting and her own bereavement.

It was recognised that Jason might have increased difficulty managing his emotions and behaviour while undertaking the bereavement work with Karen, and Desmond agreed to provide additional support to Jason and his mother during this period. All aspects of the plan were developed and agreed with Jason and his mother. The plan was written up in simple language and everyone received a copy. It was agreed that they would meet again in four weeks to review progress and that the short-term goals and interventions could be changed as long as the long-term goal of keeping Jason out of trouble and getting him engaged with activities/education was being achieved.

Conclusion

In future, there will almost certainly be further changes in our understanding of the mental health needs of young people in the justice system and also in models of care delivery. As we move towards a more needs-driven and formulation-based approach, nurses will be in a key position to take these changes forward.

References

Abram, K., Teplin, L., Charles, D., Longworth, S., McClelland, G. and Dulcan, M. (2004) Post-traumatic stress disorder and trauma in youth in juvenile detention. *Archives of General Psychiatry*, 61(4): 403–10.

Augimeri, L., Webster, C., Koegl, C. and Levene, K. (2001) *Early Assessment Risk List for Boys: EARL-20B, Version 2*. Toronto: Earlscourt Child and Family Centre.

Bevington, D., Fuggle, P., Fonagy, P., Target, M. and Asen, E. (2013) Innovations in practice: Adolescent Mentalization-Based Integrative Therapy (AMBIT) – a new integrated approach to working with the most hard to reach adolescents with severe complex mental health needs. *Child and Adolescent Mental Health*, 18(1): 46–51.

Borum, R., Bartel, P. and Forth, A. (2002) *Manual for the Structured Assessment of Violence Risk in Youth (SAVRY)*. Tampa, FL: Florida Mental Health Institute.

Briere, J. (1996) *Trauma Symptom Checklist for Children: Professional Manual*. Odessa, FL: Psychological Assessment Resources, Inc.

Care Programme Approach Association, The (2001) *The CPA Handbook*. Chesterfield: Walton Hospital.

Casswell, M., French, P. and Rogers, A. (2012) Distress, defiance or adaptation? A review paper of at-risk mental health states in young offenders. *Early Intervention in Psychiatry*, 6(3): 219–28.

Challen, M. and Walton, T. (2004) *Juveniles in Custody – A Unique Insight into the Perceptions of Young People Held in Prison Service Custody in England and Wales*. London: HM Inspectorate of Prisons.

Children's Workforce Development Council (2007) *Common Assessment Framework for Children and Young People: Practitioners' Guide: Integrated Working to Improve Outcomes for Children and Young People*. Leeds: Children's Workforce Development Council.

Chitsabesan, P., Kroll, L., Bailey, S., Kenning, C., Sneider, S., MacDonald, W. and Theodosiou, L. (2006) Mental health needs of young offenders in custody and in the community. *British Journal of Psychiatry*, 188(6): 534–40.

Coid, J., Yang, M., Tyrer, P., Roberts, A. and Ullrich, S. (2006) Prevalence and correlates of personality disorder in Great Britain. *British Journal of Psychiatry*, 188(5): 423–31.

Conners, C., Sitarenios, G., Parker, J. and Epstein, J. (1998) The Revised Conners' Parent Rating Scale (CPRS-R): factor structure, reliability, and criterion validity. *Journal of Abnormal Child Psychology*, 26(4): 257–68.

de Vogel, V., de Ruiter, C., van Beek, D. and Mead, G. (2004) Predictive validity of the SVR-20 and Static-99 in a Dutch sample of treated sex offenders. *Law and Human Behavior*, 28(3): 235–51.

Delligatti, N., Akin-Little, A. and Little, S. (2003) Conduct disorder in girls: diagnostic and intervention issues. *Psychology in the Schools*, 40(2): 183–92.

Department of Health (2009a) *The Bradley Report: Lord Bradley's Review of People with Mental Health Problems or Learning Disabilities in the Criminal Justice System*. London: Department of Health.

Department of Health (2009b) *Healthy Children, Safer Communities: A Strategy to Promote the Health and Well-Being of Children and Young People in Contact with the Youth Justice System*. London: Department of Health.

Department of Health (2008) *Refocusing the Care Programme Approach*. London: Department of Health.

Department of Health (2004) *National Service Framework for Children, Young People and Maternity Services*. London: Department of Health.

Dolan, M. and Rennie, C. (2008) The Structured Assessment of Violence Risk in Youth (SAVRY) as a predictor of recidivism in a UK cohort of adolescent offenders with conduct disorder. *Psychological Assessment*, 20(1): 35–46.

Doreleijers, T., Boonmann, C., van Loosbroek, E. and Vermeiren, R. (2011) Assessing the psychometric properties and the perceived usefulness of the BasisRaadsOnderzoek (BARO) as a first-line screening instrument for juvenile offenders. *Child and Adolescent Psychiatry and Mental Health*, 5(24): 1–7.

Douglas, K., Ogloff, J. and Hart, S. (2003) Evaluation of a model of risk assessment among forensic psychiatric patients. *Psychiatric Services*, 54(10): 1372–9.

Edens, J. (2006) Unresolved controversies concerning psychopathy: implications for clinical and forensic decision-making. *Professional Psychology: Research and Practice*, 37(1): 59–65.

Forth, A., Kosson, D. and Hare, R. (2003) *The Psychopathy Checklist: Youth Version Manual*. Toronto: Multi-Health Systems.

Golding, K. (2008) *Nurturing Attachments: Supporting Children who are Fostered or Adopted*. London: Jessica Kingsley.

Griffin, H., Beech, A., Print, B., Bradshaw, H. and Quayle, J. (2008) The development and initial testing of the AIM2 framework to assess risk and strengths in young people who sexually offend. *Journal of Sexual Aggression*, 14(3): 211–25.

Hawton, K., Harris, L., Hall, S., Simkin, S., Bale, E. and Bond, A. (2003) Deliberate self-harm in Oxford, 1990–2000: a time of change in patient characteristics. *Psychological Medicine*, 33(6): 987–95.

Hempel. I., Buck, N., Cima, M. and van Marle, H. (2013) Review of risk assessment instruments for juvenile sex offenders. *International Journal of Offender Therapy and Comparative Criminology*, 57(2): 208–28.

Henggeler, S., Halliday-Boykins, C., Cunningham, P., Randall, J., Shapiro, S. and Chapman, J. (2006) Juvenile drug court: enhancing outcomes by integrating evidence-based treatments. *Journal of Consulting and Clinical Psychology*, 74(1): 42–54.

Hughes, N., Williams, H., Chitsabesan, P., Davies, R. and Mounce, L. (2012) *Nobody Made the Connection: The Prevalence of Neuro-disability in Young People who Offend*. London: Office of the Children's Commissioner.

Kerig, P., Moeddel, M. and Becker, S. (2011) Assessing the sensitivity and specificity of the MAYSI-2 for detecting trauma among youth in juvenile detention. *Child and Youth Care Forum*, 40(5): 345–62.

Kodjo, C. M. and Auinger, P. (2004) Predictors for emotionally distressed adolescents to receive mental health care. *Journal of Adolescent Health*, 35(5): 368–73.

Kraweicka, M., Goldberg, D. and Vaughan, M. (1977) A standardised psychiatric assessment scale for rating chronic psychotic patients. *Acta Psychiatrica Scandinavia*, 55(4): 299–308.

Kroll, L., Bailey, S., Myatt, T., McCarthy, K., Shuttleworth, J., Rothwell, J. and Harrington, R. (2003) *The Mental Health Screening Interview for Adolescents*. London: Youth Justice Board.

Kroll, L., Woodham, A., Rothwell, J., Bailey, S., Tobias, C., Harrington, R. and Marshall, M. (1999) Reliability of the Salford needs assessment schedule for adolescents. *Psychological Medicine*, 29(4): 891–902.

Maughan, B. and Kim-Cohen, J. (2005) Continuities between childhood and adult life. *British Journal of Psychiatry*, 187(4): 605–17.

Meltzer, H., Gatward, H., Goodman, R. and Ford, T. (2000) *Mental Health of Children and Adolescents in Great Britain*. London: The Stationery Office.

Millon, T. (1993) *Millon Adolescent Clinical Inventory Manual*. Minneapolis, MN: National Computer Systems.

Mitchell, P. and Shaw, J. (2011) Factors affecting the recognition of mental health problems among adolescent offenders in custody. *Journal of Forensic Psychiatry and Psychology*, 22(3): 381–94.

Mitchell, P., Smedley, K., Kenning, C., McKee, A., Woods, D., Rennie, C. E., Bell, R. V., Aryamanesh, M. and Dolan, M. (2011) Cognitive behaviour therapy for adolescent offenders with mental health problems in custody. *Journal of Adolescence*, 34(3): 433–43.

National Association for the Care and Resettlement of Offenders (2007) *Effective Practice with Children and Young People who Offend – Part 2*. Youth Crime Briefing, March 2007. London: National Association for the Care and Resettlement of Offenders.

Offender Health Research Network (2014) The Comprehensive Health Assessment Tool (CHAT): Resources [online]. Available at: www.ohrn.nhs.uk/OHRNResearch/CHAT (accessed 19 February 2015).

Prentky, R. and Righthand, S. (2003) Juvenile Sex Offender Assessment Protocol-II (J-SOAP-II) [online]. Available at: www.psicologiagiuridica.eu/files/didattica/jsoap2.pdf (accessed 1 February 2013).

Print, B., Griffin, H., Beech, A., Quayle, J., Bradshaw, H., Henniker, J. and Morrison, T. (2007) *AIM2: An Initial Assessment Model for Young People who Display Sexually Harmful Behaviour*. Manchester: AIM Project.

Ramchandani, P. (2004) The epidemiology of mental health problems in children and adolescents from minority ethnic groups in the UK. In M. Malek and C. Joughin (eds) *Mental Health Services for Minority Ethnic Children and Adolescents*. London: Jessica Kingsley, pp. 66–80.

Rennie, C. and Dolan, M. (2010) The significance of protective factors in the assessment of risk. *Criminal Behaviour and Mental Health*, 20(1): 8–22.

Ryan, T. and Mitchell, P. (2011) A collaborative approach to meeting the needs of adolescent offenders with complex needs in custodial settings: an 18-month cohort study. *The Journal of Forensic Psychology and Psychiatry*, 22(3): 437–54.

Seagrave, D. and Grisso, T. (2002) Adolescent development and the measurement of juvenile psychopathy. *Law and Human Behavior*, 26(2): 219–39.

Storvoll, E. and Wichstrom, L. (2002) Do the risk factors associated with conduct problems in adolescents vary according to gender? *Journal of Adolescence*, 25(2): 183–202.

Trupin, E., Stewart, D., Beach, B. and Boesky, L. (2002) Effectiveness of a dialectical behaviour therapy program for incarcerated female juvenile offenders. *Child and Adolescent Mental Health*, 7(3): 121–7.

Vreugdenhil, C., Doreleijers, T., Vermeiren, R., Wouters, L. and van den Brink, W. (2004) Psychiatric disorders in a representative sample of incarcerated boys in the Netherlands. *Journal of the American Academy of Child and Adolescent Psychiatry*, 43(1): 97–104.

World Health Organization (1996) *ICD-10: Multiaxial Classification of Child and Adolescent Psychiatric Disorders*. Cambridge University Press: Cambridge.

Worling, J. (2004) The estimate of risk of adolescent sexual offense recidivism (ERASOR): preliminary psychometric data. *Sexual Abuse: A Journal of Research and Treatment*, 16(3): 235–54.

Youth Justice Board (2014) *Youth Justice Statistics 2012–13*. London: Youth Justice Board.

Chapter 15

CAMHS nurses as entrepreneurs

Dawn Rees

Key points

- The traditional concept of nursing as solely relating to bedside care and compassion is an anachronism; those qualities are necessary and indeed they inform the reasons why people enter the profession, but nursing roles are ripe for further development. Opportunities to innovate and to lead change continue to emerge.
- The position of nursing as a profession, the demands of nursing practice, the emerging culture of practitioner-based innovation and the individual qualities of some nurses equip them for entrepreneurial approaches. This is the case both in practice and in business. Combined with a permissive environment and pursuing opportunities inside and outside the health system, nurses with entrepreneurial qualities can establish themselves as formidable change agents, leading healthcare reform and innovation.
- Nurse entrepreneurs often experience constraint and caution in the nursing environment, which can be dominated by procedure, clinical governance and patient safety. It is frequently the experience of impenetrable procedures, red tape, lack of communication between departments and the difficulties of achieving joined-up thinking and action across a number of departments that creates inertia and impacts on creative approaches and solutions.
- Using nurses and other health professionals to innovate and act in intrepreneurial roles is a very cost-effective strategy. However, it needs to be a constituent part of workforce planning if talent and aptitude is to be retained within the health system and patient-facing capacity is not compromised.

Entrepreneur

A person who organises and operates a business or businesses taking on greater than normal financial risks in order to do so.

(Collins Dictionary)

A social entrepreneur is what you get when you combine Richard Branson and Mother Teresa – a hybrid between business and social value creation.

(Pamela Hartigan, Managing Director, Schwab Foundation)

Intrepreneurship

    employees developing new business activities for their employer

(Bosma *et al.* 2010: 3)

Introduction

Roy Griffiths, in his landmark inquiry into the management of the NHS, declared that if Florence Nightingale were carrying her lamp through the corridors of the NHS today, she would almost certainly be searching for the people in charge (Naylor 2015). If Florence Nightingale was walking the wards of the NHS today, however, she would be looking beyond them – out into general practice, into community services, into the private and voluntary sectors and out into social care and other local authority services. She would be looking for the other inspirational leaders who would help her make her wards work better. Among those to whom she would be looking would be patients. And all those other people would be looking back for exactly the same result.

More recently than the Griffiths report, The King's Fund (2011) published *The Future of Leadership and Management in the NHS: No More Heroes*. Its core message, aside from a vigorous defence of management and its role, was that the NHS needed to move beyond an outdated model based on heroic leadership of institutions by individuals to one where leaders focus on systems of care and on engaging staff in delivering results. The report argued that leadership of the twenty-first-century health system needed to be shared, distributed and adaptive. Today, the case for that style of leadership is even stronger, for myriad reasons.

The King's Fund think piece on adaptive, shared and distributed leadership and management in the NHS perfectly informs this chapter on the role of entrepreneurship in nursing. Nurses are ideally placed to lead the way in innovation, redesign and new ways of working. They represent the largest profession in health services. Over the past 15 years, their roles have changed and been enhanced; they have become more demanding, more diverse and more technical, and particularly in the last five years, they have been at the forefront of creating innovative approaches to doing more with less – implementing radical changes in patient care, improving quality and implementing evidence-based practice.

The traditional concept of nursing as solely relating to bedside care and compassion is an anachronism; those qualities are necessary – and indeed inform the reasons why people enter the profession – but nursing roles are ripe for further development. Opportunities for innovation and leading change continue to emerge.

This chapter is in two parts. The first explores what we mean by entrepreneurship and intrepreneurship and how the changing shape of the NHS and private healthcare has incrementally influenced opportunities for nurses to innovate, lead change, manage initiatives and play a major part in transformational leadership in health provision. The second part considers who the entrepreneurs and intrepreneurs in the system are, what they are doing and how they are doing it. Finally, a framework is offered for nurses to think about how to set up a business and run it efficiently, ethically and effectively.

Are entrepreneurs born or made?

The position of nursing as a profession, the demands of nursing practice, the emerging culture of practitioner-based innovation and the individual qualities of some nurses equip them for entrepreneurial approaches, both in practice and in business. Combined with a permissive environment and pursuing opportunities inside and outside the health system, nurses with entrepreneurial qualities have already established themselves as formidable change agents, leading healthcare reform and innovation.

Nurses are the largest single profession in the health sector and ideally positioned to lead and innovate. Talk to most nurses and ask them about what internal characteristics and abilities make them good at what they do and they will tell you – the confidence that comes from being well trained; possessing core competencies that help them with task completion; flexibility; an interest in people; the ability to assess and manage risk; the ability to manage people and budgets; creating opportunities for change; following through; using evidence-based practice; motivating staff, thinking strategically and planning ahead; being outcomes focused; basing actions on values and reflection; innovation; optimism; and compassion.

What hinders their effectiveness are slow and inflexible systems; the ability to influence budget allocation; lack of training in innovation and leadership; and the inevitable bureaucratic hierarchies that exist in health settings. Traynor *et al.* (2006) report on the perceptions of nurses in multidisciplinary settings and identifies three barriers to good teamwork and, by definition, the ability to use their role to influence leadership and change in teams:

- differing perceptions of teamwork;
- different levels of skills acquisitions to function as a team member;
- the dominance of medical power that influenced interaction in teams.

So, what characteristics do some of the leading business leaders and entrepreneurs demonstrate? Richard Branson of the Virgin Group says emotional intelligence, daring, working with teams, self-belief and being trustworthy, optimistic and self-aware. Karren Brady, former manager of Birmingham City Football Club, says determination, energy, ambition, an interest in innovation and a dedication to completing the task. Entrepreneur Deborah Meaden says self-belief, resilience, good judgement and planning. What other factors assist their success? The ability to set and control priorities and budgets, control of the agenda, the ability to respond quickly to market forces, leading from the front, taking risks and relative freedom from constraint are all enabling factors in the life of a legitimate entrepreneur.

Why don't we have more nurse entrepreneurs? Do we know how many innovators and entrepreneurs are nurses? Of course we do not. However, having interviewed six nurse entrepreneurs in preparation for this chapter, what is striking is that their success has been, in part, determined by what story they told themselves about themselves and due to recognition that the characteristics of good business leaders and entrepreneurs are not so different from those of good nurses who have an interest in leading and driving change, whether it be within health settings or in setting up a new business. Innovative nurses (some of whom are intrepreneurs and some entrepreneurs) are simply applying their talents and their training in a different way – often in a way that sets them apart from other nurses. They have acquired a profile as an entrepreneur even though they do not consider themselves to be one. As such, they do not always fit into a neat niche in public sector organisations.

The nurses who were interviewed to inform this chapter expressed views that broadly reflect the findings in Traynor *et al.*'s (2006) report to the National Co-ordinating Centre for NHS Service Delivery and Organisation. They were attracted to intrepreneurship and entrepreneurship because they could use their imagination effectively and had more control over what they did and how they did it; they expressed greater job satisfaction, used a variety of approaches and skills for problem-solving and had a greater sense of personal agency and influence.

Nurses said that they often experienced restraint and caution in the nursing environment, which is dominated by procedure, clinical governance and patient safety. It is frequently the nurses' experience of impenetrable procedures, red tape, lack of communication between departments and the difficulties of achieving joined-up thinking and action across a number of departments that creates inertia and impacts on creative approaches and solutions. Raup (2008) suggests that the organisational environment of the hospital itself may serve as a barrier. Organisational processes often substitute for leadership, and change is difficult due partly to the inertia of bureaucracies, norms and traditions.

The delivery of high-quality care and transformational change is peppered with examples of evidence-based innovation led by nurses. Yet implementation based on innovation is difficult. Those involved are often frustrated by the length of time it takes to implement change in the wider health system despite such innovations being implemented successfully in one location; the learning and the change often disseminates very slowly, if at all. Diffusion of the learning from innovation is a major challenge in all industries, including healthcare, suggests Berwick (2003). Nonetheless, through experiencing the inevitable frustrations of organisational inflexibility and the lack of opportunity or authority to move and change quickly, individual creativity and innovative practice can be ignited, leading individuals to develop a professional profile as a leader, an innovator – an intrepreneur – in the system. Or as an entrepreneur outwith it.

A changing environment

The nursing environment has been subject to considerable change over the past 20 years with greater levels of technology and the rise of specialist nurses, consultant nurses, nurse prescribers and nurse practitioners; in addition, the drive toward more evidence- and outcomes-based practice and the delivering of performance targets based on aspects such as access, waiting times, choice and referral to treatment times have reinforced the rise of the 'expert' to implement and evidence change.

Government policies have driven change and, therefore, the innovation agenda; these have a direct impact on organisational behaviour and responses, including innovative practice. As illustration of policies that have had an influence: in 1999, the new Health Act proposed the replacement of GP fundholding and introduced primary care groups with a role for nurses on boards; *The NHS Plan* (Department of Health 2000) reinforced the emphasis on flexible nursing roles and introduced nurse prescribing; modern matrons were introduced in 2001; *Our Health, Our Care, Our Say* (Department of Health 2006) promoted nurse-led innovation and encouraged social enterprises; the introduction of 'quality', 'choice' and national targets fed innovation schemes; *Equity and Excellence – Liberating the NHS* (Department of Health 2011) set out the radical agenda for change in commissioning and delivery and presaged the development of clinical commissioning groups (CCGs) and the shift of public health into local authorities; the Health and Social Care Act 2012 saw 152 primary care trusts replaced by 211 CCGs, all of which have clinical representation on their boards.

The NHS *Five Year Forward View* offers a clear indication that changes in structures, roles, partnership, innovation and delivery are part of its plan. This states that:

> We will invest in new options for our workforce, and raise our game on health technology – radically improving patients' experience of interacting with the NHS. We will improve the NHS' ability to undertake research and apply **innovation** – including by

developing new 'test bed' sites for worldwide innovators, and new 'green field' sites where completely new NHS services will be designed from scratch.

(NHS England 2014: 3–4)

Overall, NHS modernisation has put nurses at the centre of the agenda, while at the same time commissioning changes have resulted in a perverse incentive for a wider range of providers – social enterprises, consultancy, community interest companies and new businesses. Thus, the radical changes in both the NHS and the commissioning architecture between 2011 and 2015 have resulted in a movement toward a significantly changed and mixed health economy. However, combined with fiscal austerity, there have been redundancies of 11 per cent of Band 8 nurses and 4.5 per cent of Band 7 nurses between 2010 and 2013. These bands represent senior and experienced nurses at ward sister, modern matron and nurse practitioner level, and a total of 3,113 nurses left the system in that period. This inevitably impacts on the ability to manage risk and to implement and support innovative change while, conversely, increasing opportunities for entrepreneurial and innovative approaches internally.

Perceptions of individual risk and opportunity (which can include staying in the NHS as well as getting out of it) are influenced by opportunity, a permissive environment or a restrictive one, unemployment and a sense of individual agency. Nurses see a correlation between the principles of innovation and change management and how businesses adapt to market demands and changes. Having the mindset for growth and an environment that encourages and supports those in bespoke or nontraditional roles will often determine what career direction a nurse might take.

A recent King's Fund paper (Massie 2015) highlighted the important role of leadership in the NHS. However, more and more, nurses experience the satisfaction and challenge of leading innovation and change but find it increasingly difficult to plot a career pathway within the NHS that incorporates all they have learned in intrepreneurial roles. They frequently feel constrained by the offer of predominantly standard roles and responsibilities that tend to define traditional nursing practice. Workforce strategies must take account of this and develop career pathways for innovators and change agents if the NHS is to retain staff who are talented intrepreneurs. Not to do so will turn those intrepreneurs into entrepreneurs outside the system as nurses recognise that what they have learned about innovation is easily transferable into the business environment. The excerpt in Box 15.1 is taken from The King's Fund paper *Talent Management* (Massie 2015).

Another way of exploring the tensions and challenges experienced by nurses in leading innovation is through the application of sociological theories to the study of organisations (see Burrell and Morgan 1979; Whittington and Holland 1985; Howe 1987). These authors explore subjective and objective perspectives in the form of the sociology of regulation versus the sociology of radical change. One of the inherent tensions in the organisation of public sector delivery with its fixed systems is the relative rigidity of organisations that tend to see change being managed in terms of procedures and functions that lead to rational responses and predictable, measurable outcomes. In contrast, the paradigm of a radical, free-thinking approach to change – frequently a characteristic of change agents, innovators and intrepreneurs – creates an inevitable imbalance of form, function and governance that is a challenge to the rigid and often constraining structures of public sector organisations.

Howe (1987) further adapted models by Whittington and Holland (1985) and Burrell and Morgan (1979), describing in a personal conversation how social workers (the 'radical humanists') exhibit 'bandit-like' behaviour within their own system – spending as little time

---

Box 15.1 Developing leadership, not just leaders

NHS organisations are often described as having a high-challenge, low-support culture. If we see junior or emerging leaders as likely senior managers and leaders of the future we must ask 'what is this experience teaching them?'

The chief executive and senior leaders play an essential role in encouraging managers to share talent across the organisation to avoid thinking in siloes or assuming linear progression. You can do this by supporting stretch assignments and rotating leadership roles, giving those who have potential leadership talent the opportunity to fill gaps in a different part of the organisation or system, or lead innovation and change. For example, a director of nursing might identify a nurse who has skills that would enable them to work as a chief operating officer or a workforce specialist.

Successful deployment of workforce talent is about rethinking your view of your employees. They are not assets to be managed but rather people with options who have chosen to invest their aspirations and motivations with your organisation for a while and who will expect a reasonable return on their investment in the form of personal growth and opportunities.

Source: 'Deploying talent' in Massie (2015).

---

within the constraints of the organisation as possible and making short-term 'raids' into the opposite domain of the 'fixers' (where the resource sits, rationed and bound by rules) only when necessary and for as short a time as possible (see Figure 15.1). The radical humanist example can be adapted to apply in a similar way to nursing and the nurses' experience of intrepreneurship. In the interviews conducted prior to writing this chapter, consistent frustrations related to being an intrepreneur were voiced: 'the ability to follow through', 'getting the resource in the first place', 'being given the freedom to test things out', 'my organisation is risk-averse'.

The problem for individuals driving change within organisations, then, is how to reconcile approaches to influence and deliver change (the radical humanists) whilst also accommodating the need for and push toward stability and inflexibility within organisations that tend to support structure, order, monitoring and consistency (the fixers). If the NHS is to encourage internal innovation and intrepreneurship then it must, as The King's Fund paper (Massie 2015) suggests, look to how it supports innovation and embeds lasting change whilst developing and guiding its leaders.

One of the consistent tasks of any organisation is to manage the uncertainty out of the organisation – to keep it steady, to build internal systems that support stability and governance structures and to monitor and respond to any deviation from a stable state. The problem for intrepreneurs and entrepreneurs is that the inherent tension of uncertainty is one of the most significant drivers – they thrive on uncertainty, solving problems, creating new solutions and thinking beyond the constraints of traditional practice.

Entrepreneur or intrepreneur?

Bosma et al. (2010) found that intrapreneurs are much more likely to have intentions to start a new independent business than other employees. They are also more likely to have entrepreneurial perceptions and attitudes. Intrepreneurs, more often than other employees, personally know an entrepreneur who recently started a business, feel they have the required

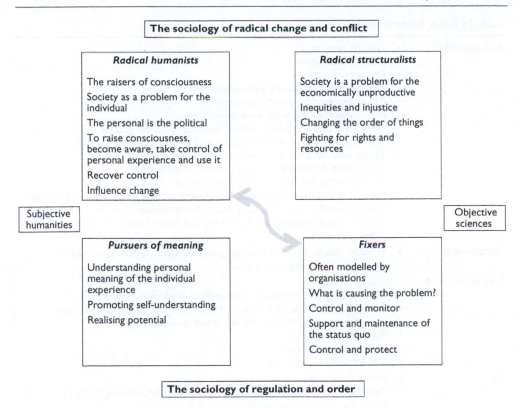

Figure 15.1 The sociology of radical change and conflict
Source: adapted from Howe (1987).

skills to start a business, see good entrepreneurial opportunities in their environment and believe that fear of failure would not prevent them from starting a business. The opportunity cost of entrepreneurship in developed countries is in opposite proportion to economic stability – intrepreneurship is more common in the developed world where the cost of failure is greater, whereas entrepreneurship is more common in emerging economies where there is less to lose (Lucas 1978).

The concepts of competition and choice set out in the Health and Social Care Act determine that there will be a mixed economy in terms of who provides services. Equally, the drive toward innovation, efficiency and shifting the balance of care from hospitals to primary care and local authority services as well as integrating provision, requiring change, collaboration and leadership, also creates a 'market'.

Market is not a popular term in modern health settings; nevertheless, it is a reality. A market is another way of describing the types of services that consumers need and want to acquire or those that government policy and/or local health trusts and providers want implemented as part of their strategic delivery plan. Consumers might be patients, clients, other organisations, other parts of your own organisation or another business.

Who are the intrepreneurs and entrepreneurs?

Tables 15.1 and 15.2 give examples of key intrepreneurial and entrepreneurial roles.

Table 15.1 Key intrepreneurial roles

Role examples	• Change leaders • Service innovators • Project managers • Clinical board members with specific roles • Those involved in service redesign • Implementation leads for new guidelines • Leads of clinical networks and/or specialist interest groups • Those who involve patients, carers and service users • Those who develop and evaluate pilot services • Those who develop the use of outcome measures • Those involved in specialist service delivery • Nurse-led initiatives (e.g. midwifery, health visiting, school nursing, sexual health and contraception, community development health visiting, crisis intervention in mental health, training and consultation models) • Commissioners
Opportunities	• In public health, primary care, targeted services, specialist services, multi-agency settings and teams
Support required	• A clear brief • A named supervisor who understands change management • A line of accountability to a steering, advisory or management group • An agreement about how the work will be financed • Budgetary authority • Outcomes measures • Time frames for delivery
Risks	• Professional isolation • Systems not sufficiently flexible to respond to fast-moving changes • Lack of a traditional network • Lack of authority in the steering or advisory group • Lack of professional supervision • Lack of patient, carer or service user involvement • Poor connection between the initiative, organisational strategic objectives and realistic financial resource • Lack of a communications strategy • Poor planning and follow-through
Reflection	• Using reflective practice as an active tool for growth • Developing opportunities for networking with people in similar intrepreneurial roles • Reading and learning about the characteristics of success in a wide range of settings
Management	• Ensuring that development, innovation and management roles are clearly defined • Regular supervision
Organisational flexibility	• Taking time to test out the risks and opportunities for the initiative and the potential enablers and disablers in the organisation • Developing good working relationships with other parts of the system affected by change or innovation to understand their reality • Establishing clear lines of reporting and accountability and seeking assurance that the organisation is able to respond flexibly to the emerging findings from the initiative

Table 15.2 Key entrepreneurial roles

Role examples	• Nursing home owners • Agency nurses and proprietors • Counsellors/therapists • Coaches and mentors • Independent midwives • Social enterprises and community interest companies • Expert witnesses • Public/private partnerships • Independent healthcare practitioners • Consultants • Trainers and advisers • Complementary therapists • Businesses outside the health/care sphere
Opportunities	• Changes in legislation, guidance or policy, revealing gaps in local provision • Capitalising on skill, expertise and reputation • Targeting the market • Providing services or hybrids that don't currently exist – spotting the gaps • Working in partnership with other experts • Freedom from constraint and ability to respond flexibly • Building capacity in specific sectors • Doing something completely different • Flexibility and control • Acting as a social entrepreneur • Forming a social enterprise • Forming a community interest company • Partnership and collaboration • Providing employment for others
Support required	• A clear business model and a business plan • Financial advice • Advice and information on registering and running a business • Managing accounts, transactions, invoicing • Marketing and business promotion advice • Sector networking • Public liability and professional indemnity insurance
Risk	• Not thinking through the implications of being self-employed • Starting a business without preparation • Over-promising and under-delivering • Naivety • Managing quality • Managing and protecting reputation • Lack of clarity about internal governance • Dealing with complaints • Managing cash flow • Professional isolation • Professional development ignored • Pension position • Managing and responding to competition
Reflection	• Building in time to reflect on process, content, delivery and quality • Building a new network of professional support • What to do if you don't like it – pathways into and out of self-employment

Table 15.2 continued

Management	• Considering whether to buy in supervision, coaching or mentoring • Staff supervision • Managing costs, cash flow, business investment, salaries, dividends, Corporation Tax • Managing time and building in time for administration as well as delivery
Organisational flexibility	• Ability to respond quickly • Ability to target and deliver services that fit your skill set • Ability to influence and/or determine the nature of contracts • Ability to work flexible hours • Potential to add capacity through Associates as well as the potential to employ more staff • Flexibility as a self-employed person is not infinite

Setting up a business

There is some basic homework to do if you are thinking about starting your own business. Running your own business – even if it is doing something very similar to that which you were doing when you were employed – is a serious undertaking. There are legal, ethical and financial aspects that you need to consider. The temptation is to let your imagination run away with you, feel that rush of adrenaline and just go for it. This approach has its place; however, if your idea is that your business will still be running in two, five, or ten years' time, you need to plan carefully whilst retaining some of that drive and adrenaline.

Business plan

You will need a business plan, but first you need to clarify the nature of your product. Write down your ideas and talk about them with other people – including people you don't know. Get them to ask you questions – the things you dare not ask yourself – such as: What will it cost to set it up? Who are your customers? How will they know what you are offering? How do you know that what you are offering is what they want? What are your fees? How will you run the office, manage the finances and pay your taxes? And what about insurance? How will you know if you are successful? What support do you have that will keep you going when times get tough?

Your business plan should be simple, honest and achievable. As a minimum, it should set out the considerations in Box 15.2.

Box 15.2 *Developing a business plan*

• How long have you been developing the idea?

• What expertise do you have in this field?

• Who will be involved in running the business?

• What is the product – how do you describe it?

• Who wants it and how will it make a difference to them?

• How will you adapt your product over time as the market changes?

- What will it cost to manufacture or deliver?
- What regulations govern the type of service or product you intend to develop?
- How will your business demonstrate compliance with quality standards for that service or product?
- What public indemnity and professional indemnity insurance is required?
- What is the market for your product?
- Do you understand the market – have you interrogated it – or are you living in the hope that yours is a 'good idea'?
- Who is currently providing the service or product, and how much of the market segment is available to you?
- How much potential for growth is there in this market?
- What is the likely response by your competitors if you enter the market?
- What is it about your product or service that will make customers choose you or your business over established businesses in this sector?
- What is different about what you provide?
- What added value can you bring?
- Do you have anyone lined up already to purchase this service or product?
- What marketing actions do you have planned to sell your product or service?
- What is the price, and is it competitive and realistic?
- How many products/services will you sell in a year/two years/four years?
- What skills do you have in relation to your idea and delivering it?
- What skills do you have in setting and managing budgets?
- What is your cash flow forecast?
- How will you ensure that there is sufficient capital in your business to survive?
- Have you considered issues such as cash flow – the level and timing of income, expenditure, debts?
- When are your predicted 'lean times'?
- Are you able to summarise a profit and loss spreadsheet across years one, two and three?
- Do you require business start-up finance, and if so, where is this coming from?
- How much do you think you need and why?
- What are the risks involved in running this business?
- How will you mediate those risks?
- How do you intend to monitor your business plan?
- Will you do it, or will someone else?
- How frequently will the monitoring take place and in what form?
- What will be the procedure if the plan deviates from your expectations?

Financial plan

Your business plan is something that should underpin your company along with a clear financial plan that sets out:

- revenue (income)
- expenditure
- cash flow
- projected growth
- profit and loss forecast
- managing debtors
- invoicing procedures
- staff costs.

The advice of an accountant is invaluable when first setting up a business. Your accountant should be registered with the Institute of Chartered Accountants in England and Wales, which is the professional body for accountants. What sort of questions should you ask your accountant? It is helpful to your accountant to understand what sort of business you want to run so she/he can advise you on the best status for your business.

Taxation

It is essential to keep records in order to provide complete financial information for your accountant. You should keep all receipts that support expenditure against the business. If you are a sole trader, you will pay Income Tax on the income you draw from the business. For a limited company, Corporation Tax will be due and any director dividends are also taxable.

National Insurance

You will need to ask your accountant and/or HM Revenue and Customs (HMRC) for advice on paying National Insurance as the rules vary according to the type of business and level of income. Remember that if you employ staff, you are responsible for deducting their Income Tax and National Insurance contributions.

Business insurance

You should consider the range of business insurance necessary for your type of business and take advice. This can include professional indemnity insurance; public liability insurance; cover for loss of earnings; and motor insurance for business use.

Pension

If you are self-employed, you should give thought to your pension requirements. You might consider moving your NHS pension across to a private pension scheme; however, you should take independent advice about pension arrangements.

Types of business

Sole trader

If you start working for yourself, you're classed as a self-employed sole trader – even if you've not yet told HMRC. As a sole trader, you run your own business as an individual. You can keep all your business' profits after you've paid tax on them. You are allowed to employ staff. The term 'sole trader' means you're responsible for the business, not that you have to work alone. You are personally responsible for any losses your business makes.

Limited company

A limited company is an organisation that you can set up to run your business – it is responsible in its own right for everything it does and its finances are separate to your personal finances. The company owns any profit it makes after it pays Corporation Tax (@ 20 per cent). The company can then share its profits with its directors.

Ordinary business partnership

In a business partnership, you and your business partner (or partners) personally share responsibility for your business. You can share all your business' profits between the partners. Each partner pays tax on his or her share of the profits.

Limited partnership and limited liability partnership

In both limited partnerships and limited liability partnerships (LLPs), you can share all the business' profits between the partners. Partners pay tax on their share of the profits. Every year, the partnership must send a partnership Self Assessment tax return to HMRC. Also all the partners must send a personal Self Assessment tax return every year, pay Income Tax on their share of the partnership's profits and pay National Insurance. You must also register the partnership if you expect your takings to be more than £83,000 a year.

Liability for business debt differs depending on whether you are in a limited partnership or a LLP. For limited partnerships, liability for debts that cannot be paid is split among partners. Partners' responsibilities differ as general partners can be personally liable for all the partnership's debts. Limited partners are only liable up to the amount they initially invest in the business. General partners are also responsible for managing the business. In LLPs, partners are not personally liable for debts the business cannot pay. Instead, their liability is limited to the amount of money they invested in the business. Partners' responsibilities and share of the profits are set out in an LLP agreement and 'designated' members have extra responsibilities.

Social enterprise

Social enterprises are businesses that trade to tackle social problems, improving communities, people's life chances or the environment. They make their money from selling goods and services in the open market, but they reinvest their profits back into the business or the local community.

Community interest company

The community interest company (CIC) was established by statute and is regulated by the Community Interest Company Regulations 2005. This is designed to provide a legal status to enterprises that provide benefit to the community or that trade with a social purpose rather than to make a profit. A CIC can be limited by shares or by guarantee. Most are limited by guarantee. If a CIC is limited by shares then it is subject to a dividend cap, which means that while investment can be generated through issuing shares, the CIC model cannot be exploited for personal gain.

Franchise

A franchise is where a franchisor provides a licensed privilege to the franchisee to run their business using an existing product and provides support and help in organising, training, merchandising, marketing and managing in return for a monetary consideration. What this means is that the owner of the product (the franchisor) effectively gets a wider distribution of the product through affiliated dealers (franchisees). It generally involves paying an initial fee and ongoing royalties to the franchisor in return for the use of the trademark.

Setting up a business is daunting but exciting. Sustaining and growing a business is time-consuming, intellectually challenging and more than a full-time job. The interviews that were conducted with nurse entrepreneurs in the preparation of this chapter revealed some common themes that emerge for many new business owners. Most business owners said they had no regrets that they had spotted a market and were ready for a change. All the nurses that were interviewed said that they had been in senior nursing or NHS development roles before they became self-employed and that they were ready for a major change. All said that their roles had equipped them for most of the challenges of self-employment and that, in the end, self-employment was a way of continuing the development roles they had undertaken within the NHS. When asked why they had switched from being employed to self-employed, every nurse said that they wanted more autonomy, a greater sense of freedom and personal agency, and the opportunity to change aspects of care or provision that seemed impossible – or was taking too long – in the NHS. Interestingly, their comments were peppered with thoughts about how their former roles had equipped them to do what they are doing now.

Summary

This chapter touches on some of the stark challenges facing the NHS. Just as patients are demanding more from services and wanting greater involvement, so too are nurses. Those with a personality type that is open to innovation and who are comfortable with uncertainty understand the experience of leading and implementing change. They may find that the paucity of career pathways for innovators, change agents and risk-takers within the system influences future decisions about where to best realise their potential. Using nurses and other health professionals to innovate and act in intrepreneurial roles is a very cost-effective strategy. However, it needs to be a constituent part of workforce planning if talent and aptitude is to be retained within the health system and patient-facing capacity is not compromised.

References

Berwick, D. (2003) Disseminating innovations in health care. *The Journal of the American Medical Association*, 289(15): 1969–75.

Bosma, N., Stam, E. and Wennekers, S. (2010) *Entrepreneurial Employee Activity: A Large Scale International Study*. Tjalling C. Koopmans Research Institute Discussion Paper Series, No. 12-12. Utrecht: Utrecht School of Economics, Utrecht University.

Burrell, G. and Morgan, G. (1979) *Sociological Paradigms and Organisational Analysis*. London: Heinemann.

Department of Health (2011) *Equity and Excellence: Liberating the NHS*. Cm 7881. London: The Stationery Office.

Department of Health (2006) *Our Health, Our Care, Our Say: A New Direction for Community Services*. Cm 6737. London: The Stationery Office.

Department of Health (2000) *The NHS Plan: A Plan for Investment, A Plan for Reform*. Cm 4818-I. London: The Stationery Office.

Howe, D. (1987) *An Introduction to Social Work Theory*. London: Ashgate.

King's Fund, The (2011) *The Future of Leadership and Management in the NHS: No More Heroes*. London: The King's Fund.

Lucas, R. E., Jr. (1978) On the size distribution of business firms. *Bell Journal of Economics*, 9(2): 508–23.

Massie, D. (2015) *Talent Management: Developing Leadership Not Just Leaders*, Leadership in Action series. London: The King's Fund.

Naylor, R. (Chair) (2015) *Ending the Crisis in NHS Leadership: A Plan for Renewal*. London: Health Service Journal.

NHS England (2014) *Five Year Forward View*. London: NHS England.

Raup, G. H. (2008) Make transformational leadership work for you. *Nursing Management*, 39(1): 50–3.

Traynor, M., Davis, K., Drennan, V., Goodman, C., Humphrey, C., Lock, L., Mark, A., Murray, S., Banning, M. and Peacock, R. (2006) *A Report to the National Co-ordinating Centre for NHS Service Delivery and Organisation of a Scoping Exercise on the Contribution of Nurse, Midwife and Health Visitor Entrepreneurs to Patient Choice (NM96)*. London: National Co-ordinating Centre for NHS Service Delivery and Organisation.

Whittington, C. and Holland, H. (1985) A framework for theory in social work. *Issues in Social Work Education*, 5(1): 25–50.

Index

Note: page numbers in italic type refer to Figures; those in bold type refer to Tables.